Developing Practice for Public Health and Health Promotion

Jennie Naidoo BSc MSc PGDip PGCE

Principal Lecturer, Health Promotion,
University of the West of England, Bristol, UK

Jane Wills BA MA MSc PGCE

Professor of Health Promotion, London South Bank University, London, UK

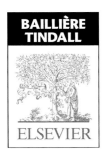

BAILLIÈRE
TINDALL

ELSEVIER

Edinburgh   London   New York   Oxford   Philadelphia   St Louis   Sydney   Toronto 2010

BAILLIÈRE
TINDALL
ELSEVIER

First edition 1998
Second edition 2005
Third edition 2011

ISBN 978 0 7020 4454 0
Formerly 978 0 7020 3404 6

British Library Cataloguing in Publication Data
A catalogue record for this book is available from the British Library

Library of Congress Cataloguing in Publication Data
A catalogue record for this book is available from the Library of Congress

Notices

Knowledge and best practice in this field are constantly changing. As new research and experience broaden our understanding, changes in research methods, professional practices, or medical treatment may become necessary.

Practitioners and researchers must always rely on their own experience and knowledge in evaluating and using any information, methods, compounds, or experiments described herein. In using such information or methods, they should be mindful of their own safety and the safety of others, including parties for whom they have a professional responsibility.

With respect to any drug or pharmaceutical products identified, readers are advised to check the most current information provided (i) on procedures featured or (ii) by the manufacturer of each product to be administered, to verify the recommended dose or formula, the method and duration of administration, and contraindications. It is the responsibility of practitioners, relying on their own experience and knowledge of their patients, to make diagnoses, to determine dosages and the best treatment for each individual patient, and to take all appropriate safety precautions.

To the fullest extent of the law, neither the Publisher nor the authors, contributors, or editors, assume any liability for any injury and/or damage to persons or property as a matter of products liability, negligence or otherwise, or from any use or operation of any methods, products, instructions, or ideas contained in the material herein.

Printed in China

Contents

PART 1 Drivers of public health and health promotion practice

PART 2 Strategies for public health and health promotion practice

PART 3 Priorities for public health and health promotion

Acknowledgements

We would like to thank all our colleagues and students who, through their ideas, experiences and debates, have contributed to this book. We would also like to thank our families for supporting our writing.

This book is dedicated to our children: Kate, Alice, Jessica and Declan.

Introduction and how to use this book

Public health and health promotion have very different origins and antecedents, yet in the modern world they are increasingly seen as two complementary and overlapping areas of practice. This has had the effect of broadening the scope of both disciplines. For historical reasons, public health, with its roots in public health medicine, tends to be seen as the senior partner, embodying the status and kudos of medicine and science. Public health is often used as an umbrella term to encompass health promotion; however, health promotion, with its diverse origins and roots, has much that is distinctive, valuable and unique to offer. One need only think of the following principles and ways of working that derive from health promotion but are now firmly embedded in public health practice: involving people and communities, working across boundaries and partnership working, empowering people, and a concern with the structural causes of health inequalities. The aim of this book is to help practitioners clarify for themselves the scope, direction and skills embodied within health promotion and public health practice.

Health promotion refers to efforts to prevent ill health and promote positive health. From a relatively narrow focus on changing people's behaviour, health promotion has become a broad and complex field encompassing policy change and community action. The central aim is to enable and empower people to take control of their own health. Promoting health is now to some extent everybody's business. It is a concern not just of health services but also of all those involved in health and social care, education and environmental protection.

Public health has been traditionally associated with public health medicine and its efforts to prevent disease. It has been defined as 'the science and art of preventing disease, prolonging life and promoting health through the organised efforts of society' (Acheson 1988). Public health includes the assessment of the health of populations, formulating policies to prevent or manage health problems and significant disease conditions, the promotion of healthy environments, and societal action to invest in health-promoting living conditions.

Our starting point in this book is to acknowledge the multidisciplinary nature of health promotion and public health; however, we argue that a social structuralist model of health remains the most helpful explanatory model. Such a model recognizes the profound effects of social structures such as income distribution, employment opportunities and social capital on health, whilst still allowing scope for individual agency and empowerment.

The twenty-first century poses enormous challenges for public health, including the major demographic change of ageing populations in the developed world; climate change, environmental threats and increased urbanization; anti-health economic forces of globalization such as tobacco and junk food; economic growth alongside increasing poverty and inequality; and the rise of chronic and degenerative diseases alongside a resurgence of infectious diseases. People have the right to healthy choices and governments have a responsibility to tackle those issues that impact on health. Public health needs to negotiate the line between individual freedom and social responsibility, which means engaging in public debates about evidence, risk and values. To be effective, public health needs to have the informed consent and support of the population.

In our companion book, *Foundations for Health Promotion*, edn 3 (Naidoo and Wills 2009), we reviewed some of the knowledge and skills with which practitioners need to be familiar if they are to promote health, and looked at some examples of differing approaches to this task. This book further explores what should inform the practice of public health and health promotion. The challenge for practitioners is to embrace the health promotion principles espoused by the World Health Organization – equity, community participation, intersectoral collaboration, and the reorientation of primary health and social care services – with the pressures of everyday practice. Many practitioners find it difficult to incorporate such a broad approach and move 'upstream' to tackle the determinants of health. Our aim in this book is to support the efforts of practitioners to achieve this task and to become committed and skilled public health practitioners.

Practitioners need to be aware of the forces that contextualize, drive and sometimes constrain their practice. These forces or drivers of public health and health promotion practice include theoretical and conceptual frameworks that inform interventions, a developing research and evidence base, and the values that underpin and feed into the policy context. These drivers of practice are discussed in Part 1 of this book.

Practitioners also need to understand core strategies for public health and health promotion practice. These strategies inform and underpin a multitude of interventions, programmes and projects spanning priority topics, key agencies and targeted client groups. Developing an understanding of, and competence in, these strategies enables practitioners to increase the impact of their health promotion and public health work. The core strategies that we identify and discuss in Part 2 of this book are: tackling health inequalities, public, patient and community participation and involvement, working in partnerships, and empowerment strategies.

Practitioners need to be familiar with current public health priority issues and how they are being addressed in practice. Priorities for public health and health promotion may be defined in different ways. Categories used in policy and strategy documents include social determinants of health: disease conditions, lifestyles and behaviours that constitute risk factors for disease, and vulnerable or marginalized groups of people. We address each of these four priority categories in Part 3 of this book. Each chapter in Part 3 discusses why these topic areas are priorities, and provides examples of the range of approaches used to tackle these issues.

This book uses a clear, user-friendly but challenging style that encourages readers to engage with the subject. The book is clearly structured and signposted for ease of reading and study. A checklist at the end of this introduction provides a tool for practitioners to interrogate their own practice and make links to relevant sections in the book. Each chapter starts with a few key points and an overview outlining the contents of that chapter and ends with a conclusion, further discussion questions and recommended reading. Interspersed throughout the text are a number of helpful features:

- Discussion point – to enable individual or small group discussion to clarify and consolidate understanding and learning.
- Example, research or case study of practice – to demonstrate good practice developments and innovative interventions.
- Practitioner talking – quotes to use as triggers to engage the reader in the topic and encourage reflection on practice.
- Activity for individual assessment – to enable the reader to reflect and make links between their own practice and relevant theory and research.

When appropriate, feedback on these features is provided in the text.

We hope that this book will enable practitioners to develop their public health and health promotion knowledge and skills, and their confidence. Public health and health promotion are constantly evolving and developing, and the speed and scope of change can be daunting for practitioners. We hope that this text will go some way towards unpacking what is included in public health and health promotion and thereby enable practitioners to identify and develop their public health role.

References

Acheson D: *Public health in England*, Report of the committee of inquiry into the future of the public health function, London, 1988, HMSO.

Naidoo J, Wills J: *Foundations for health promotion*, edn 3, Edinburgh, 2009, Baillière Tindall.

Checklist for public health and health promotion practice

Drivers of public health and health promotion	What are the key drivers for public health and health promotion? What is the relative contribution of scientific evidence versus theory and values?	**Part 1**
Theoretical perspectives and frameworks	What informs my understanding of public health and health promotion problems?	Chapter
	What is my vision for public health? What principles should underpin its practice?	Chapter
	Is my practice founded on a theoretical understanding?	Chapter
Research and evidence	Is my practice founded on research?	Chapter
	How robust is the research base for public health and health promotion?	Chapter
	Can I identify appropriate and valid sources of information/evidence to address public health questions and issues?	Chapter
	How do I know my practice is effective? How do I know it is acceptable or appropriate?	Chapter
Policy	What is the value base underpinning policies? Can I critically appraise government initiatives aimed at improving health and well-being? How can I work effectively within the existing policy framework? How am I able to influence policy?	Chapter
Strategies in public health and health promotion	What are the key strategies used to promote and protect the health of the public? What knowledge, skills and competences are needed to use these strategies effectively?	**Part 2**
Tackling health inequalities	What is the extent of avoidable health inequalities? What is the range of strategies aimed at tackling health inequalities? Is equity an underlying principle in my practice? How can I tackle inequalities, poverty and social exclusion in my practice?	Chapter

Engaging communities and individuals	How are patients and the public engaged in service/programme design and delivery? How could I involve and support different communities in assessing their own health and well-being needs? How is information about needs disseminated and responded to?	Chapter 6
Partnership working	To what extent is partnership working encouraged in my practice? Do I understand and value the contributions to public health of different disciplines, practitioners and agencies? Are the skills and resources for partnership working recognized and provided in my work practice?	Chapter 7
Empowerment	How can I empower my clients to increase control over their health? How can I provide information for my clients or the public? How do I know it meets their needs? How do I know it reaches marginalized groups? How can I encourage the public or my clients to maintain a healthy lifestyle?	Chapter 8
Priorities for practice	How do I know what the priorities for practice should be? What are the effective strategies for addressing priorities for practice? How can my practice build on and complement strategies addressing priorities at a community or national level?	**Part 3**
Social determinants of health	To what extent, and how, does my practice reflect a social perspective and understanding of the determinants of health?	Chapter 9
Major causes of ill health	What are the major priorities in terms of disease conditions?	Chapter 10
Lifestyles and behaviours	How can I address lifestyles and behaviours in a non victim-blaming manner? How do I know what the effective strategies for changing lifestyles are?	Chapter 11
Population groups	How do I reach marginalized groups without stigmatizing them?	Chapter 12

Part One

Drivers of public health and health promotion practice

Introduction

Public health and health promotion are undergoing a period of rapid change and transition. Changes in population demographics and the epidemiology of diseases, including the rise in the number of people living with long-term conditions, together with changing structures of healthcare delivery, including a focus on the primary care sector, have highlighted and expanded the role and potential of public health and health promotion to positively develop health. Various factors drive this process, including research evidence, government policy, public expectations, and practitioner expertise. These changes lead to new challenges for public health and health promotion practitioners: identifying local health needs, knowing public and patient expectations, analysing health inequalities in relation to outcomes and service provision, and determining the effectiveness and acceptability of interventions. Practitioners need the opportunity to reflect on their role, contribution and response to these challenges of the twenty-first century. The identification of a body of knowledge, theoretical frameworks and concepts that practitioners can draw upon to develop an analytical approach to a problem is central. All practitioners are called upon to base their practice on evidence, particularly evidence generated by good quality research. In addition, practitioners' interventions need to be solidly based on ethics and consensual values. An agreed-upon ethical and value base underpins policy making and implementation.

Part 1 explores in turn the key elements that enable practitioners to develop their public health and health promotion practice so that they can feel confident and justified in the decisions they make. Chapter 1 examines the body of theory and some of the key principles that inform public health and health promotion and discusses why their application to practise is difficult. Chapter 2 discusses the evidence and research that informs public health and health promotion. A reliance on epidemiology leads to a focus on addressing individual behavioural risk factors for disease, whereas a broader view of research would include collective and structural determinants of health. Chapter 3 discusses the current emphasis on evidence-based practice and the criteria for effectiveness that are used to evaluate interventions. Chapter 4 explores the ways in which policy is based on both research evidence and values. The impact of the policy context on practice in the UK, and the ways in which practitioners can affect policy, are also discussed.

Chapter One

Theory into practice

- Relationship between public health and health promotion
- Professional roles
- Process and principles
- Skills for public health and health promotion practice
- Theoretical frameworks

OVERVIEW

An understanding of the public health and health promotion theory is essential to informed practice. Yet identifying that body of theory is difficult and applying theory to practice is not straightforward. Many occupational groups claim a role in promoting health. Yet each may draw upon a different knowledge base (e.g. biomedicine, education, psychology, social sciences, organizational development) and have a different perspective on what constitutes public health and health promotion. The improvement of health and well-being may appear to be unproblematic and self-evidently a 'good thing' but it allows for a wide range of actions from efforts to change individual lifestyles, educational work with young people, to actions that change social structures. This chapter argues that practitioners should be aware of the values implicit in the approach they adopt. In so doing, practitioners begin to clarify their

view of the purpose of public health and health promotion and the strategies that are suggested by different aims. Otherwise practitioners merely respond to practice imperatives and their work is limited to narrow tasks.

Introduction

> *Public health is what we, as a society, do to assure the conditions for people to be healthy.*
> Committee for the Study of the Future of Public Health
> Washington 1988.

From the seventeenth to nineteenth centuries, public health was preoccupied with eliminating diseases such as bubonic plague, smallpox and cholera. With industrialization and rapid urbanization in the nineteenth century, public health work became focused on environmental issues such as clean water supplies, disposal of waste, and better housing, which were the province of engineers and planners. In 1842, Chadwick wrote in the *Report on the Sanitary Condition of the Labouring Population of Great Britain* that to prevent cholera 'aid must be sought from the civil engineer, not from the physician who has done his work when he has pointed out the diseases that result from the neglect of proper administrative measures, and he has alleviated the suffering of the victim'.

The epidemiological transition during the twentieth century saw the main causes of death and disability shift from infections to chronic illnesses such as heart disease, stroke, cancers, respiratory illness and accidents, where lifestyles play a causative role. Public health interventions included mass screening and vaccination and immunization programmes as well as education and advice delivered by practitioners and mass media campaigns. Public health in England can thus be divided into two periods – the Sanitary Reform period when improvements were sought through a better physical environment and the Personal Services period when the emphasis was on personal health and hygiene.

In more recent times, the political agenda in most of the Western world has been dominated by 'social responsibility' and a recognition of the importance of the wider (upstream) determinants of health. Promoting health is now recognized as a multi-agency task. Since health and well-being are affected by so many factors, health improvement cannot be delivered by the health service alone, but will arise from cross-sector action on the environmental, economic and social determinants of health such as low income, housing, transport, food supply, crime and disorder, and employment.

This chapter will explore some of the complexities involved in translating modern public health into a multidisciplinary and multiprofessional area of practice. It will examine:

- the scope of modern public health and current terminology
- the relationship of public health and health promotion

- the skills and competences of a multidisciplinary public health specialist/practitioner
- the process of modern public health
- the values and principles underpinning public health.

The scope of modern public health

What is understood to be encompassed by public health will depend on conceptualizations of health and the influences upon health and well-being, the consequent purpose and goals of improving the public's health, its scope of activities and who will be part of the associated workforce, and the values and ways of working that will underpin those activities.

Actions to improve health take different forms. If the reduction or absence of disease is the principal aim, health improvement centres around preventative medicine and influencing or persuading people to adopt healthier lifestyles. Health may be viewed more broadly as a way in which people can begin to achieve their potential; health improvement then centres around community development and involvement. Health may be seen as socially determined and a fundamental right; health improvement then centres on addressing the root causes of ill health in the physical, social and economic environment through developing integrated health strategies tackling areas such as housing, employment and nutrition.

The purpose of modern public health is to protect and promote health by:

- improving people's life circumstances (e.g. housing, employment, education, environment)
- improving people's lifestyles
- improving health services
- protecting the public from communicable diseases and environmental hazards
- developing the capacity of individuals and communities to protect their health.

The objectives of the national strategy to tackle obesity (DH 2008) illustrate the potential range of activities with which a practitioner might be involved:

Box 1.1 **Practitioner talking**

I think we have a problem with the word health, because I think health has a certain set of definitions that are attached to it. And if you ask people what would make them healthier, or what would lead to better health, what they will tell you is that we need a lot more of the NHS-type health services. So people will quite genuinely tell you 'if there were more doctors people would be healthier'.

Hunter et al 2007, p. 62

Commentary

Health is understood in many different ways but for most people it is associated with physical health. Although health is influenced by genetics, socio-economic circumstances and individual lifestyles, technical medicine, surgery and biochemical treatments receive most attention. McKeown's analysis of the historical record of medicine (McKeown 1976) has had an enduring professional and political impact in puncturing medicine's claims to importance in saving lives. The public, however, associate improvements in health not with environmental or economic change but with more medicine.

- Promoting healthy growth and healthy weight in children, for example maintaining breastfeeding.
- Promoting healthier food choices, for example provision of food in schools and nurseries.
- Building physical activity into our lives, for example school travel plans and safer routes to school.
- Creating incentives for better health, for example point of decision educational materials and workplace cycle schemes.
- Personalized support for obese individuals, for example weight management in primary care.

An increasing range of practitioners are likely to see public health goals and targets as part of their official remit. Local strategic implementation for obesity is likely to involve dieticians, teachers, school nurses, midwives, health visitors and sports development workers. Some of these (e.g. planners whose decisions regarding open spaces may influence people's walking habits) would not normally conceive of public health as part of their role.

The key elements of modern public health are seen to be:

- having a population perspective
- recognizing the role of governments in tackling underlying socio-economic causes of ill health
- working in partnership with local communities to ensure their involvement in all stages of service development and planning
- working in partnerships with other agencies and the public to develop health improvement strategies
- developing the capacity of communities, professionals and organizations to work in this way.

The relationship between public health and health promotion

If public health is 'the science and art of preventing disease, prolonging life and promoting health through the organized efforts of society' (Acheson 1988), then health promotion would appear to be subsumed under public health. Traditionally, however, public health has meant disease prevention, an approach demanding knowledge of medical conditions and an ability to assess and monitor disease trends. In many Western countries, therefore, public health has been a specialty of medicine. More recently, the term 'New Public Health' has been used to reflect a broader, social view of public health.

Health promotion was defined in the Ottawa Charter (WHO 1986) as being centrally concerned with empowering people to take greater control over their health and thus includes a range of strategies to strengthen communities, develop supportive environments and inform and educate about health issues. In many countries health promotion is well established as a field of study and area of activity with a clear ideology deriving from the World Health Organization's principles of 1984 (WHO 1984).

It is apparent that public health and health promotion are very different disciplines drawing on different bodies of theory, strategies and values:

> *The public health and health promotion professions embody – and tolerate – conflicting ideas of why and how health should and could be improved. The meaning of public health and health promotion are themselves contested and open to misunderstandings. The origins of these conflicts lie in the contested nature of health itself, of the causes of ill health, of the methods for reducing health and promoting well-being and fundamentally, in the motivation for such interventions.*
>
> Webster and French 2002, p. 11.

Partly because of the diversity of its practice and partly because of the dominance of medicine as a profession and discipline, the robustness of health promotion in the UK has been questioned (Wills and Scott Samuel 2007; Wills et al 2008). The term health promotion has been largely replaced by the term 'health improvement', one of three domains of public health alongside health protection and service improvement shown in Figure 1.1 and identified by the Faculty of Public Health (Griffiths et al 2005). Debates over appropriate terminology reflect intense differences over purpose and scope. In Canada for example, 'population health' is now the dominant discourse replacing health promotion, which like public health in England privileges an epidemiological approach to understanding. This positivist model of research and inquiry results in the de-politicization of health issues.

Box 1.2 **Discussion point**

What do you identify as the difference between public health and health promotion?

Your answer may have focused on the different scope of the activities, the different values and perceived purpose, or the different knowledge and skills required. Table 1.1 highlights some of the differences between health promotion and public health medicine.

Modern public health therefore incorporates many of the activities, strategies and principles of health promotion. The disciplines underpinning public health and health promotion have different philosophies and forms of enquiry that inform different kinds of interventions to promote health, and disciplinary battles continue to rage over the relative contribution of biomedicine, epidemiology and the social sciences to our understanding of ill health. In the UK, the term multidisciplinary public health has become a widely accepted term to describe the range of professions and fields that will make up the public health and health

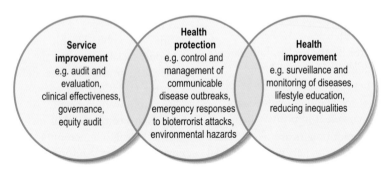

Figure 1.1 ● Three domains of public health. (Source: Griffiths et al 2005)

Table 1.1 Public health and health promotion

	Public health medicine	**Health promotion**
Focus	Disease prevention, monitoring and management	Protection and promotion of health
Knowledge base	Biomedicine Epidemiology Health economics	Sociology, social policy, education and psychology
Core tasks	Research into the aetiology, incidence and prevalence of diseases Surveillance and assessment of population health Managing outbreaks of communicable disease (and non-biological hazards) Planning, monitoring and evaluating screening and immunization programmes Planning programmes and services to improve healthcare provision	Developing policies to protect and promote health in different settings Education and information for health and behaviour change Working with communities to identify and meet needs Organizational development
Areas of practice	Health sector	All sectors where people 'work, live and play'
Process	Top down: collecting information and policy development	Bottom up: collaboration and partnerships, capacity building of communities and individuals
Values	Authority, expertise, adherence	Collaboration, partnership, advocacy, mediation, enablement

improvement field and to overcome the distinction between medically qualified public health specialists and the non-medically qualified. The challenge for modern public health then is to move beyond public health medicine and to acknowledge the role of health promotion in the overall task of health improvement.

The public health workforce

Many countries are focused on the task of clarifying the nature of the public health function, the structure of the workforce and the building of its capacity and capability, and the consequent development of appropriate competences. Promoting health has become 'everybody's business'. The Chief Medical Officer of England (DH 2001) distinguished:

- those who lead and influence public health strategy (specialists), for example directors of public health
- those whose work contributes directly to health improvement (practitioners), for example public health nurses and midwives
- those whose practice should be informed by health improvement principles, for example social workers and teachers.

Many practitioners now have public health or health promotion identified as an aspect of their role and Chapter 10 in our first book *Foundations for Health Promotion* (Naidoo and Wills 2009) reviews some of these changing roles. There is also a body of professionals who are deemed 'specialists' by virtue of their training, functions and experience. For the past 50 years in the UK, specialist public health practice was the province of doctors who chose this medical specialty although this is now open to those who are not medically qualified. Health promotion was a clearly defined function within the NHS and open to people from diverse backgrounds but this specialized workforce has been eroded due to organizational changes (DH/Welsh Assembly 2005). Many professional groups have integrated health promotion into their practice and there are numerous studies exploring attitudes to the integration of health promotion into professional roles (e.g. Long et al 2001; Maidwell 1996; McKay 2008). It has been claimed enthusiastically, particularly by nurses in moves away from a single practitioner-single patient approach to one of greater partnership with clients and more work in and with communities. Yet this shift in focus has not been easy to put into practice.

Box 1.3 **Discussion point**

Why might it be difficult for nurses to adopt a health promotion/public health role?

For most practitioners, such activities are additional to their primary role which is individual client care and disease prevention activities. Inclusion of community-based activities or education work into a practitioner's remit poses an additional burden of work and extra time, resulting in it becoming 'bolted on' rather than integral to their way of working. Many health visitors, for example, struggle to release time from caseload work and routine assessment to focus on community-based activities. It is not surprising then that in most studies nurses frequently regard communication skills and the quality of the

nurse-patient relationship as their most significant contribution to health promotion. The nursing process itself still encourages nurses to identify individual problems and therefore the ability to understand health as an interrelationship between social and political factors as well as biomedical and psychological factors is rare.

Box 1.4 **Activity**

How do you think your professional group interprets its health promotion and public health role?

How practitioners interpret their health improvement role will depend on many factors including their professional training, their role in the organization, their personal experience, interests, and social and political perspective. Environmental Health Officers (EHOs), for example, work directly within communities and as such seem ideally placed to lead local government in its role to promote health. In practice, the spectrum of activity for EHOs is limited by their statutory duties under the Environmental Protection Act 1990 which enables action to be enforced where there is risk of disease. Work pressures and statutory duties mean EHOs spend their time on population protection and enforcement work and do not have the available time or resources to work proactively with communities. The examples of nurses and EHOs demonstrate how difficult it is to prioritize public health, even though practitioners may be very positive about their role and potential. By making public health everybody's business, there is a danger that it becomes nobody's responsibility.

Skills and competences for public health and health promotion

As we have seen, an increasing range of practitioners see themselves as promoting health. This raises the question of identifying recommended skills in order to undertake the task.

Box 1.5 **Discussion point**

Consider the task of health improvement. What do multidisciplinary public health practitioners need to be able to do?

Many occupations including health promotion and multidisciplinary public health try to characterize their professional activity in terms of competences or standards for practice. In the UK, standards for public health specialists and practitioners have been developed (see Box 1.6) that relate to key functions and the competences that need to be evidenced to show achievement and in order to achieve registration to practise (currently as a specialist but practitioner registration is soon to be started). For example, to demonstrate competence in surveillance and assessment of population health, a specialist would need to have undertaken needs assessments using appropriate epidemiological and/or other approaches (see www.skillsforhealth.org.uk). Core skills in which public health specialists additionally need to demonstrate competence are strategic leadership, research and development, and ethical management.

The Public Health Skills and Career Framework (http://www.skillsforhealth.org.uk/page/career-frameworks/public-health-skills-and-career-framework) is a tool for describing the skills and knowledge needed across nine levels of the public health workforce whoever the employer and whatever the nature of the work. It provides an overview of the competences and knowledge needed in each area and at each level and links to:

- National Occupational Standards (NOS) – those for public health practice developed by Skills for Health and other sector skills councils, for example community development, health trainers.
- The NHS Knowledge and Skills Framework (NHS KSF) which specifies core competences that are linked to pay and progression.

The concept of competence has aroused much controversy. It can be seen as narrow and mechanistic, focusing on task and not enabling practitioners to acquire the value base essential for critical practice.

Box 1.6 **The functions of public health practice (Skills for health 2001)**

- Surveillance and assessment of the population's health and well-being, for example undertaking needs assessments and analysing routinely collected data
- Promoting and protecting the population's health and well-being, for example investigating disease outbreaks, monitoring and controlling communicable disease outbreaks, monitoring and evaluating the implementation of a screening programme, and setting up smoking cessation groups
- Developing quality and risk management within an evaluative culture, for example using research evidence to inform decision making about interventions

- Collaborative working for health and well-being, for example developing local partnerships to tackle health issues
- Development of policies, strategies and service, for example analyse local data on access to and uptake of primary care services
- Developing and implementing policy and strategy, for example carrying out a Health Impact Assessment on a proposed planning decision
- Working with and for communities, for example mapping local organizations and holding a community planning event

All practitioners need to be not just technicians but reflective practitioners with a professional literacy. Competences cannot cover all types of activities nor the personal processes entailed in health improvement. In specifying a range of activities in which the practitioner must perform, the role of theory and understanding is diminished. 'Knowing' becomes merely preparation for 'doing' with no requirement to reflect on theoretical bases or make sense of working practice.

Reflective practice

The professional education of many practitioners, particularly in health and education, has been illuminated in recent years by the work of Schon and the concept of the 'reflective practitioner'. Schon (1983) characterizes professional practice as the high ground of research and theory as swampy lowland that consists of the messy, confusing problems of everyday practice. Schon likens many practitioners to the jazz musician or cook who is highly skilled at what he or she does and because of his or her experience is able to improvise, but who may not know or understand the theoretical basis of musical syncopation or the emulsification of fats. Schon argues that through reflection-in-action a practitioner learns the tricks of the trade and what works in practice. This personal or experiential knowing is an essential part of a practitioner's understanding. Schon also says, however, that practitioners need to be able to reflect *on* action and to remove themselves from the swamp of practice and take a broad view. The reflective practitioner is able to integrate these two aspects.

Through this process, links are made between experience, theory and practice. Kolb (1984) argued that if we are to learn effectively, experience needs to be carefully and systematically reflected upon. Practitioners and students in classroom situations who focus on an 'experience' or a situation about which they felt uncomfortable may begin to understand the ways in which their knowledge was inadequate for the situation. Through sharing that information they can discover how others experience in a different way something they may have taken for granted. Through analysing or interpreting the issue or situation they can abstract general principles from it. By drawing on theoretical frameworks they can see what further knowledge may be required, and then apply this back to their practice, perhaps trying out new ideas or doing things in a different way. The whole process is a cycle of practice-theory-practice or PRAXIS.

Box 1.7 **Discussion point**

Think of an action which you have taken recently or a programme that you have been part of, about which you felt uncertain or confused. Figure 1.2 shows a cycle of questions to encourage you to reflect on this experience and identify any learning points from it and how other learning can help you to make sense of it.

Schon (1983) argues that 'technical rationality' dominates professional thinking. But it is important that practitioners think about *why* things are done in the way they are, *how* they could be done differently and *what* they are trying to achieve. Practitioners may believe they can apply their professional knowledge to select the best method for their purposes. But the problems of the real world (and the practice of public health and health promotion is no exception) are not presented as neatly parcelled issues. When practitioners decide the form of their health improvement activity they are also choosing to frame the issue in a particular way which may mean reconciling, integrating or choosing among different interpretations and approaches. The action they take reflects particular aims and values – particular beliefs about health, about the influences on people's health and about the role of the practitioner. In the following example, reflection has facilitated development.

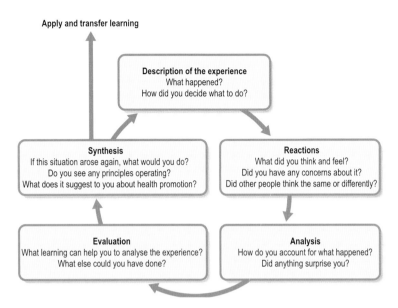

Figure 1.2 ● The cycle of reflection.

 Box 1.8 **Practitioner talking**

Many local projects are funded from pots of money allocated for specific programmes such as Sure Start or New Deal for Communities. Practitioners have to submit bids with a project proposal. One such bid allocated for regeneration was for Community Food Workers to act as local nutrition educators. The lead practitioner comments 'The community kitchens were poorly attended despite wide promotion within all the community groups. When I thought about why this might be, I realised I had been led by the possibility of getting some money and developed a project that might meet the criteria for funding. I hadn't bothered to go to the community and find out what people wanted. The idea of consultation was alien to my professional culture. The most I had done was a patient satisfaction survey. Understanding

both the principles of participation that underpin health promotion work and theories of community development have helped me to consider how I can involve the community. I now see that if we had worked with the community they would have owned the projects and may even have chosen other priorities'.

Commentary

The response of many practitioners to identified public health issues is shaped by the need to be visibly 'doing something', by funding streams and by a guiding intuition. This practice wisdom is discussed in detail in our third book on evidence-informed decision making. The guiding principles of health promotion in relation to involvement and participation may get relegated in the face of such pressures.

Values and principles for practice

All actions are value-based in the sense that we have a view about the desirability, worth or merit of a particular action. In relation to practice therefore, values are concerned with what public health and health promotion wants to achieve and how it will act to reach those goals.

Box 1.9 **Discussion point**

Think of a national or local strategy. What values are present in the strategy as represented in its aims and the interventions it proposes? To what extent do these fit with your own values?

The value or central purpose that many strategies place on health is the prevention of disease. A guiding principle may then be one of effectiveness and getting the most from available resources and identifying actions that are based on evidence. Alternatively you may have couched your answer according to the process of health improvement such as recognizing different understandings of health and the perspective of clients or building confidence and skills for people to take control of their lives. The principles guiding your practice may then be empowerment and participation. Every activity then reflects an underlying ideology or set of values that shapes how the issue is understood, the knowledge and theories used to understand it, and the strategies and ways of working that are adopted. The values for public health and health promotion traditionally derive from three key sources:

- The four classical principles of healthcare ethics – respect for personal autonomy, non-maleficence (not inflicting harm on others), beneficence (acting for the benefit of others), and justice (distributive and social) (Beauchamp and Childress 1995).
- The principles of health promotion described in Box 1.10 below (WHO 1985).

Box 1.10 **World Health Organization guiding principles for health promotion**

The World Health Organization outlined a set of guiding principles for health promotion as part of its commitment to Health for All (WHO 1985)

- equitable (guided by a concern for equity and social justice)
- empowering (to enable individuals and communities to assume more control over the factors that affect their health)
- participatory (involving all concerned at all stages)
- intersectoral (involving the collaboration of agencies to form all relevant agencies)
- holistic (fostering physical, mental, social, spiritual and sexual well-being)

Box 1.11 **Activity**

What principles guide your work? From what do these derive, for example your personal values, a professional code of conduct, health promotion principles?

- The principles relating to governance and accountability in the public sector including being evidence-informed, transparent, professional and offering value-for-money.

A characteristic of a profession is that there is a code of conduct, the purpose of which is to persuade the public that the occupation can be trusted and acts with integrity. Codes of conduct derive from the values which underpin that profession. For example, traditionally a doctor's duties to their patients are outlined in the Hippocratic Oath. Where a code of practice does not exist, many professions attempt to establish a commonality of purpose through subscription to a shared set of values and principles which increase the status of the field and help clarify the distinctive ethical dilemmas faced by public health practitioners. Although a public health profession exists, a variety of different professions who may have a different set of values – for example, epidemiologists, EHOs, nurses also practise public health.

 Box 1.12 **Example**

Principles for practice

'Show respect for all persons, and respect service users beliefs, values, culture, goals, needs, preferences, relationships and affiliations' British Association of Social Work www. basw.co.uk para. 3.1.2.2.

'Ways of working for health promotion include a commitment to sustainable development and promoting trust (delivering on what is promised to people)' SHEPS Cymru 2008.

Public health specialists (Faculty of Public Health 2001) 'practise good standards of public health make sure individuals and communities are not put at risk work within the limits of professional competence'.

Modern public health, as all health care, is about making decisions and choosing between alternative actions. In making those decisions we may draw upon:
- personal preference based on principles and values
- past practice and precedent
- professional judgement
- views of users, clients and the public
- available resources
- evidence of effectiveness from sound and rigorous research
- theoretical frameworks.

Public health and health promotion theory in practice

Within the planning and development of strategy and programmes, the explicit use of theory is not common despite Kurt Lewin's oft quoted statement that 'There is nothing as practical as a good theory' (Lewin 1952). The reality is that for most

 Box 1.13 **Practitioner talking**

We know what the principles of health promotion are but I don't think we practise them. We still do things FOR people not with them and lots of my colleagues are intent on simply finding ways to get people to change their behaviour. The only value that binds us together is equity but I suspect we interpret that differently. For me, we have a duty to work with the socially excluded to reduce health inequalities. For others though it's also about working upstream.

Commentary

Tackling inequalities is a central aspect of public health and health promotion practice. Significant inequalities in health exist in most countries based on income and ethno-cultural status and there is considerable evidence to describe these. National strategies to address such inequalities variously include actions to reduce disparities in access to health care, early interventions for specific conditions such as diabetes that disproportionately affect disadvantaged groups, and improving living standards.

practitioners theory is unrealistic and inapplicable in the face of the stark realities of day-to-day practice. Many practitioners adopt a pragmatic or common-sense approach.

 Box 1.14 **Discussion point**

What is the common sense that underpins public health and health promotion?

Look at the examples below:

'Practitioners just need to find the best ways of getting the message across'

'Middle class people are more educated and understand how to look after themselves'

'We need to understand people's attitudes so we can challenge their negative beliefs.'

But as Thompson points out: 'common sense is ideological – it serves to reinforce traditional values and the inequalities associated with these. It is based on implicit assumptions and if we rely on common sense to guide our thoughts, we are not in a position to question those assumptions' (Thompson 1995, p. 28).

 Box 1.15 **Activity**

What traditional values and associated inequalities do you think are exemplified in the above quotations?

It is often assumed, for example, that there is a healthy way of living and practitioners focus on the individual or individuals with the aim of changing their behaviour to this end. As discussed in Chapter 5, the 'healthier choice' is not available to all. Thus people may be blamed for health behaviours over which they do not have control. The simple equation that knowledge + attitudes = behaviour has also formed the basis of much health education work, yet the provision of information alone is unlikely to change behaviour. The giving of information can reinforce the expert status of the practitioner and fail to provide for the active participation of clients in an education process which addresses issues of concern to them. Middle class, educated people are often seen as 'easier' clients and so are targeted more (yet need it least). When practitioners do not derive their practice from a theoretical framework, the practice wisdom regarded as 'common sense' tends to reinforce simplistic assumptions which serve to reinforce inequalities.

Theory is perceived by many practitioners to be book learning. Many practitioners value received wisdom – 'we do it like this' – and learning on the job over an intellectual understanding of the practice process. To know 'how to' is more important than to 'know why'. This issue has been vehemently debated in recent years by those involved in professional education. Nurse educators have expressed concern that less time is spent on the wards and in hands-on work and more emphasis is being placed on research-based knowledge. Those involved in teacher education have expressed equal concern about the reverse situation – that more time is to be spent in classrooms and less on the theoretical underpinning of education! The apparent reluctance to use theoretical models for practice has led to long debates in many health and social care fields about a theory-practice gap and its implications for service provision and programmes.

 Box 1.16 **Discussion point**

Consider the following opposing viewpoints on the importance of theory. 'Which comes closest to your own view', 'What further arguments could you use to support this view'. (You might want to debate this with a colleague.)
A. Theory isn't important. Accounts of interventions show little evidence of them having been based on theory. Promoting health is just common sense and experience. The skills gained in previous training are quite adequate for this role. We just need to find out the best way of getting through to people. All this high flown stuff is unrealistic.
B. It is important that our work does derive from a sound knowledge base and logic for the intervention. We need to be able to see why we do it the way we do and to be able to explain this to others who may have a different view. Understanding theory helps to clarify purpose and effectiveness and makes it less likely to suffer contradictions.

In the complex and evolving field of public health and health promotion, an understanding of theory assumes great importance:
• To clarify the different paradigms of public health and health promotion.
• To inform programme planning and the choices made about actions to tackle major issues and to avoid simply making shots in the dark about what might improve health.
• In the absence of evidence to inform decision making, when theoretical explanations which are based on empirical reality offer a tool for logical and coherent practice.

- To give credibility to practice and give the practitioner the confidence to justify their choice of action when confronted with differing interpretations by colleagues, managers or politicians.
- To bind a discipline separating it politically and philosophically from another, and may thus contribute to a process of professionalization in which knowledge is organized and systematized.
- In the attempt to conceptualize health improvement beyond a set of activities, competences or skills which raises questions about the status of public health and health promotion as a field of study. What knowledge do practitioners draw on to practise?

 Box 1.17 **Discussion point**

Mr Jones is 76 and has leg ulcers. He is in the early stages of Alzheimer's disease and lives alone since the death of his wife in the previous year. The District Nurse visits Mr Jones daily to dress his leg and draws upon her technical knowledge to do so, regarding herself as a competent practitioner. She is aware that she must include Mr Jones' health needs in her nursing assessment.
- How does the District Nurse begin?
- What factors will influence how she 'frames' the health promotion aspects of her work?

The District Nurse might regard health promotion as integral to her care of Mr Jones or she might regard it as an additional task to be 'bolted on' to her essential work of monitoring his disease status. She might see her role as enabling Mr Jones to keep himself safe and in good health, or as preventing harm or disease from befalling him. Whichever role she prioritizes will affect her activities. If her priority is safety and good health she might advise Mr Jones about a healthy diet and home safety precautions and spend considerable time talking to Mr Jones in order to enhance his capacities. She might enlist the services of voluntary and self-help organizations and try to broaden Mr Jones' social contacts. If her priority is to prevent disease or harm, she

might focus on providing support for Mr Jones by liaising with Social Services to provide Meals on Wheels or day care and refer him to the occupational health service to assess his home for cooking and bathing aids.

This example illustrates how practitioners work in different paradigms. A paradigm can be defined as 'a way of knowing' and thereby interpreting a field of study characterized by particular beliefs and values, by particular theories and ways of problem solving and by particular methods and tools that are used in practice. The paradigm within which many practitioners work is that of Western science which has a mechanistic view of the body and views health as the antithesis of disease. Within this paradigm there are several theories or sets of propositions that explain or predict events such as theories about behaviour change or risk factors for disease. Practitioners may work in different paradigms, drawing upon different theories, and this will depend on their role, their professional background and training, and their personal beliefs and interests.

In the example above, the practitioner drew on theories from social psychology and used them as a tool to help her question her purpose and consider the factors influencing uptake of the intervention. Theory helped her to understand the variables affecting behaviour and provided insight into the strategies most likely to effect change. A reflective practitioner is constantly examining practice and adapting what to do in the light of experience. Without a theoretical base, however, they are merely technicians.

There are many different theories derived from different disciplines that practitioners may draw upon:
- How people learn.
- How diseases are caused and how they may be prevented.
- How people make decisions and change their behaviour.
- How society is organized and how social structures influence health.
- How messages are communicated and can be targeted to particular groups.
- How organizations change their focus and ways of working.

Box 1.18 **Practitioner talking**

I was part of a working group to set up a workplace health and activity programme. Based on our commonsense belief that everyone wants to protect their health, we thought that we'd get people involved by offering health checks which would then alert people to the risks to their health from lack of exercise and excessive weight. Opportunities for change were provided through a programme of exercises, monitoring of exercise recovery rates, nutrition advice, weighing and food diaries. The company even agreed to pay employees half time rates for attending the programme. The programme was quite successful but many employees did not participate, some dropped out and few managed to maintain an activity programme for themselves.

Commentary

When planning a subsequent programme, I drew particularly on social cognitive theory and the concept of value expectancy which states that people are likely to take some action if they believe the action will be effective and if they value the action's results (Ajzen 1988). I realized that a vague promise of better health in the future didn't mean as much to the employees as it did to me in my professional role even though I, too, struggle to maintain a healthy weight. Through informal discussions I learned that the participants' values related to 'feeling more attractive', 'wearing different clothes', 'being able to take part in sports and exercise'. Social cognitive theory also helped me to understand the importance of understanding their motivations and readiness to change, the support they have, and their confidence in their ability to take up and maintain an exercise programme. This resulted in the introduction of smaller targeted group sessions and personalized support through regular text messages.

These theories derive from many different disciplines. Rawson (2002) has described health promotion as a 'borrowed discipline' importing theories from other bodies of knowledge such as sociology and psychology. Alternatively public health and health promotion can be seen as disciplines in their own right with discrete bodies of knowledge and distinct theories, perspectives and methods.

Theories are organized sets of knowledge that help to analyse, predict or explain a particular phenomenon. A theory may explain:

- The factors influencing a phenomenon, for example why some parents refuse immunization for their children.
- The relationship between these factors, for example whether this is related to levels of knowledge and perceptions of risk; attitudes to interventions; beliefs about disease; levels of media attention; social norms.
- The conditions under which these relationships occur, for example do immunization rates fall when there is media attention to risk; in particular seasons; in particular social groups?

Modern public health is a complex field drawing on a range of disciplines. Inevitably then its theoretical base is equally diverse (Nutbeam and Harris 2004):

- Theories that explain individual health behaviour, for example the Health Belief model.
- Theories that explain change in communities, for example the Diffusion of Innovation.
- Theories that explain how communities can be mobilized for action, for example Achieving Better Community Development.
- Theories that guide the use of communication strategies, for example social marketing.
- Theories that explain changes in organizations, for example Force Field Theory.

Theoretical frameworks illustrate the key assumptions about how the programme will achieve the desired

Box 1.19 **Example**

Modern public health – is it multidisciplinary?

Consider the ways in which the disciplines outlined below contribute to health improvement. How, for example, would each discipline contribute to an HIV/AIDS prevention strategy?

Psychology

Psychology helps us to understand and explain human behaviour essential to health and the ways in which individuals make health-related decisions about, for example, taking up exercise, using a condom, or changing drinking patterns. Psychological theories of mass communication in the 1960s, which assumed a direct link between knowledge, attitudes and behaviour, are still widely adhered to despite the ineffectiveness of programmes based on this premise. Psychology explores lay and professional health conceptualizations and the ways this might affect decision making.

Sociology

In analysing how society is organized and the social processes within it, we can examine the social role of medicine and how health and illness have come to be defined. An analysis of power and control and an understanding of the relationship between social structures and individual action help us to consider how changes to promote health might come about. An analysis of the way in which society is stratified helps practitioners to consider how individual behaviour is constrained and influenced and how socio-economic status, gender and ethnicity influence health status.

Epidemiology

Epidemiology contributes understanding about the aetiology of disease and the effectiveness of preventive medicine. Epidemiology is based on a medical science model, although increasingly there have been calls to establish a social epidemiology of health. The study of risk factors for disease and health should, it is argued, go beyond traditional lifestyle or biomedical factors, to embrace factors such as degree of social networks and isolation and socially produced stress.

See Bunton and Macdonald (2002), Naidoo and Wills (2008).

---

outcomes. Many practitioners, however, have only vague ideas about how and why a programme may work and any theory is implicit. Yet theory enables the practitioner to identify the issue, think through alternative strategies having identified the factors influencing the issue, and identify the interventions most likely to be effective and the factors that need to be taken into consideration during implementation and evaluation.

The wide choice of interventions that might be used to promote health involving a range of practitioners and professionals in different settings makes it difficult to see what knowledge base might be used to guide practice. Practitioners are often eclectic and use different models reflecting the way in which they frame the issue. Theories of behaviour change, for example, have been widely adopted and have diffused into the design of health promotion interventions, reflecting the view that individuals are responsible for their own health.

Psychological theories such as the Health Belief Model (Becker 1974), the Theory of Reasoned Action (Ajzen and Fishbein 1980), Social Learning Theory (Bandura 1977) and the Transtheoretical Model of Change (Prochaska and DiClemente 1984) have dominated the field of health promotion as practitioners try to understand how to motivate and maintain behaviour change. Three sets of beliefs have emerged as important in determining behaviour or health change:

- Perceived benefits versus the costs associated with change.
- Perceptions about the attitudes of others to the behaviour.
- Self-efficacy or the belief in one's ability to achieve the change.

Individuals and population groups differ in their perception of the need for change and its benefits and this understanding has been critical in the adoption of more targeted and client-led approaches. Learning theory seeks to explain how behaviour is maintained. The likelihood of an individual behaving in a particular way (e.g. quitting smoking) tends to increase when that behaviour is followed by positive reinforcement (e.g. less breathlessness). A person's motivation to change will depend in part on how desirable the reinforcing factors are.

The theories described above focus on understanding how individuals can modify their health risks. A key element of modern public health is the capacity of communities to identify and act collectively on issues affecting their health. Many practitioners have been influenced by Freire (1972) whose liberation education model provided both a philosophy of education and development and a practical method of getting people actively involved, breaking through apathy and a way of developing a critical awareness of the causes of problems. Arnstein's (1969) ladder of involvement has also been influential in encouraging practitioners to review community levels of participation in decision making (see Chapter 7). Increasingly, the policy focus has been on describing a 'competent' or healthy community as a way of helping us to understand how to create safer and more productive communities that can implement local actions.

As Nutbeam and Harris (2004, p. 38) observe 'unlike the theories and models of health behaviour, community mobilization does not lend itself so comfortably to highly structured study and comprehensive theory development'. Much of the understanding about community action derives from practitioner experience and observation and much of the theoretical development focuses on identifying the process of capacity building and its elements driven by a desire to develop indicators to measure change.

Organizational contexts also play a part in achieving health improvement. Management theory has developed particularly in relation to understanding how to improve organizational performance but it also illuminates the process of change. Understanding why change occurs and the political, economic, societal and technological factors that operate on organizations and affect their development helps to remind practitioners to take account of the internal and external environment (Senior 1997). The 1990s in the UK saw, for example, a Labour administration after 18 years, low inflation, a commitment to low personal taxation and demoralized trade unions. The White Paper on the NHS introduced early in the new government (1997) stated that the status quo for the NHS was not an option and the modernization agenda has entailed torrents of change. Understanding the psychological process entailed in change is crucial to its implementation whether it be shifting the practice role of a health visitor, developing a health promoting school or being part of a changing Primary Care Organisation. Resistance to change is normal according to Lewin's (1952) Force Field Theory. During any period of change, there will be pressure to change and to maintain the status quo and a balance needs to be found. If the pressure to change is too great then resistance sets in.

These different theoretical frameworks derive from different disciplines and traditions and all provide the constructs in which the myriad tasks of public health and health promotion may be understood. In addition there are numerous models of health promotion that emerged during the 1980s in an attempt to define and clarify practice. Such models help:

* To conceptualize or map the field of health promotion.
* To interrogate and analyse existing practice.
* To plan and chart the possibilities for interventions.

Beattie's model (1996, p. 140), for example, is useful for 'charting and selecting the particular mix of approaches that make up a programme or project and also in exploring and reviewing the ethical and political tensions within an intervention in terms of the balance of social values it encompasses'. The model shows how health promotion is embedded in the sociocultural and political framework arising from the tension between expert-led, target-driven and top-down approaches and participatory and needs-led approaches. A further tension derives from the conflicting views on the determinants of health and whether these are seen as structural and demanding collective activity, or individual leading to information-giving, communication educational and counselling approaches. Health promotion is not a technical activity in which practitioners merely choose the best strategy for improved health. The field of health promotion clearly reflects the tension between different value positions about power, knowledge, responsibility and autonomy. Health promotion models are discussed in detail in Chapter 5 of our first book *Foundations for Health Promotion* (Naidoo and Wills 2009).

Conclusion

It is difficult to draw boundaries around public health and health promotion and agree who is promoting health and protecting the public and what sorts of activities this entails. Attempts to specify core competences and skills of public health specialists and practitioners reflect a professional strategy to safeguard a specific role and identity along with associated benefits, both economic and psychological. However, such attempts also risk causing division, hierarchy and competition amongst the many different practitioners who need to work collaboratively in order to gain maximum benefits for public health. Health promotion is a central aspect of public health activity that needs to be recognized and valued, instead of being assumed to be a commonsense, bolt-on task for all health practitioners. It would be easy to be side-tracked into defining and defending professional roles and competences. Perhaps the most important aspect is to reflect on what we are doing in the name of health improvement and what it is we are trying to improve.

As you will see in Part 2, it is not as simple as just getting on with it. Public health and health promotion have a close, but at times uneasy, relationship, mainly because public health medicine has traditionally been the 'senior partner', accorded a greater status and authority than health promotion. Modern public health seeks to integrate both health promotion and public health medicine into a new multidisciplinary

endeavour. Inevitably, different practitioners will have different views on the purpose of public health and health promotion and the best methods to achieve health improvement. A public health consultant may prioritize the uptake of available screening and immunization programmes locally, whereas a health promotion specialist may prioritize community development activities focusing on identifying local needs and empowering communities to address these needs. Differing roles, professional backgrounds and funding constraints as much as ideology will influence the way in which a practitioner defines the purpose of public health. Our position is that public health and health promotion need to be based on sound theoretical underpinnings and adhere to certain core principles. In the rest of this book we explore how these principles might be put into practice and the sorts of dilemmas this throws up. It is from these dilemmas and trying to apply theory to practice that practitioners can learn and contribute to a developing field.

Further discussion

- A reflective practitioner is one who is capable of improving practice by being sceptical about practice wisdom and questioning the approach taken. In what ways are you incorporating reflective practice into your work?

- Consider a health improvement intervention with which you have been involved. What theoretical assumptions underpinned this activity? How would it be influenced by a consideration of other theoretical perspectives?

Recommended reading

- Bunton R, Macdonald G, editors: *Health promotion: disciplines and diversity*, edn 2, London, 2002, Routledge.

    An important book which traces the theoretical roots of health promotion in disciplines such as psychology, sociology, education, politics, genetics and epidemiology.

- *Critical Public Health* 18(4), 2008.

  A special issue of this journal devoted to health promotion in the twenty-first century. It includes discussions of the development of health promotion in Australia, Canada, Southern Africa and England.

- Davies M, MacDowall W, editors: *Health promotion theory*, Maidenhead, 2006, Open University Press.

- Macdowall W, Bonell C, Davies M, editors: *Health promotion practice*, Maidenhead 2007 Open University Press.

  Two short introductions to health promotion theory and practice

- Naidoo J, Wills J: *Foundations for Health Promotion*, London, 2009, Baillière Tindall.

  Part 1 of our companion volume that provides more detail on many of the issues discussed in this chapter including the development of health promotion and its theoretical approaches.

- Earle S, Lloyd C, Sidell M, et al, editors: *Theory and research in promoting public health*, London, 2007, Sage.

- Douglas J, Earle S, Handsley S, et al, editors: *A reader in promoting public health: challenge and controversy*, London, 2007, Sage.

- Lloyd C, Handsley S, Douglas J, et al, editors: *Policy and practice in promoting public health*, London, 2007, Sage.

  A series of texts to support an Open University course that examines debates and issues involved in multidisciplinary public health. Through the varied chapters and articles, these books provide an interesting review of the complexity of the field.

- Scriven A, Orme J, editors: *Health promotion: professional perspectives*, Buckingham, 2001, Open University.

- Watterson A, editor: *Public health in practice*, Basingstoke, 2003, Palgrave/Macmillan.

  These two texts examine the public health and health promotion roles of a range of professionals and explore the organizational and policy contexts and disciplinary approaches that influence practice.

References

Acheson D: *The future of public health in England*, London, 1988, HMSO.

Ajzen I: *Attitudes, personality and behaviour*, Maidenhead, 1988, Open University Press.

Ajzen I, Fishbein M: *Understanding attitudes and predicting social behaviour*, Englewood Cliff, 1980, Prentice Hall.

Arnstein S: Eight rungs on the ladder of citizen participation. In Cahn SE, Passelt BA, editors: *Citizen participation: effecting community change*, New York, 1969, Praeger.

Bandura A: *Social learning theory*, Englewood Cliffs, 1977, Prentice Hall.

Beattie A: The health promoting school: from idea to action. In Scriven A, Orme J, editors: *Health promotion: professional perspectives*, Basingstoke, 1996, Macmillan.

Beauchamp TL, Childress JF: *Principles of biomedical ethics*, Oxford, 1995, Oxford University Press.

Becker MH: *The health belief model and personal behaviour*, Thorofare, NJ, 1974, Slack.

Bunton R, Macdonald G, editors: *Health promotion: disciplines and diversity*, edn 2, London, 2002, Routledge.

Committee for the Study of the Future of Public Health: *The future of public health. Division of health care services/institute of medicine*, Washington, 1988, National Academy Press.

Department of Health: *The report of the Chief Medical Officer's project to strengthen the public health function*, London, 2001, DH.

Department of Health: *Healthy weight healthy lives: a cross government strategy*, London, 2008, DH.

Department of Health/Welsh Assembly Government: *Shaping the future of public health: promoting health in the NHS*, London, 2005, Department of Health.

Faculty of Public Health: *Good public health practice – general professional expectations of public health physicians and specialists in public health*, London, 2001, Faculty of Public Health Medicine.

Freire P: *Pedagogy of the oppressed*, Harmondsworth, 1972, Penguin.

Griffiths S, Jewell T, Donnelly P: Public health in practice: the three domains of public health, *Public Health* 119:907–913, 2005.

Hunter DJ, Marks L, Smith K: *The public health system in England: a scoping study*, Durham, 2007, Centre for Public Policy and Health, Durham University. Available at http://www.sdo.nihr.ac.uk/files/project/150-final-report.pdf.

Kolb DA: *Experiential learning – experience as the source of learning and development*, New Jersey, 1984, Prentice Hall.

Lewin K: *Field theory in social science: selected theoretical papers*, London, 1952, Tavistock.

Long A, Smyth G, Smyth A: Community nurses, midwives and health visitors' views of their role in promoting the health and social well-being of the population in Northern Ireland, *All Ireland J Nurs Midwifery* 1(5):176–183, 2001.

Maidwell A: The role of the surgical nurse as health promoter, *Br J Nurs (BJN)* 5(15):898–904, 1996.

McKay K: An exploration of student midwives' perceptions of health promotion in contemporary practice, *MIDIRS Midwifery Dig* 18(2):165–174, 2008.

McKeown T: *The role of medicine: dream, mirage, or nemesis?*, London, England, 1976, Nuffield Provincial Hospitals Trust.

Naidoo J, Wills J, editors: *Health studies: an introduction*, edn 2, Basingstoke, 2008, Macmillan/Palgrave.

Naidoo J, Wills J: *Foundations for Health Promotion*, edn 3, London, 2009, Baillière Tindall.

Nutbeam D, Harris E: *Theory in a nutshell: a guide to health promotion theory*, London, 2004, McGraw Hill.

Prochaska JO, DiClemente C: *The transtheoretical approach: crossing traditional foundations of change*, Harnewood, IL, 1984, Done Jones/Irwin.

Rawson D: The growth of health promotion theory and its rational reconstruction: lessons from the philosophy of science. In Bunton R, Macdonald G, editors: *Health promotion: disciplines and diversity*, edn 2, London, 2002, Routledge.

Schon D: *The reflective practitioner*, London, 1983, Temple Smith.

Scott Samuel A, Wills J: Health promotion in England, sleeping beauty or corpse? *Health Education Journal*: 66(2):115–119, 2007.

Senior R: *Organizational change*, London, 1997, Pitman.

SHEPS Cymru: *The principles and practice and code of professional conduct for health education and promotion specialists in Wales*, 2007.

Skills for Health: *National standards for specialist practice in public health*, Bristol, 2001, Skills for Health.

Thompson N: *Theory and practice in health and social welfare*, Maidenhead, 1995, Open University Press.

Webster C, French J: The cycle of conflict. In Adams L, Amos M, Munro J, editors: *Promoting health: politics and practice*, London, 2002, Sage.

WHO: *Health promotion: a discussion document on concepts and principles*, Geneva, 1984, World Health Organization.

WHO: *Targets for health for all*, Copenhagen, 1985, World Health Organization.

WHO: *Ottawa Charter for Health Promotion*, Copenhagen, 1986, World Health Organisation.

Wills J, Evans D, Scott Samuel A: Politics and prospects for health promotion in England, *Critical Public Health* 18(4):521–531, 2005.

Chapter Two

2

Research for public health and health promotion

Key points

- Nature of research
- Positivist and interpretivist paradigms
- Research for public health and health promotion:
  - Lived experience
  - Participatory research
  - Mixed methods research
- Using research in practice

OVERVIEW

Research is a link between theory and practice. It should, and does, inform practice, but using such knowledge and applying it can be difficult. The greater emphasis on accountability in the NHS has led to calls for practice to become more evidence based and, therefore, for practitioners to develop skills in conducting and appraising research. Evidence-based practice is the subject of Chapter 3. This chapter looks at the nature of the research that informs public health and health promotion, and argues that such research should contribute towards tackling the social causes of ill health and disease. This suggests the need for research that is qualitative (explores people's lived experience and understanding of their own health) and participatory (uses research methods that involve both the researchers and the researched working together). The chapter concludes by looking at the ways in which practitioners can use research in practice.

Introduction

In Chapter 1, we discussed the importance of practitioners becoming critical and self aware. A reflective practitioner will be looking closely at his/her professional practice, asking 'what is the best way of doing this?' or 'why do we do it this way?'. It may be that a practitioner acts on the basis of tradition or an intuitive 'knowing in action' which derives from experience (Schon 1983) but a reflective practitioner will wish to be informed about his decisions.

The shift from an occupation to a profession, which has taken place in nursing and multidisciplinary public health, is characterized by an increased focus on research as the foundation for professional knowledge and practice. There is considerable pressure for all health and social care practitioners to be aware of relevant research and to base their practice on research findings. Practitioners may be aware of this, yet be unable to pinpoint any specific relevant findings. This may be because practitioners are not aware of the relevant research journals, or are unable to access journals and conferences, or lack the opportunity, skills and time to keep up-to-date with research. The weight of new information, even though it may be more readily available through the internet, means practitioners may suffer from information overload and be unable to sift out what is useful and relevant. Practitioners may not use research because they lack the critical appraisal skills and confidence to assess the quality and relevance of published studies. Practitioners may also be sceptical of the value of research because it is difficult to institute any change in their practice or organization.

 Box 2.1 **Practitioners talking**

The following practitioners, when asked to identify research that had made an impact on them, were all able to cite a particular study:

Paula, a nurse

'Marmot's (2003) research into social status and health made me realize how important it is for people to feel in control of their lives and exercise autonomy. Instead of going in and telling people what to do, I now make time to find out their priorities and preference, and work together with them to achieve their goals.'

Penny, a health visitor

'I read Putnam's (2000) book on holiday, and the notion that social capital could be linked to health was an eye opener for me. The fact that improving community relationships and trust had a direct and positive effect on life expectancy and infant mortality, meant I could justify working with communities and this could become a legitimate part of my work.'

Peter, a health promotion specialist

'I remember reading the official report on tackling inequalities in health (DH 2003) and being so relieved to know that this was a national priority, and that proper resources were going to be allocated to it. And then reading the progress report (DH 2008), and realizing there was still so far to go. It made me think twice about the need to target and prioritize messages about healthy lifestyles like healthy nutrition, physical activity and stopping smoking. It made me consider how to promote healthier lifestyles to people whose living conditions make it difficult for them to change.'

Pat, a teacher and counsellor

'When I first came across Mellanby et al's (2000) review of research indicating that peer education was at least as effective – and maybe more effective – than teachers, it gave me lots of food for thought. Apart from it ringing true – after all, that's how I learnt about sex when I was a teenager – it made me think about developing peer education programmes about personal relationships, instead of giving the usual "I'm the expert, here's the information" talk about sex and personal relationships.'

Few practitioners see research as an integral component of their practice. It is seen as 'out there', separate from the knowledge base that informs practice, which is often received wisdom passed on from practitioner to student. However, practitioners often have questions relating to their practice, which can be answered by appropriate research studies. Examples of practitioners' questions include the Macmillan nurse who wants to know why women choose not to come for mammography screening, the health promotion specialist who wants to know whether a safety education programme for young children has made any difference to the accident rate, and the midwife who wants to find out the needs of prospective fathers from the antenatal services. If we see research as providing information to guide the planning and carrying out of interventions, then research ceases to be seen as a remote activity but becomes an extension of everyday work.

This chapter aims to help you reflect on what distinguishes research in public health and health promotion. It looks at the social context in which research for public health and health promotion takes place and the kind of information that informs practice. It is not a tool kit to make you a better researcher. Some excellent texts are recommended at the end of the chapter which can provide guided tours of research methods and the fine-tuning in using particular methods. Above all, being a researcher involves doing research and 'getting your hands dirty'; it cannot be learnt from a book.

 Box 2.2 **Discussion point**

What do you think distinguishes research from everyday findings about things that interest you?

What is research?

Health promotion is based on theories about what influences people's health and what are effective interventions or strategies to improve health. Such theories are based on research. The term 'research' refers to any systematic information-gathering activity used to describe, explain or explore an issue in order to generate new knowledge.

Research:
- is the investigation of the real world
- is informed by values about the issue under investigation

- follows agreed practices and ethical guidelines
- is guided by theory and assumptions about the presumed relations between different phenomena
- asks meaningful questions
- is systematic and rigorous
- is transparent.

There are several ways in which research informs public health and health promotion and contributes to its development. It may help, for example, to determine priorities for action from a seemingly endless list of possibilities. Epidemiological research or a needs assessment exercise may be the starting point for deciding which issues should be tackled. Evaluative research may determine the effectiveness or acceptability of particular interventions. A research audit may examine which resources and systems are in place for the purpose of improving the performance of an organization or project. Research can also support, challenge or generate new theory. The studies cited by the practitioners in the example above illustrate how research contributes to the body of knowledge informing public health and health promotion.

Research has achieved a much higher profile in health organizations in recent years. Policy, service provision and professional practice are expected to be based on evidence derived from rigorous research. For example, in 2009 NICE (National Institute for Health and Clinical Excellence) launched NHS Evidence, a web-based service disseminating research-based best practices (www.nice.org.uk). Professional judgement and the preferences of users and clients may also influence decision making but the cultural shift to evidence-based health care that is explored further in Chapter 3 represents a major challenge for practitioners. A large body of research for public health and health promotion derives from public health medicine and epidemiology. Epidemiology analyses patterns of disease and risk factors in populations, and seeks to identify and quantify the effect of different causal factors (genetic, lifestyle, environmental) on health.

Box 2.3 **Example**

Methods used by epidemiologists

- Cross-sectional studies to determine prevalence, or patterns of conditions, or behaviours in populations, or groups at one point in time – for example since 1991, there has been an annual Health Survey for England (National Centre for Social Research). In addition, every 2 years, a specific theme is identified for further study; for example in 2009, the theme was crime and safety.
- Case-control studies to investigate the causes of a condition by comparing a group with the condition with a control group – for example research into the effect of exposure to radon in homes on lung cancer rates in Europe (Darby et al 2005).
- Cohort or longitudinal studies to observe a group over time to see if there is any association between particular behaviours or characteristics and patterns of disease – for

example the Framingham (Massachusetts) Heart Study began in 1948 and is now studying the third generation of participants. Many risk factors for heart disease linked to diet and exercise were identified in this study. More recently, data from this study have been used to study the link between social networking, happiness and health (Fowler and Christakis 2008).
- Randomized control trial (RCT) compares a group experiencing an intervention with a similar control group which does not – for example an RCT of a workplace health promotion programme in Norway (Tveito and Eriksen 2009) found that, whilst there were no statistically significant effects on sick leave rates or health-related quality of life, the intervention group reported significant positive effects on well-being and work experience.

Epidemiology is generally acknowledged as a core scientific method underpinning public health. For example, the Whitehall I study tracked a large cohort of 18,000 men employed in the Civil Service since 1967, and has been influential in establishing the link between social status and health (Marmot et al 1984).

The Whitehall II study has followed up a cohort of 10,308 male and female civil servants since 1985. The Whitehall II study found no diminution in the links between social status and health (Marmot et al 1991), and is now examining inequalities in health in an ageing population (Adler et al 2008; Britton et al 2008).

 Box 2.4 **Example**

The uses of epidemiology

- *To observe the effects of social factors on health* – for example linking the rise in the number of cars on the road with the incidence of asthma.
- *To provide a 'map' of the distribution and size of health problems in the population* – for example infant mortality rate being distributed unequally among social classes.
- *To estimate the risks to an individual of suffering a disease* – for example the risk to

a post-menopausal woman taking hormone replacement therapy, of contracting breast cancer.
- *To assess the operation of services and the extent to which they meet the population's needs* – for example the take-up rate for the breast cancer screening programme and the effect on breast cancer incidence and outcomes.

Source: adapted from Ashton (1994)

Epidemiology therefore has many uses to public health and health promotion; however, it is not the sole means of acquiring information and knowledge. As with all research, epidemiological findings need to be interpreted within the specific theoretical framework in which they are grounded. Epidemiology reflects the dominance of the medical science paradigm. This approach seeks to identify the risk factors of disease and is informed by a belief that research needs to be objective and scientific.

Positivist and interpretivist paradigms

Knowledge is structured by the context in which a question is framed and the methods used to obtain, analyse and interpret data. The same topic can give rise to many different questions and thus be investigated from many different angles. The dominant research tradition in health and social care derives from a positivist approach which uses the methods and principles of the natural sciences. Positivism is based on the premise that there are objectively real phenomena or 'facts' which can be studied in a neutral scientific manner. However, this claim for objective neutrality has been questioned and it has been asserted that all knowledge production is influenced by values, ideologies and funders' agendas.

In contrast to positivism, the interpretivist tradition aims to explore and describe the meaning of phenomena as experienced and perceived by the individual person or people. This tradition derives from the concern of social sciences to understand the subjective meaning of human experience, which in turn rests on the premise that reality is a social construct that is always mediated by subjective meanings and contexts. Resulting knowledge is therefore always contextual and never absolute. The difference between these two approaches to research and knowledge is illustrated in the following example.

 Box 2.5 **Example**

Positivist and interpretivist research into ageing

Ageing is an important issue in the developed world, largely because a rapidly ageing population means an increase in the costs of providing medical and social care.

Positivist research views ageing as a real phenomenon, measurable through objective scientific tools, for example measurement of bone loss associated with the ageing process. Positivist research into caring for the elderly might produce projected population profiles and extrapolate the possible extent of certain age-related diseases (e.g. dementia, arthritis) in the future. Positivist research might also attempt to measure the projected costs of caring for an ageing population in the future. Research findings are viewed as objective and generalizable.

Interpretivist research, by contrast, seeks to explore the meanings and context of ageing amongst elderly and younger populations. Positive (e.g. wisdom) and negative (e.g. dependency) connotations of ageing might be identified and explored. The significance and meaning of ill health associated with ageing would be researched, and the factors that help or hinder people's coping mechanisms (e.g. social networks, religious beliefs) might be studied. Research would study the perceived benefits (e.g. grandparents providing childcare for working parents) as well as the disadvantages of an ageing population. Research findings are specific to the population (in terms of gender, social class, ethnicity) being studied, although findings might be transferable to other similar populations.

Positivism is associated with quantitative research methods – the gathering of 'hard' data which can be quantified in some way. Quantitative research attempts to measure aspects of a phenomenon and explain any differences in variables between groups or over time. Quantitative research tests a hypothesis, which is a suggested explanation of why differences occur. The experiment is the main method. In experimental studies, one aspect in two matched groups is varied to see if it makes any difference to the result. Any difference can then be attributed to that variable. Randomized controlled trials, in which participants are randomly allocated to a control or experimental group, are used to assess the effectiveness of interventions. In research involving people and their lives, it is impossible to control for all the factors which may influence outcomes. There may also be ethical concerns about withholding a potentially beneficial intervention from one group of participants; or conversely of carrying on with an intervention that appears to be harmful. There is further discussion about the role of randomized controlled trials and their contribution to the understanding of the effectiveness of interventions in Chapter 3.

 Box 2.6 **Example**

Randomized controlled trials of exercise-based cardiac rehabilitation programmes

A systematic review and meta-analysis of 48 randomized controlled trials investigating the impact of exercise-based cardiac rehabilitation programmes in patients with coronary heart disease was undertaken. Results showed that such programmes were associated with reduced all-cause mortality and reductions in some associated risk factors, for example cholesterol levels, systolic blood pressure, and smoking rates. The study concluded that exercise-based cardiac rehabilitation programmes had demonstrable benefits.

Source: Taylor et al 2004

Interpretivism is associated with qualitative research methods which focus on understanding the ways in which an issue is perceived by the people whom it affects. Thoughts, feelings and meanings are viewed as real phenomena which can be studied by the researcher. Using methods such as interviews, observation and case studies the researcher can come to understand the perspective of the participants. In contrast to the positivist tradition, there is no assumption about what are the important phenomena which are then measured. Interpretivism gathers 'rich' data and then derives plausible theories and explanations from analysing that data. This approach has also been called 'grounded theory' (Glaser and Strauss 1986) because the mode of analysis (deriving codes and categories from the data until 'saturation point' is reached and no new codes or categories emerge) leads to theory that is grounded in, and emerges from, real life experience.

If we use the example of research into sexual health we can see how different paradigms or schools of thought determine what is to be studied. Most research into the spread of HIV/AIDS has been concerned with discovering the incidence, prevalence, and distribution of HIV in the population over time. By comparing the proportion of infected people engaging in different risk activities, attempts are made to correlate the risk of infection with behaviour. This knowledge can be used in the targeting and design of health education messages. Epidemiologists can also evaluate the effectiveness of health promotion activities by charting rates of HIV infection against interventions.

Gary Dowsett, who designed research programmes for the WHO Global Programme on AIDS, commented on the need for more close-focus research which looks at contexts and social situations in which people make sexual decisions:

Utilizing precious research resources to maximize the measurement of HIV infection and AIDS in any one country will not greatly enhance the prevention and care/support response. A less exact and more general idea of HIV/AIDS prevalence/incidence will, when coupled with a well-theorized understanding of sexual and drug use cultures or contexts, offer far more useful starting points for action than all the surveillance data in the world.

(Dowsett 1995, p. 28)

Box 2.7 **Discussion point**

What contribution do you think qualitative research could make to HIV prevention?

Quantitative and qualitative research derive from different epistemological perspectives or views about the nature of knowledge and so are often presented as diametrically opposed. Table 2.1 summarizes the two philosophically divergent positions.

Table 2.1 Quantitative and qualitative research

	Quantitative	Qualitative
Paradigm	Positivism	Interpretive/naturalistic
Epistemological base	Science Knowledge is part of an objective reality separate from individuals	Humanities Knowledge is based on how individuals perceive experiences through 'individual lenses'
Researcher's role	Objectivity and detachment	Subjectivity and engagement
Aim	To progress towards the truth and verify knowledge	To understand multiple realities
Purpose	To understand causality	To interpret and reveal complexity
Methodology	To isolate and study discrete variables, for example experimental study	To understand the issue in context, for example ethnography, phenomenology
Methods	Less detailed information from larger number of participants, for example questionnaire To measure size of an effect Uses standardized measuring instruments	More detailed information from smaller number of participants To measure why effects occurred Uses a variety of methods, for example interviewing focus groups to find out participants' reality, concepts and meanings
Values	Validity, reliability	Validity, trustworthiness, credibility, confirmability, transparency
Presentation	Analysis of numbers and systematic quantification and analysis	Analysis of words and meanings, for example thematic content analysis, discourse analysis
Contribution to theory	Falsification (to disprove hypothesis) and test theory Deductive Generalization	To build theory, for example grounded theory emerges from the data Inductive Understanding complexity

In recent years, this apparent divide between these research traditions has been disputed. As Watterson and Watterson (2003, p. 26) point out, 'Public health methods are essentially eclectic'. Most health issues are so complex that different methods are suitable for different tasks and one method may illuminate or inform another.

Those using quantitative methods are often advised that it is good practice to inform their study with exploratory qualitative research. Different methods can, in addition, tap multiple realities and thus arrive at more valid findings. Triangulation refers to the use of multiple methods as a means of increasing validity. 'Triangulation in surveying is a method of finding out where something is by getting a fix from two or more places. Analogously, Denzin (1988) suggested that this might be done in social research by using multiple methods, investigators, or theories' (Robson 2002, p. 290).

Despite such arguments about interdependence, we would argue that there remains an epistemological divide. Qualitative research is often seen as subjective and lacking in rigour because researchers inevitably carry their own baggage with them when conducting research. Observations or interviews are not neutral data collection processes, but will depend in part on what researchers brings to the task – their training and knowledge, and also their own experiences, values and life history. Bias can be minimized by acknowledging the researcher's perspective, being open about all aspects of the process (transparency), and reflection on the researcher's role and contribution to the findings (reflexivity). Qualitative research findings are not generalizable as samples are usually too small and unrepresentative to be statistically significant. Yet enough should be known about the sample being studied to be able to judge the extent to which the findings are applicable elsewhere (transferability). Because qualitative research does not require any particular statistical expertise, it is often assumed that anyone with a modicum of interpersonal skills can do it. However, qualitative research requires specific skills, for example reflectiveness, neutrality and empathy, and is no less rigorous than quantitative research.

What counts as research?

 Box 2.8 **Discussion point**

Why do a high proportion of women stop breastfeeding within 2 weeks of their return home after delivery?

Consider the following two research studies and decide which of the two studies is more likely to get research funding and why.

Which of the two studies is more likely to get published in a nursing, midwifery or medical journal?

Study 1

A cohort study to compare breastfeeding rates at 2 and 4 months after delivery in women discharged 48 h after delivery and women discharged more than 72 h after delivery. A statistical package was used to compare length of time on the maternity ward with the length of time breastfeeding.

Study 2

An ethnographic study using participant observation in which the midwife's interaction with breastfeeding mothers was observed and their conversations with them about breastfeeding were noted in field notes. Mothers' views about breastfeeding and their perceptions of the support received from midwives were collected by semi-structured interviews.

Although this is a very simple example, you probably concluded immediately that the first study would be more likely to get funding and to be published. Public health researchers seeking funding often find that there is a methodological status hierarchy whereby qualitative research is deemed less legitimate than quantitative biomedical or epidemiological research (Green and Thorogood 2004). When seeking to get work published, the format many journals require – of hypothesis or question, method, results and discussion – reflects the type of research which will be deemed acceptable.

Multidisciplinary public health seeks to utilize and integrate the insights and knowledge produced by both quantitative and qualitative research. As such, it spans the biomedical and social science paradigms of health. To use the example above, it is as important to know why there is resistance to breastfeeding as it is to quantify the impact of a supportive environment on breastfeeding rates.

In recent years, there has been a significant emphasis on monitoring and evaluation. The World Health Organization recommends that at least 10% of financial resources for any initiative should be allocated for evaluation (WHO 1998). Evaluation methods encompass both quantitative and qualitative approaches. Although there is a large degree of overlap between research and evaluation, the two are separate: 'Evaluation is the systematic examination and assessment of features of a programme or other intervention in order to produce knowledge that different stakeholders can use for a variety of purposes' (Rootman et al 2001, p. 26). Evaluation is essentially value-driven, because it is appraising an intervention in terms of pre-determined criteria (Douglas et al 2007). Positivist research, by contrast, would claim to be neutral and an exercise in fact finding.

The definition of the issue to be studied, the research design, the methods used to carry out the research, the interpretation of the results and the dissemination of findings all reflect the way in which health improvement is perceived. So when we think about research for health improvement we need to think about what sort of information we need and what paradigm we are working in.

 Box 2.9 **Activity**

Can you think of an example of research relating to issues of interest or significance to a particular group which has not been taken up or funded?

Research for public health and health promotion

Public health and health promotion span many different disciplines and do not fit neatly into any existing disciplinary paradigm. Biomedicine, epidemiology and social sciences all contribute valuable knowledge and insights into the field of public health and health promotion. This leads to a complex situation regarding research, since biomedicine, epidemiology and social sciences use very different notions of research methodology and methods and have varying degrees of 'respectability'. Quantitative methodology has what is viewed as a solid grounding and has a track record in providing valuable insights. This knowledge may be characterized as providing answers to the 'what?' and 'when?' questions. To take the example of immunization, quantitative research can provide answers to questions about how communicable diseases spread in communities, and how effective immunization programmes are. Qualitative methodology, by contrast, is seen as less useful and less rigorous, and its insights are often dismissed as being very specific and not generalizable to other groups and populations. However, we would argue that qualitative research is invaluable in providing answers to the 'how?' and 'why? questions. For example, knowledge about unimmunized groups in society, and whether this is a deliberate choice or not, may be gleaned from qualitative research, and then used to provide effective 'top up' immunization campaigns. Quantitative and qualitative research methodologies therefore each contribute vital knowledge and insights, and both need to be included as contributing to the research base for public health and health promotion.

Qualitative research covers a vast array of methodologies and methods, which may be categorized in many different ways, including according to philosophical orientation, ideological affiliation, or practical methods. Park (1993) identified three different ways of knowing about a social issue:
- Instrumental (traditional science).
- Interactive (lived experience).

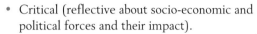

- Critical (reflective about socio-economic and political forces and their impact).

Bryant (2002) argues that all three types of knowledge are meaningful and should feed into the public health and health promotion policy process.

There are several excellent textbooks on qualitative and quantitative research methodologies and methods (see recommended further reading at the end of this chapter for details). This chapter does not seek to replicate this material, but instead to focus on what is unique and contested concerning the research base for public health and health promotion. Therefore this section will examine three contentious areas: the contribution to public health and health promotion of research into the lived experience, participatory research and mixed methods research.

The lived experience

Biomedicine and epidemiology focus on the statistics and facts about disease patterns in populations, and this knowledge is the bedrock of public health medicine. However, the newer concept of multidisciplinary public health stresses the need to explore how people construct concepts of health and illness and make sense of their experiences.

One of the claims of scientific knowledge is that it is objective and impartial. Lay knowledge represents another way of knowing. Although unrepresentative in

Box 2.11 Example

Living with diabetes

Campbell et al (2003) conducted a meta-ethnography of seven qualitative research studies on lay experiences of living with diabetes. Six key concepts were identified as contributing to well-being and a positive outlook:

- time and experience
- trust in self
- a less subservient approach to care providers
- strategic non-compliance with medication
- effective support from care providers
- an acknowledgement that diabetes is serious.

This suggests that empowerment, which includes non-compliance with medical advice, is vital to maximizing well-being. This in turn suggests a need to move away from the traditional model of 'doctor knows best' to a more egalitarian relationship between practitioners and patients.

a statistical sense, studies of lay beliefs do draw upon ideas that are general and shared. They thus present other discourses which need to be acknowledged and which compete with and contest the truth-claims of scientific knowledge. An illustration of this is provided by Allotey et al's (2003) study comparing the experiences of people suffering from paraplegia from Australia and

---

Box 2.10 Practitioner talking

I remember during training we were standing at the bedside of an elderly woman with diabetes, and a nurse telling us "This patient knows more about her disease than I do". At the time I wondered what was the point of telling us that, as it made it sound not worthwhile training to become a nurse. Now I appreciate the wisdom of that remark.

Commentary

A concern with lay knowledge and the lived experience of health, ill health and being a patient also underlies several policy strands.

For example, the Expert Patient programme is based on the recognition of patient knowledge and expertise about living with chronic disease (Donaldson 2003). Previous research had demonstrated that educating and empowering patients with arthritis led to an improvement in health status and social functioning (Lorig et al 1999). The Expert Patient programme uses trained lay volunteers to provide education in order to empower people living with chronic disease, and hence improve their quality of life.

Source: Campbell et al 2003

Cameroon. The DALY (disability adjusted life year) is a universal measure of the overall burden of disease. One DALY is equal to one year of healthy life lost. However, Allotey et al (2003) found significant national differences inthe extent to which paraplegia impacted on people's lives. The use of the DALY significantly under-represents the burden of living with chronic disease in developing countries. Allotey et al (2003) argue that, whilst socio-economic determinants of disease are widely recognized, we need to also acknowledge the importance of socio-economic determinants on the severity of disease.

Qualitative research is important in helping to 'unpack' complex phenomena such as living with chronic disease. Whilst quantitative research can itemize functional loss, the actual impact of chronic disease on people's lives is much more diverse and wide-ranging. For example, Hwang et al's (2004) study into Korean women living with rheumatoid arthritis identified eight major themes: severe pain, self-esteem, negative feelings, reflecting on the past life, concentrating on recovery from disease, a comfortable mind in pain, support of family and others, and new life. These themes provide valuable information for service providers wishing to provide appropriate and relevant services for their patients.

Acknowledging and using lay knowledge and insights drawn from people's lived experiences inevitably means working in partnership. This involves quite a radical departure from the traditional model of expert professional and ignorant patient, and necessitates a shift in perception, values and practice on the part of both practitioners and patients. Partnership working is discussed in more detail in Chapter 7.

 Box 2.12 **Discussion point**

Reflect on your experience of caring for people with chronic conditions. In what areas (if any) do you think they are more knowledgeable about the disease than you are, and in what areas (if any) do you think you are more knowledgeable? How can you as a practitioner make the best use of your own knowledge, and that of your patients?

Participatory research

One of the core principles of health promotion, according to the World Health Organization (WHO 1986), is that people have a right and duty to participate in the planning of their health care. If research forms the basis for this, then people also have a right to be active and equal participants in that research process and its dissemination. Research from whatever paradigm is often seen as 'expert' knowledge. It is often produced by and for other experts and can be intimidating and inaccessible to the lay person.

 Box 2.13 **Discussion point**

What might be the advantages and disadvantages of conducting participatory research rather than traditional research?

Traditionally research involves an expert researcher and passive subjects. Participatory research views the research participants as equal partners in the research process. This means that participants or communities are involved in all stages of the research process, from identifying areas to study, to the choice of appropriate methods, and the interpretation and application of results. The research process therefore becomes a means of empowerment as well as a means of producing knowledge. Community-based participatory research (CBPR) has become increasingly popular in public health and health promotion circles. This has been attributed to the fact that CBPR is both ethical and effective. Participatory research is empowering and supports people's autonomy, and may therefore be seen as a health promoting process in its own right. At the same time, such research produces relevant knowledge regarding real life issues of current concern to communities. This knowledge may then contribute to the design and implementation of effective interventions. Participatory research that taps into community agendas and concerns is therefore eminently practical and is likely to lead directly to appropriate and relevant action (Cook 2008). An example of CBPR is Horn et al's (2008) study of developing smoking cessation programmes for American Indian teenagers. Horn et al (2008) attribute the success of this intervention to the use of values-driven and community-based principles, including integrating the community's cultural knowledge and building capacity within the community.

Most researchers who have used a CBPR approach are enthusiastic about its usefulness and ethical robustness. However there are some drawbacks. CBPR involves a large commitment in terms of time and resources in order to access community views and to facilitate genuine partnership working across the community/researcher divide. The issues that are identified may include social factors (e.g. racism, homophobia) that are embedded in various social institutions and phenomena, not all of which are amenable to action by the research partners. Despite these caveats, the overall evaluation of participatory research is very positive. Participatory research has been hailed as providing the blueprint for a new type of research that is both ethical and practical, and which leads directly to effective action.

Mixed methods research

One obvious solution to the dilemma of whether to choose quantitative or qualitative methods to research public health issues is to use both. Mixed methods research has become increasingly popular as a pragmatic response to the dilemmas of what to focus on in research (Tashakkori and Teddlie 2003). Mixed methods research has evolved as a means of triangulation – the use of different perspectives or data to provide insights about a phenomenon. Using both quantitative and qualitative methods means that a variety of questions about a topic may be addressed (see Example below). Whilst enthusiasts claim mixed methods research provides valuable corroborated insights and knowledge, detractors claim that the enterprise is flawed, because it is attempting to unite fundamentally different ideological and theoretical perspectives. There are also practical challenges facing any researcher wishing to adopt a mixed methods approach. Quantitative and qualitative methods require different skills and expertise and traditionally

have been taught and used in different disciplines. Using a mixed methods approach means recognizing and valuing both methods equally. However, the benefits of adopting a mixed methods approach are increasingly being recognized and promoted, not least in the field of public health and health promotion. The evolution of mixed methods research has been heralded as a third research paradigm (alongside qualitative and quantitative paradigms) (Johnson et al 2007), and its 'coming of age' is signalled by the launch of a new journal in 2007 – the Journal of Mixed Methods Research.

 Box 2.14 Example

Mixed methods research into smoking

A study into the incidence of smoking amongst young people used mixed methods to address the following questions:

How many young people smoke? (quantitative method – survey)

What is the gender, socio-economic, and ethnic profile of smokers and non-smokers? (quantitative method – survey)

Why do young people smoke? (qualitative method – interviews)

What might persuade young people to quit smoking? (qualitative method – interviews)

By using mixed methods, the research study was able to identify the demographic profile of young people most at risk (smokers) as well as the factors influencing their decision to smoke or quit. This information was used to design a targeted smoking cessation intervention.

Using research in practice

Providing research that everyone agrees is relevant is an important step towards the effective use of research in practice. However, there are many other obstacles to using research in practice.

The utilization of research depends on effective dissemination. Practitioners have access to a large volume of research, evidence and guidance through electronic databases, evidence syntheses and journals. Unless the recommendations arising from these studies are incorporated into practice, such research initiatives are wasted. Practitioners need to become critical consumers of research, knowing the research in their area and being able to evaluate it with confidence (see Chapter 3 on evidence-based practice). Merely knowing about research findings is rarely, however, sufficient to change practice. The diffusion and adoption of innovation takes years, not months.

Often it requires practitioners to change long-held patterns of behaviour – and at what point research justifies a change in practice is debatable.

Box 2.15 **Activity**

Can you identify any changes or innovations in practice in your area of work? To what extent has research contributed to these changes? What other factors were involved?

Examples of midwifery and health visiting practice changing in response to research findings might include the change in advice to parents about the sleeping position of babies who should not be laid down on their fronts; or the routine enquiry into domestic violence during antenatal visits. Both these shifts in practice are attributable to research findings which led to a higher profile of the issues and new professional guidelines.

Research can challenge taken-for-granted assumptions and therefore being research-minded is a crucial part of reflective practice. But it is also important to be critical: how does one decide which evidence is sufficiently convincing to influence practice? Because this is difficult, and because knowledge is never a given but is always changing, practitioners often resort to their 'knowing-in-action' and ignore new

findings. There may also be a delay in the diffusion and adoption of interventions because they are not widely known. The publication of effectiveness reviews and meta-analyses (see Chapter 3) may help to diffuse knowledge but they need to be more user-friendly and adopt wider criteria than the randomized controlled trial as the 'gold standard' if they are to help practitioners directly.

Box 2.16 **Discussion Point**

What would it mean for you as a practitioner to be more 'research-minded'?

Most training courses for health and social care practitioners now include research appraisal skills and alert students to ways in which research studies can lack rigour. Common problems include making claims that are not substantiated by the data, or claiming that findings from exploratory studies can be generalized, or providing selective data to support a particular point of view. It is also important to be able to identify when research has been conducted rigorously. For quantitative research, rigour is achieved through representative samples which ensure that the findings can be generalized. Statistical manipulation of the data must be appropriate for the kind and quality of data obtained. For qualitative research, rigour is achieved through being systematic and open in the methods used and applying critical reflection to the research process. Rigorous qualitative research achieves relatability; or the discovery of insights which can be used in similar situations.

In the following chapter, we look at the strict criteria which are used to classify studies of effective public health and health promotion interventions. For practitioners, reading about research is a key component of developing research expertise both substantively and practically. Making a reasoned judgement about the value of a research study takes skill and practice but analysing strengths and weaknesses in the work of others helps practitioners in the design of their own studies.

Published papers are usually refereed by external reviewers in the field but this does not guarantee that the research is trustworthy. There is also a mass of needs assessment and evaluation studies, which practitioners routinely carry out but which are not published and so remain invisible. This body of research is termed 'grey literature'. It is important that practitioners do share their findings and experiences by bringing them into the public domain through reports, articles and conference papers. In this way the body of knowledge and theory about the relatively new field of multidisciplinary public health can be developed. Evaluating practice is discussed in greater detail in Chapter 20 in our companion volume *Foundations for Health Promotion* (Naidoo and Wills 2009). As well as being a critical consumer of research, there is an increasing emphasis on practitioners being accountable for their practice and therefore engaging in reviews of its effectiveness. They are called upon to demonstrate the health gain from any intervention and to base decision making on research.

Conclusion

The wider context for public health and health promotion is dominated by a positivist research paradigm, which quantifies and objectifies reality. Attempts to integrate an interpretivist research paradigm have often floundered under the charge of being too subjective and not rigorous enough. Multidisciplinary public health and health promotion face a challenging task in attempting to bring together both research traditions. However, the benefits of doing so are considerable, including insights into the 'why?' and 'how?' questions as well as the 'what?' and 'when?' questions.

The principles of research are ones that all practitioners can use – being aware of the way in which an issue is being defined, the philosophical principles which underpin the chosen methodological approach, the need to reflect on theory, and the ability to scrutinize and analyse available information. This practice of enquiry is an addition to the kind of

knowing that an experienced practitioner already has and it adds to common sense and intuitive problem-solving (Robson 2002).

In addition to the argument that research is a tool for practice there is also the view that research activity should promote the values and principles of public health and health promotion. Hence the calls for research to go beyond the scientific paradigm and embrace participatory research directed towards the social determinants of health and qualitative research which seeks to understand people's health experience.

Further discussion

- How can public health and health promotion research be translated into action and policy? What processes and partners are involved?

- What importance do you give to research in your work? Should your practice be more research linked? If so, how could you do this?

- Which research paradigm (quantitative, qualitative or mixed) would you favour for conducting research in your specialist field, and why?

Recommended reading

- Bowling A, Ebrahim S: *Handbook of health research methods*, Maidenhead, 2005, Open University.

  A comprehensive introduction to research methods with a focus on their applicability to health issues.

- Creswell JW, Clark VLP: *Designing and conducting mixed methods research*, London, 2007, Sage.

  A comprehensive guide to the use of mixed methods in research.

- Earle S, Lloyd CE, Sidell M, et al, editors: *Theory and research in promoting public health*, 2007, Milton Keynes, Open University Press/Sage.

A comprehensive overview of the theory and research base for multidisciplinary public health. Both quantitative and qualitative methodologies are explored and appraised.

- Gomm R: *Social research methodology: a critical introduction*, edn 2, Basingstoke, 2008, Palgrave Macmillan.

  An expert, comprehensive and readable guide to qualitative and quantitative research methods. The research process is unpacked and illustrated with real life examples, and research terms and concepts are fully explained.

- Green J, Thorogood N: *Qualitative methods for health research*, London, 2004, Sage.

A practical guide to carrying out qualitative research in health fields. This text follows the whole research process, from gaining ethical approval, through data collection and analysis, to writing up, dissemination and critical appraisal. Case studies illustrate key points.

- Silverman D, editors: *Qualitative research: theory, method and practice*, London, 2004, Sage.

  A comprehensive account of different qualitative methods of data collection and analysis, including visual and internet data. The use of case studies and practical examples helps the reader to fully engage with themes and issues.

References

Adler NE, Singh-Manoux A, Schwartz J, et al: Social status and health: a comparison of British civil servants in Whitehall-II with European- and African-Americans in CARDIA, *Soc Sci Med* 66(5):1034–1045, 2008.

Allotey P, Reidpath D, Kouame A, et al: The DALY, context and the determinants of the severity of disease: an exploratory comparison of paraplegia in Australia and Cameroon, *Soc Sci Med* 57(5):949–958, 2003.

Ashton J, editors: *The epidemiological imagination*, Buckingham, 1994, Open University.

Britton A, Shipley M, Singh-Manoux A, et al: Successful aging: the contribution of early-life and midlife risk factors, *J Am Geriatr Soc* 56(6):1098–1105, 2008.

Bryant T: Role of knowledge in public health and health promotion policy change, *Health Promot Int* 17(1):89–98, 2002, Oxford University Press.

Campbell R, Pound P, Pope C, et al: Evaluating meta-ethnography: a synthesis of qualitative research on lay experiences of diabetes and diabetes care, *Soc Sci Med* 56(4):671–684, 2003.

Cook WK: Integrating research and action: a systematic review of community-based participatory research to address health disparities in environmental and occupational health in the USA, *J Epidemiol Community Health* 62:668–676, 2008.

Darby S, et al: Radon in homes and risk of lung cancer: collaborative analysis of individual data from 13 European case-control studies, *Br Med J* 330:223, 2005.

Denzin N: *The research act: a theoretical introduction to sociological methods*, edn 3, New Jersey, 1988, Prentice Hall.

Department of Health (DH): *Tackling health inequalities*, London, 2003, The Stationery Office.

Department of Health (DH): *Tackling health inequalities: 2007 status report on the programme for action*, London, 2008, The Stationery Office.

Donaldson L: Expert patients usher in a new era of opportunity for the NHS, *Br Med J* 326(7402): 1279–1280, 2003.

Douglas J, Earle S, Handsley S, et al: *A reader in promoting health: challenges and controversies*, Buckingham, 2007, Open University Press.

Dowsett G: Focus on HIV/AIDS research, *Healthlines* 28:1995 December.

Fowler JH, Christakis NA: Dynamic spread of happiness in a large social network: longitudinal analysis of the Famingham Heart Study social network, *Br Med J* 337:a2338, 2008.

Glaser B, Strauss A: *The discovery of grounded theory: strategies for qualitative research*, Chicago, 1986, Aldine.

Green J, Thorogood N: *Qualitative methods for health research*, London, 2004, Sage.

Horn K, McCracken L, Dino G, et al: Applying community-based participatory research principles to the development of a smoking-cessation program for

American Indian teens: "Telling our story", *Health Educ Behav* 35(1):44–69, 2008.

Hwang EJ, Kim YH, Jun SS: Lived experience of Korean women suffering from rheumatoid arthritis: a phenomenological approach, *Int J Nurs Stud* 41(3):239–246, 2004.

Johnson RB, Onwuegbuzie AJ, Turner LA: Toward a definition of mixed methods research, *J Mix Methods Res* 1(2):112–133, 2007.

Lorig K, Sobel DS, Stewart AL, et al: Evidence suggesting that a chronic disease self-management program can improve health status while reducing hospitalization. A randomized trial, *Med Care* 37:5–14, 1999.

Marmot MG: Understanding social inequalities in health, *Perspect Biol Med* 46(3):S9–S23, 2003.

Marmot MG, Davey Smith G, Stansfield S, et al: Health inequalities among British civil servants: the Whitehall II Study, *Lancet* 337:1387–1393, 1991.

Marmot MG, Shipley MJ, Rose G: Inequalities in death-specific explanations of a general pattern? *The Lancet* 1(8384):1003–1006, 1984, May 5.

Mellanby AR, Rees JB, Tripp JH: Peer-led and adult-led school health education: a critical review of available comparative research, *Health Educ Res* 15(5):533–545, 2000.

Naidoo J, Wills J: *Foundations for health promotion practice*, edn 3, London, 2009, Baillière Tindall.

Park P: What is participatory research? A theoretical and methodological perspective. In Park P, Brydon-Miller M, Hall B, Jackson T, editors: *Voices of change: participatory research in the United States and Canada*, Toronto, 1993, Ontario Institute for Studies in Education Press.

Putnam R: *Bowling alone: the collapse and revival of American community*, New York, 2000, Simon and Schuster.

Robson C: *Real world research: a resource for social scientists and practitioner-researchers*, edn 2, Oxford, 2002, Blackwell.

Rootman I, Goodstadt M, Hyndman B, et al, editors: *Evaluation in health promotion: principles and perspectives*, Copenhagen, 2001, World Health Organization.

Schon D: *The reflective practitioner*, London, 1983, Temple.

Tashakkori A, Teddlie C, editors: *Handbook of mixed methods in social and behavioural research*, Thousand Oaks, CA, 2003, Sage.

Taylor RS, Brown A, Ebrahim S, Jolliffe H: Exercise-based rehabilitation for patients with coronary heart disease: systematic review and meta-analysis of randomized controlled trials, *Am J Med* 116(10):682–692, 2004.

Tveito TH, Eriksen HR: Integrated health programme: a workplace randomized controlled trial, *J Adv Nurs* 65(1):110–119, 2009.

Watterson A, Watterson J: Public health research tools. In Watterson A, editor: *Public health in practice*, Basingstoke, 2003, Palgrave, pp 24–51.

WHO: *Health promotion evaluation: recommendations to policy-makers report of the WHO European Working Group on health promotion evaluation*, Copenhagen, 1998, World Health Organization.

WHO: *Ottawa charter for health promotion*, Copenhagen, 1986, World Health Organization.

Chapter Three

3

Evidence-based practice

OVERVIEW

Evidence-based practice and policy have become the new mantra in health care. Yet there is no clear consensus about what defines the information that can be described as 'evidence', or how it should be used to drive changes in practice or policy. The traditional 'hierarchy of evidence' has very clear limitations when used to evaluate practice in areas such as policy change, community development or individual empowerment. This chapter outlines current thinking about evidence, the reasons for pursuing evidence-based practice and policy, and the skills practitioners need to acquire in order to become evidence-based. Evidence-based policy and practice are similar in many ways. Both are activities which take place in a complex context where other factors, such as custom, acceptability or ideology, may be more important than evidence in determining outcomes. This chapter focuses on evidence-based practice and the challenges this poses for practitioners. Many of the issues relating to evidence-based policy are discussed in Chapter 4 on policy. Specific dilemmas which arise when applying evidence-based practice to broad public health and health promotion goals are identified and discussed. This chapter concludes that evidence-based practice in health promotion and public health needs to go beyond the scientific medical model of evidence to include qualitative methodologies, process evaluation, and practitioners' and users' views. Evidence-based practice is a useful tool in the public health and health promotion kitbag, but it is not the only or overriding criterion of what is effective, ethical and sound good practice.

Introduction

Box 3.1 **Activity**

Think of an example of your practice where you have changed what you do. Has this change been brought about by:
- policy and/or management imperatives
- colleagues' advice
- technological advances
- cost
- evidence-based practice recommendations
- your own assessment and reflection
- users' requests and feedback.

Chapter 1 explored how evidence, theory and ethical values shape decision making in public health and promotion. Figure 3.1 illustrates some of these influences, indicating that evidence is just one among many drivers.

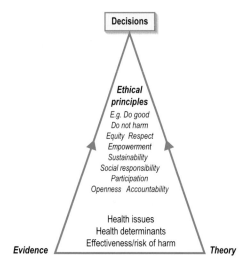

Figure 3.1 ● Influences on health promotion decision making (from Tannahill 2008).

Other factors which affect current practice are tradition, management directives concerning policy targets, performance and service users' views. Muir Gray (2001) argues that most healthcare decisions are opinion based and driven principally by values and available resources.

Box 3.2 **Discussion point**

What is meant by evidence in the context of decision making to improve health?

Evidence may refer to relevant facts that can be ascertained and verified. These facts may refer to incidence of disease; effectiveness and cost-effectiveness of interventions and preventive services; the views of service providers and users.

Chapter 1 highlighted how good practice requires the use of explicit research evidence and non-research knowledge (tacit knowledge or accumulated wisdom). The process is uncertain and frequently no 'correct' decision exists, especially in the complex field of public health where there are few conclusive outcomes. Evidence-based practice (EBP) claims to provide an objective and rational basis for practice by evaluating available evidence about what works to determine current and future practice. It was first applied to medicine, when Sackett defined it as: 'The conscientious, explicit and judicious use of current best evidence in making decisions about individual patients based on skills which allow the doctor to evaluate both personal experience and external evidence in a systematic and objective manner' (Sackett et al 1996, p. 71). As such, it is clearly differentiated from:
- tradition ('this is what we've always done')
- practical experience and wisdom ('in my experience, this approach is the most effective one')
- values ('this is what we should do')
- economic considerations ('this is what we can afford').

Many professions have embraced the advantages of an evidence-based approach to decision making.

EBP offers the promise of maximizing expenditure by directing it to the most effective strategies and interventions. The exponential rise of information technology and almost instant access to a multitude of sources of information makes EBP a more realistic possibility. However, it is unrealistic to expect practitioners to track down and critically appraise research for all knowledge gaps. It can be difficult for individual practitioners to know what is happening in the research world and pre-searched, pre-appraised resources, such as what the systematic reviews of the Cochrane Collaboration can offer an already synthesized and aggregated overview of the most up-to-date research findings for the busy practitioner.

 Box 3.3 **Activity**

What are the opportunities and barriers for evidence-based practice in your organization?

The opportunities for EBP may include:
- a current policy environment that values evidence
- links between service providers and universities to offer guidance and support
- new systems of clinical governance, audit and accountability that offer rigour and consistency in assessing outcomes
- greater emphasis on service users' views and feedback
- education and training that prepares practitioners to be reflective, to critically appraise research findings, and to use and evaluate EBP
- multiprofessional working that encourages collective debate and consensus regarding EBP.

Barriers to EBP include:
- reliance on the dominant positivist scientific model of evidence that may undervalue alternative sources of evidence
- increased workload and expectations with limited time for reflection
- limited research data in non-medical, non-pharmacological areas

- patchy access to information services
- shortage of critical appraisal skills
- pre-existing targets and performance indicators.

Whilst policy makers and practitioners may have their own agendas, and practice may be determined by factors such as protectionism, self-interest or ideological commitments as well as resource constraints, EBP offers the attraction of being above these concerns and offering definitive and neutral answers as to what constitutes best practice.

The conventional approach to finding, reviewing and assessing evidence has been imported from medicine and clinical decision making. It has established a 'gold standard' of evidence that privileges systematic reviews of randomized controlled trials (RCTs). Such reviews cover only a small proportion of public health issues, namely a small set of specific questions that can be answered by experimental methods, for example, do hip protectors reduce fractures from falls? As we have seen in our earlier book *Foundations for Health Promotion* (Naidoo and Wills 2009), and as we shall discuss further in Part 3 of this book, health outcomes are influenced by complex and interrelated factors. These include social, economic and environmental factors, as well as specific health-related behaviours, interacting with psychological, genetic and biological factors. Evidence that we may seek to guide public health and health promotion interventions is not always available – not because health promotion is ineffective but because of a paucity of evaluations. In order to understand 'what works' to improve health, we need to use evidence from a variety of sources, including qualitative and context-specific types of information or evidence.

Chapter 2 discussed how qualitative research is often denigrated as being 'soft', biased and not generalizable. However, there are accepted standards for rigour in qualitative research, and finding out about people's perceptions, beliefs and attitudes is crucial to successful health promotion and public health interventions. Investigating the complex processes involved in health improvement programmes, or measuring a range of effects, including people's views, provides vital knowledge for practitioners.

Such evidence may not conform to the scientific model, but does offer a more realistic and useful assessment of how in practice interventions lead to outcomes.

 Box 3.4 **Example**

Types of evidence

'Scared Straight' is a programme in the USA that brings at-risk or already delinquent children, mainly boys, into prison to meet 'lifers'. Inmates, the lifers themselves, the juvenile participants, their parents, prison governors, teachers and the general public were very positive about the programme in all studies, concluding that it should be continued. However, in a systematic review, seven good quality randomized control trials showed that the programme increased delinquency rates among the treatment group (Petrosino et al 2000 cited by Macintyre and Cummins 2001). Participants may not tell the same story as the outcome evaluation for many reasons, but their views on the process are valid and important data in their own right. Participants' views on the appropriateness and accessibility of the programme are essential in deciding whether or not to adopt programmes. The ideal programme will be both effective in terms of achieving desired outcomes, and acceptable to participants.

As Davies et al (2000, p. 23) observe, 'There is a tendency to think of evidence as something that is only generated by major pieces of research. In any policy area there is a great deal of critical evidence held in the minds of both front-line staff in departments, agencies and local authorities and those to whom the policy is directed'. This broader range of evidence from government advisers, experts and users needs to be included in decision making about health improvement. This more inclusive approach to evidence is advocated by many commentators and forums. For example, the 51st World Health Assembly urged all member states to 'adopt an evidence-based approach to health promotion policy and practice, using the full range of quantitative and qualitative methodologies' (WHA 1998).

What does it mean to be evidence based?

For the health practitioner, becoming evidence based means building practice on strategies which research has demonstrated are the most effective means for achieving stated aims. In theory, this would mean swapping uncertainties and traditional practices for specified techniques and strategies in the knowledge that they would lead to certain outcomes. In reality, there is never such absolute certainty, and research is not always totally reliable and valid, even if it is available for the particular issue of concern. So EBP is a journey towards more reliable and effective practice, and one that involves the practitioner becoming open-minded and flexible. To become evidence based, one has to be willing to change one's practice. This refers to organizations as well as individuals or professions. Individual practitioners' attempts to become more evidence based may flounder due to organizations' entrenched practices and inability to change.

Decision making in public health and health promotion demands information or evidence about the nature of the problem to be addressed, including its magnitude and whom it affects, as well as evidence about possible interventions. When considering the evidence that has been 'tested' in an intervention practitioners need to know:

- does it improve health, that is, is it effective?
- is it cost effective compared to other interventions or doing nothing, that is, is it efficient?
- is it acceptable to users or the public?
- can it be implemented safely, consistently, and feasibly and will it strengthen practice?
- will it tackle injustice and contribute to reducing inequalities?

Box 3.5 **Practitioner talking**

I work in Southern Africa and we need to find ways of reducing HIV transmission and continue to promote the condom. One company offered to supply us with female condoms but rather than just go ahead and distribute them on an ad hoc basis we wanted to know if there was any evidence supporting the use of the female condom in Africa. In particular, we wanted to know:

- *How many women use female condoms?*
- *What are their experiences and what would be the barriers to their acceptability?*
- *What are the sociocultural issues influencing acceptability in African contexts?*
- *How have they been implemented in other health settings?*
- *Would there be political support within our sexual health strategy for the promotion of the female condom?*

We did a simple internet search and found lots of scholarly papers but they reported information from African American women in the USA or STD clinic users which didn't seem relevant. One person had reported at the 2004 AIDS conference in Bangkok about a programme distributing female condoms in a district. We did find one paper in the South African Medical Journal (Beksinska et al 2001) but we could only read the summary online and so don't know whether this study is relevant or comprehensive.

Commentary

This practitioner had access to the internet and search skills both of which often constitute barriers to EBP. The access for full text papers is limited for most practitioners especially in low-income countries. Most evidence on the female condom relates to its effectiveness in reducing STI transmission and not its acceptability.

Many public health and health promotion interventions have been introduced without good evidence that their outcomes meet stated objectives. For example, breakfast clubs in schools have been widely introduced and promoted as part of a drive to improve healthy eating and to tackle inequalities in child health. Evaluation shows that they provide children with a nutritional start to the day, can therefore improve concentration and performance, and promote social interaction. However, there is only limited evidence of their effectiveness in promoting healthy eating amongst children, or of their ability to target the most disadvantaged children (Lucas 2003).

It is this uncertainty that has led to the production of evidence-based briefings that appraise current evidence of effective interventions in a digestible form for practitioners and policy makers. Evidence-based briefings select recent, good quality, systematic reviews and meta-analyses and synthesize the results. Clinical guidelines are a top-down strategy to produce practice in line with available evidence of what works

and to ensure comparable standards and reduce variations in practice. Clinical guidelines translate evidence into recommendations for clinical practice and appropriate health care that can be implemented in a variety of settings. Recommendations are graded according to the strength of the evidence and their feasibility. So recommendations supported by consistent findings from RCTs that use available techniques and expertise would be graded more highly than recommendations supported by an expert panel consensus that rely on scarce expertise and resources. The National Institute for Health and Clinical Excellence (NICE) publishes guidance on public health interventions (see www.nice.org.uk/guidance/PHG/published.) Such guidance makes recommendations for populations and individuals on activities, policies and strategies that can help prevent disease or improve health. The guidance may focus on a particular topic (such as smoking), a particular population (such as schoolchildren) or a particular setting (such as the workplace).

Box 3.6 **Discussion point**

If guidelines are 'systematically developed
statements to assist decision making
about appropriate interventions for specific
circumstances', is it feasible to produce them for
public health and health promotion?

Health promotion and public health practitioners
face particular difficulties in becoming more evidence based. These include:

- the complexities of searching for primary studies
  which are sparse
- assessing evidence from non-randomized studies
  (including qualitative research)
- finding evidence relating to process and how an
  intervention works
- synthesizing evidence from different study
  designs
- transferability of results to other contexts which
  differ from those used in the original research.

Skills for EBP

Adopting an evidence-based approach follows five
key stages:

- turning a knowledge gap into an answerable
  question
- searching for relevant evidence
- extracting data/information for analysis
- appraising the quality of the information/data
- synthesizing appraised information/data.

Box 3.7 **Activity**

What knowledge or skills do you need to be an
evidence-based practitioner?

Being evidence based means having both the knowledge and the confidence to tackle issues effectively.

To become an evidence-based practitioner means
adopting a critical view with regards to research and
evidence, and being willing to change your practice if
the evidence suggests this is worthwhile. The practitioner who seeks to become evidence based needs
to acquire the knowledge and skills to find out and
access, critically appraise, and synthesize and apply
relevant evidence. Evidence includes research as well
as more anecdotal and developmental accounts linking inputs to outputs.

Being evidence based includes the ability to separate evidence from other drivers of practice, including politics, custom and ethical considerations.
Above all, being evidence based requires an open
and critical mind to reflect on your own knowledge
about an issue, and assess competing claims of knowledge. Many interventions are implemented despite a
lack of certainty about the evidence for their effectiveness because practitioners act on intuition or
respond to pressures to do something. Cummins and
Macintyre (2002) refer to 'factoids' – assumptions
that get reported and repeated so often that they
become accepted. They describe the way in which
food deserts (areas of deprivation where families
have difficulty accessing affordable, healthy food)
have become an accepted part of policy because they
fit with the prevailing ideological approach, although
there is little evidence to support their existence.
Equally, some interventions are not implemented
despite evidence of their effectiveness because they
are not politically or socially acceptable.

Asking the right question

There are now many 'short-cuts' to evidence in systematic reviews, evidence briefings and guidance but
knowledge gaps remain. For example, NICE recently
published guidance on promoting physical activity for
children and young people (NICE 2009) but there
was little evidence on what works to promote activity in pre-school children. Being clear about what
you need to know is a vital first step. It is this process that starts the search for relevant evidence and
the process of appraisal. Asking the right question

means finding a balance between being too specific (asking a question that is unlikely ever to have been researched), and being too vague (asking a question that will produce a mass of research studies, many of which will be inapplicable to the context and circumstances you are interested in).

 Box 3.8 **Discussion point**

A smoking cessation coordinator is concerned at the rising rates of smoking among young women. The coordinator wants to extend the service to young people who wish to quit. The coordinator thinks that a cessation group could be established in one of the local secondary schools but is not sure how to proceed or whether the accepted model of cessation would work with young people. What does she need to know?

The coordinator will be interested in those factors that facilitate young people to quit and the factors that might act as barriers. The coordinator will search for research on the impact of the school setting on smoking, smoking cessation interventions in schools and its efficiency in relation to other methods such as health education and its acceptability to young women. If insufficient research is available, they may look at other research on young people's attitudes to quitting and cessation studies in other settings.

What counts as evidence?

Evidence may be of many different types, ranging from systematic reviews and meta-analyses, to collective consensual views, to individual experiences and reflections. All types of evidence have their uses. EBP traditionally reifies science above experience but as we have seen in Chapter 1, experiential reflection is an important part of informed practice. Similarly, the expertise of users is vital to developing acceptable interventions. Most EBP relies on:

- written accounts of primary research in refereed academic and professional journals
- academic and professional texts (reviewed)
- independently published reports
- unpublished reports and conference papers and presentations (grey literature).

Evidence may be defined as data demonstrating that a certain input leads to a certain output. However, the use of evidence to inform practice is broader than this, and encompasses:

- information about an intervention's effectiveness in meeting its goals
- information about how transferable this intervention is thought to be (to other settings and populations)
- information about the intervention's positive and negative effects
- information about the intervention's economic impact
- information about barriers to implementing the intervention (SAJPM 2000, p. 36, cited in McQueen 2001).

The scientific medical model has gained dominance in the debate about defining evidence. This model states that evidence is best determined through the use of scientific methodologies which prioritize quantitative objective fact finding. The use of scientific models of evidence leads to a search for specific inputs causing specific outputs, regardless of intervening or contextual factors such as socio-economic status, beliefs or a supportive environment. Such intervening factors, which mediate and moderate the effect of inputs, are viewed as 'confounding variables' and study designs try to eliminate their effect. The RCT, using the experimental method, is viewed as the most robust and useful method for achieving results which qualify as evidence and is viewed as the 'gold standard'. The criteria relevant for RCTs include:

- The intervention is experimental, with a control group which does not experience the intervention.
- There is random allocation of individuals to the experimental or control group.
- Allocation is double-blind; that is, neither patients nor practitioners know which group is the experimental or control group.

- There is a baseline assessment of patients to ensure that the experimental and control groups do not differ in any significant ways.
- There is a full follow-up of all patients.
- Assessment of outcomes is objective and unbiased.
- Analysis is based on initial group allocation.
- The likelihood of findings arising by chance is assessed.
- The power of the study to detect a worthwhile effect is assessed.

Box 3.9 **Discussion point**

What drawbacks, if any, can you identify regarding the use of this rigorous methodology?

The RCT methodology is appropriate for the analysis of alternative treatments or therapies for medical conditions affecting individual patients. Even in these cases, RCTs cannot take account of significant differences in practitioner input, such as level of enthusiasm, technical skills or knowledge. There may also be ethical concerns if one treatment looks markedly better or worse than another at an early stage. For interventions that are group or population based, it becomes very difficult if not impossible to adopt an RCT methodology. Groups differ according to geography, demographic and socio-economic factors, so finding a true control group is very difficult. It is impossible to isolate groups so there may be 'leakage' of relevant variables (such as information) from one group to another.

There is now a well-established 'hierarchy of evidence' shown below which grades research findings according to how valid and reliable the research methodology is deemed to be. Valid means that appropriate methods to answer the question are selected and correctly performed, and therefore the results are generalizable to other populations. Reliable means that the research methodology is transparent and unbiased and could be replicated, with the same results, by other researchers.

Box 3.10 **Example**

The hierarchy of evidence

The hierarchy goes from the most reliable evidence (Type 1) to the least reliable evidence (Type 5).

- *Type 1 evidence*: Systematic reviews and meta-analyses, including two or more RCTs.
- *Type 2 evidence*: Well-designed RCT, for example, prospective experimental trial of treatment where subjects are randomly assigned to the experimental or control group.
- *Type 3 evidence*: Well-designed controlled trial without randomization, for example, retrospective study comparing a control and intervention group.
- *Type 4 evidence*: Well-designed observational studies, for example, case studies.
- *Type 5 evidence*: Expert opinion, expert panels, views of service users and carers.

Box 3.11 **Activity**

How appropriate is the hierarchy of evidence for public health and health promotion?

The hierarchy of evidence has evolved in the context of individual care and treatment carried out within one disciplinary paradigm – scientific medicine. Public health and health promotion, which focus on communities and populations, provide a very different subject for research. They are multidisciplinary bodies of knowledge, and the evidence they draw upon is correspondingly varied. The use of evidence within health promotion has been likened to the judicial notion of evidence, which is typically a mixture of witness accounts, expert testimony and forensic science (McQueen 2001). Using this concept of evidence, individual stories which relate processes, interpretations and outcomes are as valid as scientific trials which seek to determine the effect of single causal factors.

This more inclusive notion of evidence, with its combination of accounts which vary in terms of what they construct as the truth, seems more appropriate to public health and health promotion. The scientific model of evidence could be viewed as disabling multidisciplinary practice through its prioritization of scientific evidence and its discounting of other forms of evidence. Using a more inclusive notion of evidence does not mean abandoning the concept of methodological rigour and quality. As we saw in Chapter 2, research studies that use qualitative methodologies may still be assessed for rigour.

 Box 3.12 **Discussion point**

What criteria of methodological validity (aspects of research design which would lead you to be confident that the results are meaningful and generalizable to other populations) would you stipulate if you were conducting a review of the effectiveness of health promotion interventions to initiate and maintain breastfeeding?

Desirable methodological characteristics of research into effectiveness include:
- The intervention is described in sufficient detail so that it could be replicated by others.
- The target audience is fully described.
- The size and effect of non-respondents is included.
- There are clear outcomes or health status measurements.
- These outcomes are compared to a comparison group that has not received the intervention.

Finding the evidence

The key to EBP is that evidence is collected systematically. This means that a full search of all available sources of information is undertaken, and full details are given of how the search has been conducted. This includes citing:
- key words
- databases that have been accessed
- criteria used to include or exclude research studies.

Systematic reviews, for example, typically exclude large numbers of studies that fail to meet their criteria for rigour. Such criteria include full details of non-respondents, before and after measurements, and the use of a control group. Searches for evidence are also usually only undertaken for English language materials and are often confined to research carried out in developed Western countries. It has been claimed that this omission leads to systematic bias and lack of relevance for developing countries (McQueen 2001).

The internet has greatly expanded the amount of information that can be accessed, and it is easy to waste time collecting information which is not relevant. In order to avoid this, systematic searches should be:
- explicit – use key terms, record your search, ensure it is transparent so others can assess its value and it can be repeated
- appropriate – look where the evidence is likely to be
- sensitive – collecting all the information which is relevant to your question
- specific – collecting only information that is relevant to your question
- comprehensive – include all available information.

There are a number of valuable sources of evidence that can be used to guide practice. Bibliographic databases such as Medline or Cinahl gather together articles and give short extracts. Databases such as these, however, only hold a small proportion of relevant literature. Other databases are more like libraries of information, for example, the Cochrane Collaboration. Systematic searches involve a number of stages. These are:
- Identifying sources of information, sweeping as widely as possible at the start in order not to exclude any relevant studies.
- Using a protocol to plan your approach so that your search is transparent and can be reproduced by others. Protocols typically include a number of stages starting with the best available evidence and moving towards less reliable evidence. For example, a search might start with meta-analyses,

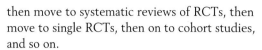

then move to systematic reviews of RCTs, then move to single RCTs, then on to cohort studies, and so on.

- Doing the search, using relevant terms and combinations of terms including abbreviations and filters. The ways in which words are linked together to search is called Boolean logic.
- Searching for quality, or narrowing the search by excluding the least useful sources. This may involve restricting the search to high quality studies or restricting the search by specifying time limits or certain combinations of terms.

In addition to the online databases listed in Example 3.13, there are many other means of searching sources of evidence. These include:

- searching online databases of unappraised primary research
- online searching of relevant websites for unpublished articles and information
- library searches of indexed and non-indexed sources
- manual searching of academic and professional journals
- manual searching of theses and independently published reports
- contacting dedicated information clearing houses and acknowledged experts.

All searches need to be systematically carried out, using consistent keywords or phrases, and these need to be made transparent in order for others to gauge their suitability and comprehensiveness.

 Box 3.13 **Example**

Searching for evidence

Obesity in children is a recognized and increasing problem. While there is considerable research into predisposing factors, most interventions that aim to control and reduce weight gain are poorly evaluated. In the USA residential weight-loss 'fat' camps have been introduced. In order to ascertain whether to introduce 'fat' camps in the UK evidence is needed on:

- their effectiveness in reducing weight in children
- their efficiency in relation to other family-centred methods
- their acceptability to children and parents
- the factors that influence their success.

One of the main problems in searching for evidence is being too broad in the search of online databases. A search using the keywords 'child' and 'obesity' would be likely to yield an excessive amount of 'hits'. Successful searching systematically limits and combines key terms and may use exclusion criteria such as English language and a year period. A search using key

words of fat – and camp – and residential revealed the following published papers:

Gately PJ, Cooke CB, Butterly RJ, et al: The acute effects of an 8-week diet, exercise and educational camp program on obese children. *Paediatr Exerc Sci* 12:413–423, 2000.

Gately PJ, Cooke CB, Butterly RJ, et al: The effects of a children's summer camp programme on weight loss with a 10 month follow up. *Int J Obes* 24:1445–1452, 2000.

Payne J, Capra C, Hickman I: Residential camps as a setting for nutrition education of Australian girls. *Aust N Z J Public Health* 26: 383–388, 2002.

Walker LLM, Gately PJ, Bewick BM, et al: Children's weight-loss camps: psychological benefit or jeopardy? *Int J Obes* 27:748–754, 2003.

Gately PJ, Cooke CB, Barth JH, et al: Children's residential weight-loss programs can work: a prospective cohort study of short-term outcomes

Box 3.13 **Example—cont'd**

for overweight and obese children, *Pediatrics* 116(1):73–77, 2005.

The Cochrane Library may yield a systematic review – in this case there is a recent review on interventions for preventing obesity in children but it does not refer to fat camps (Campbell et al

2004). A hand search of journals might include the *International Journal of Human Nutrition and Dietetics* or the *International Journal of Obesity*. A web search using a search engine such as 'Google' for key experts in this example, provided a link to Carnegie International Camp – Britain's first international weight loss summer camp.

Appraising the evidence

Not all evidence is useful for planning public health and health promotion activities. Some interventions have not been evaluated in a rigorous way and so it is difficult to know if they are worth employing elsewhere. Assessing the value of evidence is a skilled task and is termed critical appraisal. Traditionally critical appraisal in EBP determines the quality of the research study. Assessing the validity and reliability of research is used when deciding whether or not the findings are generalizable and can be applied elsewhere.

Appraising the evidence can seem a daunting prospect when there are so many sources of evidence available in various formats. It is important to obtain the relevant information from research reports:

- identification (title, date, authors, publishers, funding)
- the population, settings and activities (what, how, where, when and with whom was the intervention carried out?)
- the outcomes
- techniques of data collection and analysis.

Critical appraisal for public health and health promotion may be defined as the systematic and structured evaluation of the relevance of a study. Its purpose is 'to find in the evidence anything of value that will help you make a better decision' (Hill et al 2001: 86). Five key questions are:

- What did the research set out to find? (Are there specified aims or questions?)
- With whom was the study conducted? (Is there a clear rationale for the sample?)

- What methods were used? (Were the methods appropriate for the question? Were the methods carried out correctly?)
- What were the findings? (What methods were used to analyse the data and is this adequately described? Are the findings reported in full? Can you trust them?)
- What does it mean? (Are the findings relevant to your problem? Are they applicable to your setting?)

 Box 3.14 **Discussion point**

How do you decide if evidence should inform your decision making?

Do you agree with the following definition?

The term 'best quality' evidence should refer to evaluative research that was matched to the stage of development of the intervention; was able to detect important intervention effects; provided adequate process measures and contextual information, which are required for interpreting the findings; and addressed the needs of important stakeholders.

Hill et al 2001: 86

There is a large body of literature on critical appraisal skills as well as several useful guides (e.g. CASP – for details see Further Reading at the end of this chapter). Critical appraisal guides provide questions that enable the appraiser to assess the methodological rigour of different types of research study. Questions are grouped under three main headings:

- Are the results of the study valid?
- What are the main results?
- Will the results help locally?

Critical appraisal therefore seeks to identify useful, rigorous, high quality research and exclude irrelevant or flawed research. This is a question of degree, for it is usually possible to identify flaws in published research studies and ways in which the context of the research and one's own practice differ. Critical appraisal is then a pragmatic process whereby research is screened so that only studies that reach a certain standard of rigour and relevance are taken into account.

Synthesizing the evidence

Systematic reviews and meta-analyses are both forms of secondary research that take primary research studies as their object of study. A systematic review identifies all the relevant information available on a specific topic, critically appraises its quality, and summarises its results using an appropriate scientific methodology. The 'systematic' aspect of the review means that it is undertaken in a structured, objective and thorough manner, and that it is written up in such a way that those methods are clear enough for someone else to reproduce and come to the same results. Such reviews then go on to synthesize research findings in a form which is easily accessible to those who have to make policy or practice decisions. In this way, systematic reviews reduce the bias which can occur in other approaches to reviewing research evidence. The 'Gold Standard' methods of a systematic review are those recommended by the Cochrane Collaboration. A Cochrane review is often a time-consuming piece of research using dedicated researchers working full time. Organizations such as the Centre for Reviews and Dissemination at York and the National Institute of Health and Clinical Excellence (NICE) use very similar methods to those of the Cochrane Collaboration.

Despite the widespread and recognized value of qualitative studies, the criteria for inclusion within systematic reviews of health promotion have tended to be similar to those used by evidence-based medicine, with a dominance of experimental studies. Inclusion tends to be based on the quality of the study rather than the quality of the intervention. Their usefulness for public health and health promotion practitioners and policy makers can be limited because, as Tilford (2000) notes, reviews give insufficient information about the process of implementing an intervention and often focus on a narrow range of outcomes rather than the complexity of the programmes with which practitioners are engaged.

A systematic review should:

- specify the inclusion and exclusion criteria
- describe and use comprehensive and systematic search methods to locate all relevant studies
- assess the quality of primary studies in ways which can be replicated
- explore the consensus and variation between the findings of different studies
- synthesize primary studies.

The Cochrane Library is expanding the reviews relating to public health and health promotion (www.vichealth.vic.gov.au/cochrane). Those relating to cardiovascular health, for example, currently include reviews on dietary modification, smoking cessation, physical activity promotion, weight reduction, and compression stockings for airline passengers.

Techniques for the synthesis of qualitative research studies do exist and are developing rapidly. Meta-ethnography is the term used to describe the systematic synthesis of qualitative research studies (Noblit and Hare 1988). Meta-ethnography provides an interpretive synthesis rather than the aggregative, quantitative synthesis of meta-analysis. Meta-ethnography identifies, codes and summarizes themes from the literature until saturation point is reached, and further integration of themes is considered invalid. Attempts are made to preserve individual observations and nuances. Meta-ethnography has been used to systematically review evidence about patient and lay perspectives (Campbell et al 2003) and its use is expanding.

Box 3.15 **Example**

Sources of evidence

- *Campbell Collaboration* http://www. campbellcollaboration.org. An international collaboration which produces systematic reviews of studies researching the effectiveness of social and behavioural interventions.
- *Cochrane Collaboration* http://www.cochrane. org/. An international collaboration which produces systematic reviews of the effects of healthcare interventions. The collaboration covers a wide range of healthcare topics, for example, brief alcohol interventions in primary care Kaner et al 2007. There is health promotion and public health field, http://www. vichealth.vic.gov.au/cochrane, which seeks to provide evidence to guide practice in health promotion and public health. This field explicitly encourages collaboration and wide participation as well as the minimization of bias and ensuring quality.
- *Evidence for Policy and Practice Information Centre* http://www.eppi.ioe.ac.uk. A UK centre using innovative methods for systematic

reviews mostly related to health promotion interventions for young people.
- *The UK National Electronic Library for Health* http://www.library.nhs.uk/publichealth. A national database containing summaries of the best available evidence on topics such as alcohol, tobacco, mental health, sexual health and children and young people.
- *UK Economic and Social Research Council Evidence Network.* A UK network reviewing research into social, community and policy interventions.
- *Effectiveness Matters* http://www.york.ac.uk/ crd. Provides summaries about research evidence.
- *National Institute for Health and Clinical Excellence* (NICE) http://www.nice.org.uk. NICE is a UK organization that collates and disseminates evidence on effectiveness and cost-effectiveness.
- *Health Evidence Bulletins Wales* http://hebw. cf.ac.uk/. Provides summaries and links to research evidence.

Widening the evidence base

Reviews of evidence privilege certain forms of knowledge and information over others. However, to achieve practical results, practitioners and users need to be persuaded that the outcomes they value will be affected by an intervention. This means incorporating their views in the evidence base.

Box 3.16 **Discussion point**

How can expert, practitioner and user views be incorporated into evidence-informed decision making?

There are a number of ways in which practitioner and user views can feed into this process, including

evaluations of user views, inputs into research design and representation on committees and bodies that construct and use evidence. For example, INVOLVE (www.Invo.org.uk) examines the ways in which research is prioritized, commissioned, undertaken and disseminated.

Box 3.17 **Example**

Smoking in pregnancy

A systematic review reported increases in birth weight and a reduction in still-births following smoking cessation in pregnancy programmes. A letter to the author of the review commented on: 'the need for trials to address broader outcome measures such as the impact on other

Box 3.17 **Example—cont'd**

family members, the benefits to women's health, whether non-smoking is sustained, the impact of failing to stop smoking, stress levels, the emotional impact of having a low birth weight baby after taking part in a strategy to stop smoking and self-esteem'. Oliver (2001) reports that, as a result, the revised review incorporated observational and qualitative research, and small-scale consultations with health promotion practitioners and health service users, which broadened the content of the work and influenced the criteria by which the effectiveness of programmes was judged. To be persuasive in changing practice, evidence on programme effects and outcomes needs to be acceptable and relevant to those delivering and receiving such programmes.

Source: Oliver (2001)

Putting evidence into practice: Issues and dilemmas

Box 3.18 **Discussion point**

What, if any, problems can you foresee in becoming an evidence-based practitioner?

Although evidence-based public health and health promotion is often portrayed as the key to effective professional practice, there remain significant questions and dilemmas for practitioners seeking to incorporate evidence into their everyday practice, not the least being how to evaluate any evidence found (Rychetnik et al 2002). Common dilemmas for practitioners include:
- how much evidence is required before introducing an intervention
- does the research describe situations that are comparable to their own (including comparable caseloads or communities, organizations, staff and resources)

- does the evidence include the views of all relevant stakeholders
- what to do when the evidence goes counter to personal intuition, judgement or values
- whether evidence can ever claim to be objective or neutral
- how to identify cost-effectiveness.

Some of these dilemmas are discussed in greater detail below.

Using EBP to determine cost-effectiveness

In any discussion about effectiveness, the issue of resources is likely to crop up. Real life decisions take place within an economic context, being made with reference to costs and competing claims. It is not enough simply to argue that an intervention is effective; it also has to be cost-effective (the optimum means of producing given outcomes at least cost). The expanding field of health economics addresses these issues and seeks to provide rational tools for evaluating interventions by comparing costs with benefits. Traditionally this has taken the form of costs and benefits per individual patient, and the field of public health and health promotion, with its emphasis on social costs and benefits, has been neglected. There are now moves to address this deficit and define new constructs and frameworks which focus on public health in its broadest sense (Kelly et al 2005; Powell 2007).

Economic evaluation examines whether limited resources are used in the best possible way. The most rigorous economic evaluations examine both costs and consequences for two or more alternatives (one of which may be the existing status quo). There are five main types of economic evaluation (Donaldson et al 2002; Sefton et al 2002):

1. Cost-minimization analysis – used when there is strong evidence that two or more interventions are equally effective. This technique compares the costs to determine the least cost alternative.

2. Cost-effectiveness analysis – investigates the best way of achieving a single objective (e.g. life

years gained, improved social capital) through measuring costs and benefits to arrive at a measure of cost per unit of benefit. The least cost intervention is then determined and prioritized.

3. Cost-consequences analysis – similar to cost-effectiveness analysis but used to evaluate interventions with more than one outcome.

4. Cost-utility analysis – measures the effects of an intervention in terms of utilities (e.g. the quality adjusted life year, or QALY), focusing on minimizing costs or maximizing benefits.

5. Cost-benefit analysis – examines the costs and benefits, expressed in monetary terms, of an intervention in order to determine its desirability. A desirable intervention is one where benefits exceed costs.

 Box 3.19 **Example**

Cost-effectiveness of smoking cessation interventions

Smoking cessation interventions are very cost-effective. Overall the cost per life year gained for smoking cessation interventions is tiny, at £212–£873. This compares very favourably with the National Institute of Health and Clinical Excellence benchmark of acceptable cost-effectiveness, which is £30,000 per life year saved. Campaigns with a high level of awareness and penetration, such as the annual No Smoking Day media campaign, are even more cost-effective. Almost one million people have stopped smoking because of No Smoking Day since it first began in 1984. The estimated cost-effectiveness of No Smoking Day is around £21 per life year saved. Campaigns that target groups with high smoking prevalence may also be more cost-effective than general population campaigns. A campaign targeted at London's Turkish community, who have above average smoking rates, estimated the cost-effectiveness of this intervention was £105 (range £33–£391) per life year gained.

Sources: Parrot et al (1998), Stevens et al (2002), Flack et al (2007) www.nosmokingday.org.uk

Is the evidence comparing like with like?

It is often assumed that evidence is comparing like with like but in reality this is unlikely to be the case. In real life, interventions, even if they are following the same design or protocol, tend to vary depending on the context in which they are implemented.

 Box 3.20 **Discussion point**

What factors might account for the different outcomes of studies examining the same intervention?

Contextual factors, such as the enthusiasm or commitment of organizations and practitioners, population characteristics, for example, social stability and cohesion, and geographical factors, for example, declining or renewing areas, will all have a significant impact on outcomes. The criteria used to appraise evidence refer to the research rather than the intervention. This means that key aspects of the intervention may vary widely from study to study. For example, research into the effectiveness of brief interventions on alcohol in primary care used a definition of brief intervention that ranged from 5 to 15 minutes and possibly longer if conducted by a nurse. It could be argued that there is a significant difference between 5 and 15 minutes of one to one consultation and advice. This example demonstrates the importance of investigating processes as well as outcomes in order to identify factors leading to success. This in turn makes the case for including different kinds of evidence, qualitative as well as quantitative. A useful framework is the realistic evaluation framework proposed by Pawson and Tilley (1997). Realistic evaluation recognizes that key features of an intervention relate to the specific context which needs to be taken into account. A mechanism is only causal if it leads to an outcome within a context. The context therefore needs to be identified and evaluated as well as the intervention.

Whose definitions count?

In any public health or health promotion intervention there are a number of stakeholders who will hold very different ideas of what counts as a successful outcome, or what constitutes evidence.

 Box 3.21 **Discussion point**

How might the following view the nature of the evidence for funding a community safety programme: policy maker; health promotion/ public health practitioner; local population; academic researcher?

Views will vary significantly and cannot be accurately predicted, although it is known that factors such as occupation, socio-economic status, disciplinary background, and ideological and political beliefs will all have an impact. In order to support partnership working, different concepts of evidence need to be recognized and valued. Lay beliefs regarding evidence may be unscientific according to an epidemiological framework, but they are a valid point of view. If the recipient of a service does not value the outcome, there is little point in continuing the service. Equally, if partners include people with a background in social sciences who are constantly being told by medical scientists that their view of evidence and effective practice is misinformed, misguided or just wrong, they are unlikely to form an effective partnership. Evidence-based public health and health promotion needs to seek to embrace inclusive definitions of success that relate to the values and views of all stakeholders.

What if the evidence goes against my better judgement?

Finding and appraising evidence is a skilled task, and the findings may go counter to one's better judgement, intuition or custom. Midwives used to advise parents to put babies to sleep in the prone (tummy down) position because it seemed plausible that this was similar to the recovery position. Research has since shown that this sleeping position is associated with increased risk of sudden infant death syndrome. This research led to a major public media campaign to change practice called 'back to sleep'. This is an example where the evidence was sufficient to prompt practitioners and the public to change their custom and practice. Failure to change is attributed to lack of knowledge or appreciation of the strength of the evidence.

The government advice to use the triple vaccine for measles, mumps and rubella is founded on strong research evidence, yet many parents reject this vaccine and opt for single vaccines, even if they have to pay. The reason for this rejection of expert advice appears to lie in the many factors which impact on a parent's decision to actively treat their child. Giving a child a vaccination which might have harmful effects may be viewed as more unacceptable than taking no action and the child contracting the disease. The difference would seem to lie in the action/omission dichotomy, whereby an action is seen as more blameworthy than an omission. A parent's decision on what is best for their child takes into account factors that are invisible in large trials of treatments. So an individual child's risk of an adverse reaction to MMR might be assessed using previous history of allergic reactions, any unusual syndromes, or the reactions and behaviour of siblings. The undoubted benefits to the population of adequate levels of MMR vaccination do not apply to each individual. In addition, the severe effects of contracting measles, mumps or rubella are often downplayed because they are so infrequently seen nowadays. Parents who reject the triple vaccine would undoubtedly argue they are making a better judgement, based on their knowledge of individual circumstances, than the blanket advice of health professionals to accept the MMR vaccination.

Is evidence objective and neutral?

Social scientists accept that some degree of bias and subjectivity is inherent in qualitative research, but argue that this does not invalidate findings. As we saw in the previous chapter, they propose, instead, that transparency and reflexivity, documented as part of the research process, assist readers and researchers in determining the validity, rigour or robustness of the research. However, in traditional quantitative research fields claims are still made regarding the objectivity of quantitative methods, such as RCTs. Often the assumption is that, because these methods involve counting real phenomena – a process that can be verified – they are more objective, reliable and therefore 'better' or more 'desirable' than qualitative methods.

A more realistic view is that all research involves both the 'facts' and the theoretical frameworks that determine which facts count, and how they are interpreted. This stance may be termed the inclusive approach to research and evidence. Subjectivity is a matter of degree, not an either/or phenomenon. Denying subjectivity is no more realistic than accepting its inevitability and then seeking ways to allow for its effects. And even though quantitative research claims to be objective, commentators agree that there is no such thing as complete objectivity, and that pre-existing values and beliefs exert a powerful influence when conducting or interpreting research (Kaptchuk 2003). Although evidence may never be completely objective or neutral, it is still important to assess its validity, reliability and robustness according to appropriate criteria. The subjectivity involved in a researcher's decisions about which studies to include and exclude in a systematic review can, for example, be limited by using more than one researcher and a common data extraction form.

How can practice change in the light of evidence?

A number of initiatives are helping to facilitate access to evidence, for example, guidance from NICE. Easier access to evidence is just one hurdle to be overcome if practice is to change and become more evidence based. Changing practice involves commitment and resources as well as evidence. Practitioners need to be persuaded of the evidence but also to believe that they can change their practice in the recommended ways, and that their clients

will find this acceptable. Any change in practice is disruptive and likely, at least in the short term, to be resource-intensive. For many practitioners, operating within severe constraints and with large caseloads, this poses an additional barrier. However, as EBP becomes more embedded and applied to a variety of disciplines and practices, organizations and practitioners will become more used to adapting practice to conform to evidence. Critical appraisal skills and adaptiveness will become part and parcel of every practitioner's repertoire.

Box 3.22 **Activity**

What are the organizational and professional opportunities and barriers to implementing evidence-based approaches in public health and health promotion?

Conclusion

There has been some resistance to applying the principles of EBP to health promotion and public health. Part of this is due to the medical scientific origins of evidence-based medicine and the way in which quantitative methodologies have been privileged over qualitative methodologies. Health promotion and public health are multidisciplinary and recognize the validity of differing types of evidence, including context-specific and subjective views. Their multidisciplinary nature leads to complexity and uncertainty in the search for evidence, as different disciplines have their own rules of evidence, and attempting to consolidate these differences into an over-arching holistic body of evidence is a challenging, if not daunting, prospect (McQueen 2001).

One means of consolidating available evidence would be to use the hierarchy of evidence that privileges the RCT as providing the best evidence. However, there is on-going debate about whether or not RCTs should remain the 'gold standard' for public health and health promotion interventions.

Proponents of the RCT argue that they are feasible in the area of health promotion and do provide the best available evidence on which to base practice (Oakley 1998). Critics respond by arguing that RCTs are inappropriate for population-based, multi-component interventions where there may be a considerable time lag between the interventions and the outcomes (Nutbeam 1998). There is also a strong argument that, in line with underlying health promotion and public health values of equity, participation and autonomy, the views of practitioners and users deserve to be valued as a source of evidence in their own right.

The most useful stance for practitioners to take appears to be the inclusive concept of evidence that acknowledges and values a range of different kinds of evidence including RCTs, qualitative process research, and user views and accounts. Adopting the inclusive concept of evidence facilitates the involvement of different partners, including the public, and seeks to persuade people to implement interventions because they lead to valued outcomes. There is an important role here for the evidence-based practitioner to liaise between clients and the research community. Practitioners can disseminate, to clients and communities, knowledge and skills about the evidence gathering process as well as the evidence itself, and feed back lay concerns to researchers, organizations and colleagues. In order to undertake this role, practitioners need to be confident about their critical appraisal skills. The term evidence-informed is beginning to be used in recognition of the fact that decision making in health promotion is informed by evidence, not directed by it. The move to evidence-based, or evidence-informed, practice is already well under way, and offers practitioners the prospect of greater confidence and effectiveness. For clients, it offers the prospect of interventions based on the best available knowledge and evidence, rather than the preoccupations or biases of individual practitioners. However, evidence will always be one of several drivers of practice. The role of ethics, ideology, theory and resources as independent drivers of practice will remain, alongside evidence.

Further discussion

- What are the opportunities and barriers to your profession becoming more evidence based?

- What would you include as evidence in relation to health promotion and public health interventions, and why?

- How important do you think evidence is as a driver of public health and health promotion practice? How important do you think it should be?

- Take a recent example from your own practice and use the five stages of the EBP process to find the best evidence to guide your decision making.

Recommended reading

- Craig JV, Smyth R L, editors: *Evidence based practice manual for nurses*, edn 2, Edinburgh, 2007, Churchill Livingstone.

   An accessible and easy to follow guide to becoming an evidence-based practitioner.

- Davies HTO, Nutley SM, Smith PC: *What works? Evidence-based policy and practice in public services*. Bristol, 2000, The Policy Press.

   This readable and comprehensive book provides a useful analysis of the theoretical context in which evidence-based policy and practice are promoted. It also goes on to consider how evidence-based policy and practice are being created and disseminated in different health and welfare fields including health and social care, transport, education, housing, urban renewal and criminal justice.

- Oliver S, Peersman G, editors: *Using research for effective health promotion*, edn 2, Maidenhead, 2001, Open University Press.

   A comprehensive and readable edited book that guides the reader through the processes involved in appraising research. The problems and dilemmas of using research and evidence in the field of health promotion are debated.

- Petticrew M, Roberts H: *Systematic reviews in the social sciences: a practical guide*. Oxford, 2006, Blackwell.

    This is a readable introduction to the principles and practice of systematic reviews as well as a very useful resource of a practical how-to-do-it guide.

- Sefton T, Byford S, McDaid D, Hills J, Knapp M: *Making the most of it: economic evaluation in the social welfare field*. York, 2002, Joseph Rowntree Foundation.

An interesting and readable introduction to economic evaluation in the social welfare field. Different ways of conducting economic evaluations are outlined and illustrated using relevant case studies including community development.

- www.casp.org.uk

    The website for the Critical Appraisal Skills Programme provides checklists for how to evaluate different kinds of research studies.

References

Beksinska ME, Rees VH, McIntyre JA, et al: Acceptability of the female condom in different groups of women in South Africa – A multicentred study to inform the national female condom introductory strategy, *S Afr Med J* 91(8):672–678, 2001.

Campbell R, Pound P, Pope C, et al: Evaluating meta-ethnography: a synthesis of qualitative research on lay experiences of diabetes and diabetes care, *Soc Sci Med* 56(4):671–684, 2003.

Campbell K, Waters E, O'Meara S, et al: Interventions for preventing obesity in children. Cochrane Database Systematic Review 2002 (2):CD001871.

Cummins S, Macintyre S: 'Food deserts' – evidence and assumption in policy making, *Br Med J* 325:436–438, 2002.

Davies HTO, Nutley SM, Smith PC: *What works? Evidence-based policy and practice in public services*, Bristol, 2000, The Policy.

Donaldson C, Mugford M, Vale L: *Evidence based health economics*, London, 2002, BMJ.

Flack S, Taylor M, Trueman P: *Cost-effectiveness of interventions for smoking cessation: mass media interventions*, London, 2007, NICE/York Health Economics.

Hill A, Brice A, Enock K: Appraising research evidence. In Pencheon D, Guest C, Melzer D, Muir Gray JA, editors: *Oxford handbook of public health practice*, Oxford, 2001, Oxford University.

Kaner EF, Dickinson HO, Beyer FR, et al: Effectiveness of brief alcohol interventions in primary care populations, Cochrane Database of Systematic Reviews, Issue 2, 2007.

Kaptchuk TJ: Effect of interpretive bias on research evidence, *Br Med J* 326:1453–1455, 2003.

Kelly MP, McDaid D, Ludbrook A, et al: *Economic evaluations of public health interventions*, London, 2005, Health Development.

Lucas P: 2003, Breakfast clubs and school fruit schemes: promising practice, What Works for Children group Evidence Nugget at http://www.barnardos.org.uk/breakfast_clubs_report.pdf.

Macintyre S, Cummins S: Good intentions and received wisdom are not enough, Conference speech Evidence into Practice: Challenges and Opportunities for UK Public Health, London, April 2001, King's Fund/Health Development Agency, 2001, Available at www.hda.nhs.uk/evidence/key.html#eip.

McQueen D: Strengthening the evidence base for health promotion, *Health Promot Int* 16(3):261–268, 2001.

Muir Gray JA: *Evidence based healthcare: how to make policy and management decisions*, edn 2, Edinburgh, 2001, Churchill Livingstone.

Naidoo J, Wills J: *Foundations for health promotion*, edn 3, London, 2009, Baillière Tindall.

NICE: Promoting physical activity for children and young people (PH 17), 2009, http://www.nice.org.uk/nicemedia/pdf/PH017Guidance.pdf.

Nutbeam D: Evaluating health promotion: progress, problems and solutions, *Health Promot Int* 23:27–44, 1998.

Oakley A: Experimentation and social interventions: a forgotten but important history, *Br Med J* 317:1239–1242, 1998.

Oliver S: Making research more useful: integrating different perspectives and different methods. In Oliver S, Peersman G, editors: *Using research for effective health promotion*, Buckingham, 2001, Open University.

Parrot S, Godfrey C, Raw M, et al: Guidance for commissioners on the cost-effectiveness of smoking cessation interventions, *Thorax* 53(Suppl 5 Part 2): S1–138, 1998.

Pawson R, Tilley N: *Realistic evaluation*, Sage London, 1997.

Petrosino A, Turpin-Petrosino C, Finckenauer JO: Programs can have harmful effects!: lessons from experiments of programs such as scared straight, *Crime Delinq* 46(1):354–379, 2000.

Powell J: Health economics and public health. In Orme J, Powell J, Taylor P, Harrison T, Grey M, editors: *Public health for the 21st century: new perspectives on policy participation and practice 2nd edn*, Maidenhead, 2007, Open University Press/McGraw-Hill.

Rychetnik L, Frommer M, Hawe P, et al: Criteria for evaluating evidence on public health interventions, *J Epidemiol Community Health* 56:119–127, 2002.

Sackett DL, Rosenberg WM, Gray JA, et al: Evidence-based medicine: what it is and what it isn't, *Br Med J* 150:1249–1255, 1996.

Sefton T, Byford S, McDaid D, et al: *Making the most of it: economic evaluation in the social welfare field*, York, 2002, Joseph Rowntree.

Stevens W, Thorogood M, Kayikki S: Cost effectiveness of a community anti-smoking campaign targeted at a high risk group in London, *Health Promot Int* 17(1):43–50, 2002.

Supplement to American Journal of Preventive Medicine (SAJPM): Introducing the guide to community preventive services: methods, first recommendations and expert commentary, *Am J Prev Med* 18:35–43, 2000.

Tannahill A: Beyond evidence to ethics – a decision making framework for health promotion public health and health improvement, *Health Promot Int* 23(4):380–390, 2008.

Tilford S: Evidence based health promotion, *Health Educ Res* 15(6):659–663, 2000.

World Health Assembly (WHA): Resolution WHA 51.12 on Health Promotion, *Agenda Item 20, 16 May 1998*, Geneva, 1998, WHO.

The policy context

- Defining policy
- The policy process
- The role of values and ideology
- Stakeholders' impact on policy
- The 'implementation gap'
- Policy agendas
- Policy debates and dilemmas

OVERVIEW

The previous chapter has shown how influential the available evidence is in affecting practice. Values and the policy context affect practice in an equally profound way. Although policy may sound remote from practitioners' daily concerns, policies formulated at the national, regional, local and organizational levels have a major impact in determining practitioners' priorities and ways of working. For example, many practitioners are aware of performance targets they need to meet, duties to work in certain ways, for example involving other agencies and the public as partners, and general principles of transparency and accountability. These issues have all been highlighted by policy making and implementation. Policy formation is a complex process affected by many different factors including political ideology and stakeholders'

agendas. Policy implementation is often thought of as an unproblematic administrative matter. However, this is not the case. Policy implementation is affected by frontline workers' values and practices, and the same policy is often implemented in diverse ways with a variety of different outcomes. This chapter discusses the range of values underpinning policy formation and implementation, the policy process and key stakeholders, and some of the resulting dilemmas that affect practitioners.

Introduction

'Policy' is a vague term used in different ways to describe the direction of an organization, a decision to act on a particular problem, or a set of guiding principles directed towards specific goals (Titmuss

1974). The policy-making process has been defined as 'still the only vehicle available to modern societies for the conscious, purposive solutions for their problems' (Scharpf p. 349 cited in Hill and Hupe 2002, p. 59). The concept of policy therefore operates at different levels, describing both a specific input on a specific topic, and the values and ethos (the policy context) that inform specific goals and targets. The policy context includes values that are broadly consensual, such as democracy, and also values that are contested, such as managerialism versus professionalism. The policy context is therefore dynamic, charting public debates and the views of different lobbying and interest groups. Traditionally, public health policies are related to medical policies of disease surveillance and control. The programme of pre-school childhood immunizations and vaccinations and cervical and breast cancer screening programmes are examples of traditional public health policies. The broader concept of 'healthy public policy' has been defined by the World Health Organization (WHO 1988) as the creation of 'a supportive environment to enable people to lead healthy lives'. This broader concept means that most policy areas are implicated in the goal of better health for all. This is a reflection of the many different and complex factors that influence health and illness. The consequences of this are discussed in Chapter 11 in our companion volume (Naidoo and Wills 2009). Policy areas that impact on health include education, employment, neighbourhood renewal and regeneration, environmental issues, for example clean air, transport, food security and quality, and housing. At the international level, policies on an equally broad range of topics have a profound impact on health.

Box 4.1 **Example**

International policy on climate change: The Kyoto Protocol

The Kyoto Protocol (United Nations 1997) updated the United Nations Framework Convention on Climate Change (UNFCCC), which was adopted in 1992. The UNFCCC treaty was focused on

stabilizing greenhouse gas in order to combat global warming. The Kyoto Protocol established legally binding commitments to reduce greenhouse gas emissions by an average of 5.2% (using 1990 as the baseline). The Kyoto Protocol was adopted in 1997 and implemented in 2005. By 2008, 183 parties had ratified the protocol. The USA, the most significant producer of carbon emissions, has signed but not ratified the protocol. Many industrialized countries can achieve their agreed targets by offsetting their carbon emissions against carbon reduction projects in developing countries. This is done by developed countries purchasing carbon credits from other countries. For example, developing countries may initiate emission reduction projects such as sustainable forestry which can then be traded or bought by developed countries in order to meet their targets.

The policy context and broad macro-economic, environmental and demographic changes are major drivers of public health and health promotion. Practitioners tend to see public policy as beyond their remit, but policy exerts a powerful influence on practice.

Box 4.2 **Activity**

In what ways is your practice influenced by national or local policy?

Box 4.3 **Example**

The effect of policy on practice: The Victoria Climbie Inquiry Report

The official Inquiry Report (2003) into Victoria Climbie's death from neglect and abuse whilst in the care of her great aunt and her cohabitee identified a 'widespread organizational malaise' amongst the health and social services involved. The Inquiry Report found a failure of all the key agencies involved to follow recommended procedures when child abuse is suspected. The Report made many recommendations regarding organizational structure, management, resourcing,

Box 4.3 Example—cont'd

procedures, practice and training. However, the death of Baby P in 2007 suggests that these recommendations and lessons have not yet been adopted and embedded in practice. In 2008, an inquiry into the death of Baby P was ordered by the Children's Secretary. The inquiry found a failure to follow recommended procedures and many failings of management, supervision and practice.

Practitioners have to meet specified targets or requirements which have been identified in policy documents, for example to reduce waiting times in hospitals, or the requirement on health trusts and boards to work in partnership with local authorities. In some cases, this may mean diverting resources from established and effective practices, or innovative but well thought out strategies, to meet the new targets or goals. In other cases, the direction of an organization may be changed because of a new priority. For example, Primary Care Trusts (PCTs) in England now have a duty to oversee public health.

As we outlined in our companion book *Foundations for Health Promotion* (Naidoo and Wills 2009, Chapter 7), the development of health policy is an agreement on how health problems should be addressed, which involves a compromise between the following factors:

- ideological beliefs and values
- economic considerations
- political acceptability
- evidence-based research about 'what works'.

Box 4.4 Discussion point

What opportunities are there for practitioners to influence policy?

In the UK, opportunities for practitioners and the public to influence policy have increased as a response to the government pledge for more open government. Consultation is invited on public health policies and strategies. For example, Every Child Matters: Change for Children, published in 2004, proposed joined up working between all the different agencies (educational, health and social) involved in children's welfare. In 2005, the first Children's Commissioner for England was appointed, with a brief to support and empower children and young people in all areas of life including health and economic well-being. As part of this process, the Commissioner is committed to giving children and young people a say in government and public life.

Policies are also informed by rational economic and evidence-based principles. For example, the Wanless (2002) Review on funding the NHS outlined three possible future scenarios. The third scenario, the 'fully engaged' model, posits services and a population which is informed and enthusiastic about protecting and promoting its health, and where research is productive in identifying effective communication and implementation of messages. Crucially, this fully engaged model is proposed within the Review as the most effective and lowest cost scenario in the long term. Within this scenario, public health investment is sound economic good sense, because better health leads to more productive employees and a stronger economy.

There have been calls for policy to be based on sound evidence about what works (Cm 4310 1999). However, there is a lack of evidence about effective public health and health promotion interventions (Macintyre et al 2001). For example, there is a solid research basis about the existence of inequalities in health, but very little research into comparing the effectiveness of different kinds of intervention aimed at tackling inequalities in health. A UK review of evidence-based health policy reported that only 4% of public health research focused on interventions, of which only 10%, or 0.4% of the total, focused on the outcomes of interventions (Milward et al 2001). In part, this is due to a traditional model of evidence based on individual cases and randomized controlled trials (see Chapter 3). This model is inappropriate for macro policies that are targeted at populations or communities. The evaluation of such policies is complicated because finding control populations that are not exposed to policy is difficult. Evidence-based policy is still in its infancy, due to competing influences and the lack of appropriate evidence.

As we have seen in earlier chapters, practitioners need a solid base on which to practise. The drive to evidence-based practice, quality standards and theory-driven interventions should make practitioners feel competent and secure. Yet many feel buffeted by policy initiatives and constant change. Policy takes place in a political arena, and many practitioners feel politics is removed from their core concerns. This may mean they do not engage with the political debates and feel policy makers are divorced from the reality of service delivery. People responsible for implementing policy may not be enthusiastic, and their frontline decisions may be crucial in dissipating the intended effect of policy. Conversely, enthusiastic and committed practitioners who feel they have had a valued input into policy formation can play a key role in achieving the intended outcomes of policies. To have a voice and be able to impact on policy making and implementation, practitioners need to be familiar with, and able to understand, health policy – its origins, its goals, the process, and its effects, both intended and unintended.

Box 4.5 **Activity**

Do you regard yourself as a political practitioner?

Understanding the policy process

Policy making has been defined as 'the process by which governments translate their political vision into programmes and actions to deliver "outcomes" – desired changes in the real world' (Cabinet Office 1999). National governments set the fundamental policy direction, while locally, policies develop incrementally. Walt (1994) identifies four phases in policy making that may occur at any level, whether national or local, and also shape any policy analysis:

1. *Problem identification and issue recognition.* Why issues get onto the policy agenda; which issues do not get addressed.

2. *Policy formulation.* The goals of the policy; different options are identified and analysed; costs and benefits of alternative policies are weighed; determining who formulates policy; how and where the initiative comes from.

3. *Policy implementation.* How policies are implemented; what resources are available; how implementation is enforced.

4. *Policy evaluation.* How progress is reviewed; setting up monitoring systems; how and when adaptations are made.

There is an assumption that policy is the result of rational decision making in which choices are evaluated and a solution is chosen to achieve objectives. Yet this rational process rarely takes place. As Simon (1958) argued, real world decision makers are not 'maximizers' who select the best possible course of action but 'satisfiers' who look for the course of action that is good enough for the problem at hand. Sutton (1999) also refers to other models of policy making:

• The incrementalist model, where policies which represent the least possible change are preferred, and policy is a series of small steps which do not fundamentally challenge the status quo.

• The mixed-scanning model, which represents a middle position where a broad view of possibilities is considered before focusing on a small number of options for more investigation.

Another way of theorizing the policy-making process is to distinguish between 'top down' and 'bottom up' models. Top-down theories propose a linear policy process whereby commands from higher up are seamlessly translated into practice on the ground (Buse et al 2005). Bottom-up theories recognize that practitioners are constantly modifying and creating policy on the ground, and that the policy process is collaborative and iterative rather than linear (Walker and Gilson 2004).

Dunsire (1978) first coined the phrase 'implementation gap' to describe the gap between planned policy and real life outcomes. The implementation gap is another way of describing the power of street level bureaucrats, and lends support to bottom up theories of the policy-making process.

Box 4.6 **Example**

Implementation of the single assessment process for older people

The single assessment process (SAP) is intended to reduce duplication of effort and facilitate seamless care across a range of agencies for older people. Dickinson (2006) studied a range of stakeholders involved in SAP and found many barriers to its implementation. These barriers included staff reporting a sense of disengagement from the process, finding the tool itself hard to use, feeling it involved activities beyond their area of practice, a lack of clarity about the role of others, and insufficient support from managers in recognizing the additional time SAP would take. Although the SAP was intended to reduce time and ease the assessment process, many practitioners did not carry out the process in the way in which it was intended.

None of these models describes the policy-making process accurately, although each model refers to elements of the process. Policy making mixes the scientific and the pragmatic; the broad vision with the narrow. The degree to which each element contributes to policy making differs according to the general political environment and the specifics of the policy under consideration.

Policy development

To understand the policy process, it is important to be familiar with the structure of the government. There is a complex process for the development of national policy in many countries based on democratic constitutions (e.g. England, Canada, Australia and the United States of America). In England, a new policy is signalled by the publication of a Green Paper for public consultation and discussion. After consultation and amendment, a White Paper, which is the government's plans for legislation, is published. The policy then enters the parliamentary or legislative process, when the bill is scrutinized and amended by, first, the House of Commons and then the House of Lords. If the bill is not thrown out at any stage, it goes on to receive the royal assent, and the bill becomes an Act of Parliament. The policy has now become a legislation, which agencies are legally bound to follow. This process is illustrated in detail in Figure 4.1.

Numerous factors affect the way in which policy is finally developed and implemented:
- situational: local or timely factors
- cultural: the values and ideologies dominant in the political environment
- structural: the political system and its processes.

Box 4.7 **Example**

Alcohol pricing

Excessive alcohol consumption is linked to health, criminal and social harm, and associated costs. Despite strong evidence (Meier et al 2008) that alcohol consumption is linked to pricing, the UK government has stated that it does not see alcohol duty as a means of tackling problems associated with alcohol consumption. The government is, however, committed to introducing a new mandatory code to improve responsible retailing, for example halting happy hours and two-for-one promotions. The alcohol industry has lobbied against tax increases on alcohol, whilst publicans have launched a campaign for a minimum price of 50p per unit (to stop supermarkets' loss-leading special offers). Campaigning groups such as Alcohol Concern have lobbied against price reductions and special offers, citing the harmful effects of increased alcohol consumption.

Figure 4.1 ● The policy process. Source: Blakemore (2003).

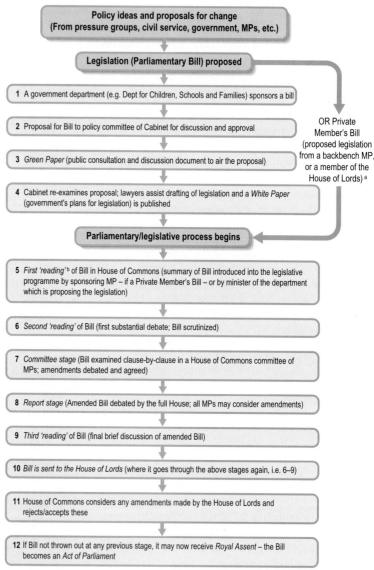

Policy ideas and proposals for change
(From pressure groups, civil service, government, MPs, etc.)

Legislation (Parliamentary Bill) proposed

1   A government department (e.g. Dept for Children, Schools and Families) sponsors a bill

2   Proposal for Bill to policy committee of Cabinet for discussion and approval

3   *Green Paper* (public consultation and discussion document to air the proposal)

4   Cabinet re-examines proposal; lawyers assist drafting of legislation and a *White Paper* (government's plans for legislation) is published

OR Private Member's Bill (proposed legislation from a backbench MP, or a member of the House of Lords)[a]

Parliamentary/legislative process begins

5   *First 'reading'*[b] of Bill in House of Commons (summary of Bill introduced into the legislative programme by sponsoring MP – if a Private Member's Bill – or by minister of the department which is proposing the legislation)

6   *Second 'reading'* of Bill (first substantial debate; Bill scrutinized)

7   *Committee stage* (Bill examined clause-by-clause in a House of Commons committee of MPs; amendments debated and agreed)

8   *Report stage* (Amended Bill debated by the full House; all MPs may consider amendments)

9   *Third 'reading'* of Bill (final brief discussion of amended Bill)

10 *Bill is sent to the House of Lords* (where it goes through the above stages again, i.e. 6–9)

11 House of Commons considers any amendments made by the House of Lords and rejects/accepts these

12 If Bill not thrown out at any previous stage, it may now receive *Royal Assent* – the Bill becomes an *Act of Parliament*

Notes:
[a] a Private Member's Bill may be introduced to either the House of Commons or the House of Lords, but must be passed by both Houses irrespective of where it starts. Government-proposed legislation almost always begins in the House of Commons
[b] Bills are not literally read out clause-by-clause.

This example illustrates the way in which policy reflects a pluralistic society of multiple interests where groups exercise influence. Some decisions are incremental, muddling through adaptations to circumstances, rather than contributions to strategic direction.

Issue recognition

For policy to be approved and enacted, an issue has first to become relevant and identified as a problem. In general there are three ways in which issues can get onto an agenda:

- following action by community groups leading to a groundswell of public opinion
- initiated by organizations or agencies concerned with the issue
- by key political figures who then mobilize support.

In addition, key incidents may also provide the trigger for gaining support and momentum for a policy, especially if they receive widespread media coverage and spark off a public debate.

Issue recognition, or agenda setting, relies on:

- problem definition
- receptive environment
- policy proposal.

Box 4.8 **Discussion point**

The UK government, in common with many other developed countries (e.g. the Australian Government 2006) has identified obesity as a major issue and developed a national strategy (DH 2008). Why was this identified as a policy problem?

Current trends indicate that by 2050 nearly 60% of the UK population will be obese (Foresight Report 2008). Obesity is linked to a variety of health problems including hypertension, diabetes, high cholesterol levels, asthma, arthritis and poor health (Mokdad et al 2003). These health effects not only impact on quality of life, but have significant economic implications for society as a whole. The causes of overweight and obesity are complex and include the increase in availability, marketing and low pricing of high energy-dense foods, and the increase in car use and sedentary leisure-time pursuits. Strategies to address these issues, adopted by both the English and Australian governments, emphasize the role of individual responsibility for health, and the importance of individual lifestyles in addressing problems. Getting obesity onto the policy agenda is a complex task that involves negotiating with powerful commercial interests and balancing contrasting ethical and ideological values relating to individual freedom and social responsibility.

Box 4.9 **Discussion point**

What examples are there where increased globalization has acted against national goals for healthy eating?

There is an increasing international dimension in which the European Union and World Health Organization may set international agreements. For example, the World Health Organization's first public health treaty, the Framework Convention on Tobacco Control, was agreed upon in 2003 (WHO 2003). It covers taxation, illicit trade, advertising and sponsorship.

Globalization may offer new opportunities for cooperation in public health, but it can also inhibit healthy public policy. Globalization has led to increased production of food and also enhanced the power of manufacturers and retailers at the expense of primary producers. Food producers are reliant on selling their products to a dwindling number of global companies, who can set their own terms and conditions. This has led to a loss of biodiversity as companies specify a limited number of crops for world markets. Whilst food scarcity is no longer an issue for the developed world, developing countries may still face food scarcity as the demand for cash crops means a loss of land available for subsistence farming. The concentration of power in the hands of a small number of global food outlets, such as McDonalds, has been blamed for contributing to an increase in unhealthy diets and the loss of home grown and home cooked products.

Globalization therefore has ambiguous effects on national goals for healthy eating. While the 5-a-day programme is facilitated by the year-long availability of fruit and vegetables, the increased reliance on manufactured and pre-cooked food with high levels of sugar, salt and saturated fats contributes to the rise of obesity and associated health problems. Yeatman (2003) argues that local food projects such as community gardens or lunch clubs are popular with local practitioners but marginal to mainstream political concerns. Local projects are acceptable and serve to divert interest away from significant issues such as the influence of global commercial food companies. Globalization has more negative effects on developing countries, for while it may foster economic growth and trade, local capacity to feed people may be lost.

The public policy environment inevitably involves struggles for power and influence in which politicians, civil servants, the media and pressure groups may try to achieve their preferred ends. One problem with public health policy is that it is not usually seen as being newsworthy. Long-term investments in health which prevent illness or disability are not as attractive to the media as topical scandals or 'feel-good' stories focused on high technology medical services and individual patients. For example, the coverage of the introduction of congestion charging in London, intended as a public health measure to reduce car use, has focused on local objections to the extra 'taxation' and stories of the effect on livelihoods. An exception

to this type of coverage is the resurgence of interest in public health protection and hazard management in the wake of the 9/11 terrorist attacks in the USA in 2001 and the war in Iraq in 2003.

Baum (2001) has shown how power is exercised in various ways and how the decision-making process can be manipulated so that certain issues are not even raised. In Australia the professional medical lobby and the private health insurance lobby are so powerful that they can ensure that the concept of an exclusively public health insurance scheme is not raised. In other cases, powerful stakeholder groups may present arguments that tap into popular sentiments and lobby support for resisting public health measures.

 Box 4.10 **Discussion point**

Consider Table 4.1. What political and social drivers for each group's position can you identify? Why do you think evidence-based policy is not always introduced?

Table 4.1 Reducing alcohol related harm: Strategies supported by different key stakeholders

Evidence-based practitioners	English government policies	Alcohol Concern (voluntary sector lobbying group)	Portman Group (alcohol industry lobbying group)
Blood alcohol concentration laws and minimum legal drinking age	Revision of licensing hours Brief interventions	Alcohol awareness campaign Education for young people	Information provision Education for vulnerable groups
Peer-led prevention programmes	Treatment programmes for alcoholics	Resources for counselling	Tighter controls restricting children's access to alcohol
Alcohol screening in hospital accident and emergency departments	Control of drinks promotions, for example happy hours	Training retailers to prevent sales to under-aged young people	Inclusion of alcohol education in the national curriculum
Brief interventions by primary healthcare staff	Control of advertising	Ban on glass bottles in pubs	
Employee assistance programmes		Lowering of the blood alcohol driving limit Fewer price promotions	

Powerful interest groups, such as the drinks industry, have lobbied successfully against the introduction of alcohol control policies. Appeals to individual choice and against a 'nanny state' have led to an emphasis on sensible drinking plus targeted interventions for vulnerable groups.

Policy formulation

Once an issue is on the public agenda, there is an opportunity for stakeholders to influence any resulting policies. There is no single method of doing this. Baggott (2000) identifies three models of stakeholder influence on the policy process:

1. Institutional politics – policy results from the interaction of different institutions and policy networks that include pressure groups as well as government agencies. This suggests a process where consensus is arrived at through negotiation and compromise.

2. Pressure-group politics – policy results from different stakeholders and pressure groups which seek to mobilize public support through the media and direct action. Policy is not a result of consensus but more a product of the most powerful vested interests. For example, the extension of drinking hours in licensed premises has been supported by commercial licensing bodies and alcoholic drinks manufacturers, although many civic groups fear the consequences for public order and public health practitioners predict an increase in alcohol-related problems.

3. Policy knowledge and policy learning – policy results from the knowledge and experience of experts and interested parties. An example is expert committees which are set up to gather evidence to input into the policy process. This suggests a rational, scientific process driven by a clear evidence base. For example, an independent expert committee reported in 1999 to ministers, who in 2000 published the *Review of the Mental Health*

Act 1983 (DH 2000) which sought to balance the need to protect the rights of individual patients with the need to ensure public safety. This review led to the Mental Health Act 2007 which includes various provisions designed to further safeguard the rights of patients.

 Box 4.11 **Discussion point**

How might practitioners have a say in policy formulation?

Practitioners may be involved in professional, civic or voluntary pressure groups lobbying for particular public health policies. Lobbying may involve individual action (e.g. writing to MPs), collective action (e.g. local demonstrations or petitions) or coordinated and funded media campaigns. Professional associations, such as the Royal College of Nursing, the British Medical Association and the Royal Society of Public Health, will have an expert view that is often sought and represented to government at the policy consultation stage.

Policies occur at many different levels. The UK government has stressed the need for 'joined up' or cross-cutting policy to tackle health and social issues. The government's policy direction is underpinned by an understanding of the wider determinants of health and that the well-being of the population does not lie solely within the remit of the health services. Addressing public health requires a cross-government, cross-departmental focus, and cross-cutting policies which relate to sectors as varied as agriculture, economics, education, transport and the environment. Colebatch (1998) has suggested that policy may be vertical – where those in positions of authority transmit decisions downwards for implementation – or horizontal, where those outside authority are important in mobilizing opinion and lobbying. Much of the government's public health policy is focused on interagency working and partnerships between different agencies to tackle health problems (see Chapter 7).

Policy implementation

Once a policy has been made, it is often assumed that the implementation stage is a non-problematic, administrative matter. However, many commentators have pointed out that implementation is a separate activity where policies are reinforced, changed or even sabotaged by frontline workers – the street level bureaucrats identified by Lipsky (1980). Street level bureaucrats are relatively low level employees who have considerable discretion in how they operate and who act as an interface between the public and the organization. Examples of street level bureaucrats are teachers, police officers, social workers, environmental health officers and health practitioners. Street level bureaucrats tend to be public service employees working in organizations with the following characteristics:

- demand outstrips supply
- resources are inadequate
- goals are ambiguous, vague or conflicting
- measuring employee performance to meet goals is difficult or impossible
- clients are typically non-voluntary and therefore are not a primary reference group for the organization.

In such situations, 'the decisions of street level bureaucrats, the routines they establish, and the devices they invent to cope with pressure, effectively become the public policy they carry out' (Lipsky 1980: xii).

 Box 4.12 Practitioner talking

Many organizations are committed to anti-discriminatory practice. One practitioner comments,

'We provide individual advice and counselling on benefits and housing issues, and our services are not well used by our local Black and Asian communities. Everyone knows that's because people from these communities like to look after their own and deal with things within the family. When someone from these communities does come through the door, they're treated the same as anyone else. That to me is being non-discriminatory; not even noticing if they're White, Black, whatever. Then we had a training session, and were told we had to treat people from Black and minority ethnic groups differently, provide interpreters, give them extra time, do outreach work. To me, that is discriminatory and not being fair to our local White population. I still treat everyone as an individual and they all get the same service'.

Commentary

The example above illustrates how, unless frontline practitioners are persuaded of the need to change their practice, they can effectively derail an organization's stated policies and intentions. Evaluation of the training session should have shown that additional inputs were required if staff were to be persuaded by the argument that, in order to provide an equal service for all, inputs to different communities may need to be unequal. Staff also need to be made aware of research findings that show people from Black, Asian and minority ethnic groups do want access to services but are put off by barriers such as language and not knowing what is available.

 Box 4.13 Discussion point

What function, if any, does the implementation gap serve?

The division between policy formation and implementation – the implementation gap – is useful to both practitioners and policy makers. It allows practitioners to retain a degree of freedom and autonomy which is valued as part of their professional identity.

In reality, practitioners may still refer to experience and hands-on knowledge to inform their practice rather than the latest policy directive or evidence. The implementation gap is also useful to policy makers as it allows them to blame any failures of policy on those responsible for its implementation.

Resources are crucial to the success or otherwise of policies. Most policies depend on the allocation of resources to enable their successful implementation. Setting policies without adequate resourcing means failure or other policies not being implemented as resources are diverted from them. Cross-cutting policies, such as tackling inequalities that affect several different services, may be hindered through the separation of service budgets and budget allocation to specific priorities. The breadth of the tackling-inequalities policy agenda demands partnerships spanning different decision making and performance systems. Having a common agenda and long-term commitments through structures such as Local Strategic Partnerships may ease the implementation of such policies.

There has been a plethora of health policies implemented during the past decade. This has led to the phenomenon of 'interventionitis' whereby practitioners are deluged by the number of new interventions, each with its own funding, criteria and targets.

Box 4.14 **Activity**

In your practice area, is the phenomenon of 'interventionitis' familiar? If it is, how do people respond and cope with the demands this makes?

Box 4.15 **Practitioner talking**

Everywhere I go senior management tell me of progress, of targets reached and objectives met, of value for money and of real change. Everywhere I go, I also see another world – a world of daily crisis, of staff under pressure, of people working with few resources and services struggling to deliver. In this world of everyone else, there is stress and low morale.

Commentary

There is often a profound implementation gap between policy and practice with a difference on the ground between senior enthusiasts who are the change agents, sceptics who tend to be the managers with a history of working in a different way, and those on the front line who may feel overloaded and unable to cope with the sheer volume and pace of change. One response is to retreat into protectionism or a silo mentality whereby practitioners seek to protect their own sphere of influence and existing areas of autonomy.

Box 4.16 **Activity**

Is there any formal evaluation (as opposed to audit) of policies affecting your work?

Policy evaluation

In principle, policy is assessed before implementation for its likely costs (e.g. through new targets); its sustainability; its risks; EU treaty obligations; environmental impact; equity impact and consumer impact. Carrying out a health impact assessment (see HIA gateway at http:///www.apho.org.uk) is intended to help make decisions by predicting the health consequences if a policy is implemented. Following implementation, policies should be evaluated to determine their impact, and this evaluation should feed back into the policy-making process. It is sometimes argued that the evaluation stage is often lacking. Policy implementation and impact may be audited, but long-term in-depth evaluation of policies is unusual. This is partly due to the complexities and difficulties of trying to evaluate policies that are intended to change practice everywhere and in a wholesale manner.

Values and policy

Policy is not primarily an empirical or pragmatic process of assessing evidence and identifying effective options, although such rational concerns may feed into the policy process. Instead, policy is clearly driven by underlying values. A value is 'an enduring belief that a specific mode of conduct or end-state of existence is personally or socially preferable' (Rokeach 1973, p. 5). In *Foundations for Health Promotion* (Naidoo and Wills 2009) we discussed the way in which certain values may influence the way in which people practise. In Chapter 1 we showed how assimilation of specific professional values (e.g. respecting service users; appreciating people's quality of life) is included within professional training and the adoption of a professional identity. In any society, but especially in a diverse democracy such as Britain, there will be a broad range of values that people hold with regard to these specific issues. Different groups will hold different values with respect to these topics, and often (but not always) there will be coherent groupings of value positions. Ideology is the term used to describe a coherent body of interrelated ideas and values.

The development of public health reflects different political ideologies and political systems. (These

are discussed in Naidoo and Wills 2009, Chapter 7.) There are alternative positions on:

- the role of the individual and that of the state
- the nature and extent of the ties that bind communities
- whether or not the economy should be managed or controlled
- the extent of legitimate state intervention in people's lives.

The spectrum of political values which underpin policy has been characterized in many different ways, and ranges from socialist to individualist, and from *laissez-faire* economics to green environmentalism to managed economies (Baggott 2007). At one end (the far right) of the spectrum are those advocating free market economics, individual liberties and minimal state regulation. At the opposite end (the far left) are those supporting a regulated economy, collective responsibilities and active state intervention. The middle ground that the Labour government in the UK tried to colonize as the 'third way' embodies values of individual rights, duties and responsibilities, as well as social justice and fairness. In the field of economics, a generally free economic market is tempered by social constraints and welfare expenditure on key services and the encouragement of joint private-public initiatives. Public sector services are to be strengthened by firm performance management coupled with a simultaneous move to devolved services, a shift from the centralized hierarchical structure or market competition of the late twentieth century.

 Box 4.17 **Example**

The third way – key values

- *Active civil society* – to combat political indifference suggested by low voter turnout, for example teaching citizenship in schools.
- *Communitarianism* – to try to rebuild societal links, for example New Deal for Communities.

- *Democratic family* – to give stability, for example more generous paternity and adoption leave as well as maternity leave.
- *Mixed economy* – to encourage private funding of public services, for example Private Finance Initiative and foundation hospitals within the NHS.

Box 4.17 **Example—cont'd**

- *Equality as inclusion* – equality of opportunity rather than equality of outcome, for example support for looked-after young people and children.
- *Positive welfare* and opportunity rather than the over-dependency fostered by a commitment to protect citizens from

the cradle to the grave, for example the establishment of the minimum wage.
- *Cosmopolitan nation* – celebrating diversity, for example organizations committed to equal opportunities and anti-discrimination policies.

Source: Giddens (1998)

These values give rise to specific strategies or policies:

- public involvement with greater user participation and involvement in services
- increased investment in public services
- mixed economy with a growing involvement of the private sector in public services
- devolved services allowing local flexibility and freedom, with additional 'earned autonomy' for best performing services
- quality assurance through clear standards and performance criteria
- partnership working to erode professional barriers and enable the delivery of seamless services
- a positive focus on disadvantaged or excluded groups
- community focus to build capacity and encourage communities to be active providers as well as users of services
- leadership qualities of vision, flexibility and adaptability are valued above the old style of bureaucratic managerialism.

 Box 4.18 **Activity**

How many of these terms are you familiar with from your workplace? How are they interpreted and used within your workplace?

Contemporary debates and dilemmas

One way of viewing policy is as the arena where competing ideological values jostle for dominance (George and Wilding 1985; Malin et al 2002). There are several areas where currently different ideological values compete for dominance in the policy arena. An understanding of these helps the practitioner to identify an individual policy's drivers in terms of values, ideology and natural advocates. This will help the practitioners to reflect on their own value position and the logical interconnectedness (or not) of different policies. In practical terms the practitioner may then be better able to lobby for support for a preferred policy. Such reflection will also enable practitioners to identify those policies to which they feel most motivated and committed, and able to implement in an effective manner.

Individual responsibility versus collectivity

- To what extent are people in charge of their own destiny?
- To what extent are people bound together through ties of kinship and community?
- What are the proper limits to individual self-determination and agency?
- How can the needs of individuals and communities be balanced?

Neoliberal politics emphasize the role of individual free will in determining health. Recognition of socially patterned inequalities in health and seeing individuals as one partner amongst many (including communities and the state) is a hallmark of Labour's ideological standpoint. In many policy initiatives relating to health behaviour there is an assumed 'contract' between the individual (whose responsibility is to make healthy choices) and the state (whose responsibility is to provide the opportunities for the individual to make healthy choices).

Box 4.19 **Example**

Choosing health – an individual or social responsibility?

Choosing Health: Making Healthy Choices Easier (DH 2004) embraced an individual and community focused policy that aimed to promote better health. Six main action areas were identified: health inequalities, smoking, obesity, sexual health, mental health and well-being, and sensible drinking. In 2006, the House of Commons voted for legislation for smoke-free zones in all public and work places. It was argued that besides protecting people from second-hand smoking, the ban would also enable many smokers to quit. The policy has been welcomed by many stakeholders as a means of reducing deaths and ill health arising from smoking (ASH 2007), and tackling health inequalities, since social class differences in smoking rates is a key driver of social class differences in health status (Jarvis and Wardle 2005). This example demonstrates that even when there is a focus on individual choice, policy is vital to ensuring that people are empowered to make healthy choices. Policy also has a role to play in protecting the public from the detrimental effects of some people's unhealthy choices.

Equality versus inclusion

- Should the policy focus be on equal outcomes, or equal opportunities to participate?

A fundamental tenet of social democracy in the UK is to focus on equal opportunities. The current emphasis is to stress the need to combat social exclusion and develop an active citizenship. Equal outcomes through, for example, greater entitlement to more generous benefits have been rejected as creating welfare dependency. Instead, the focus has been on strategies designed to bring marginalized and excluded communities (e.g. homeless people, minority ethnic groups or indigenous populations) into the mainstream of society. There are numerous policies aimed at doing this, including economic and

employment policies that make employment more economically beneficial than welfare. The employment of specialist workers is one strategy designed to include marginalized groups.

Box 4.20 **Discussion point**

What are the advantages and disadvantages of focusing on equal opportunities to participate rather than equal outcomes?

Proponents of inclusive policies argue that such an approach is empowering and enables people to fulfil their own potential and make choices about their lives. A criticism of such policies is that they do not necessarily reduce inequalities. The section on poverty and income in Chapter 5 discusses the problems associated with a strategy of inclusion that uses geographical targeting based on socio-economic indicators.

Consumerism versus empowerment

- To what extent should the public be viewed as consumers of services?
- To what extent should consumers' views shape the services we have?
- To what extent should service users be viewed as empowered?

Box 4.21 **Activity**

Do you think your workplace subscribes to a consumerist or empowerment view of service users? What policies or practices support your view?

Chapter 6 discusses the drive to involve patients and the public and the emergence of the concept of the service user. One explanation for this is to see services as more accountable and their users as having market choices, as do consumers of other products. Services need to provide information which enables consumers to make a choice in healthcare – hence the plethora of comparative data showing how services perform in relation to set targets. Services need to be responsive to local views so that they are appropriately used. However, critics argue that such information does not provide an adequate basis on which to compare quality of service, merely number crunching statistics. Genuine empowerment, such as service users' decision making at the executive level, is often resisted by organizations and professionals on the grounds that service users have specific concerns and lack the necessary strategic overview. A consumerist notion of health service users underpins the establishment of the Patients' Advocacy and Liaison Service (PALS) and the scrutiny role of local government.

Partnership versus professionalism

- Should professional identities and skills be protected?
- Or should there be moves to inter-professional working and strategic partnerships?

Chapter 7 discusses the challenges of partnership working. Partnerships require partners to respect each other's views and skills and recognize that each brings equal value to the partnership. However, many professionals are unclear as to the role and skills of other professionals, especially if they are employed by different organizations. Professionals may also feel uneasy about acknowledging service users as equal partners, leading to defensiveness about their own territory and remit.

 Box 4.22 **Activity**

What is your experience of strategic partnerships? What factors contribute to the success of such partnerships?

The drive for partnership working may be interpreted as another attack on professionals' expertise in a situation where they already feel beleaguered by managerialism, evidence-based practice and shifting policy imperatives. However, the arguments for partnership working – to provide coherent and seamless services that meet clients' needs without duplication – are very sound. Genuine partnership working need not mean a dilution of professional expertise. What partnership working does require is the recognition and valuing of areas of knowledge and expertise of other professionals, practitioners and service users.

 Box 4.23 **Practitioner talking**

I came into community nursing to make a difference, to help people, but no one seems to acknowledge or respect this. I'm surrounded by different initiatives requiring me to do x y and z before getting stuck into the real business of caring. There's so many boxes to tick, not just about clinical practice and targets, but consultation, and with so many different parties … it's exhausting, and I feel it detracts from the real business of nursing.

Commentary

Service user involvement has become an essential part of healthcare practice. Public consultation and engagement became a duty for Primary Care Trusts and NHS Trusts under the Health and Social Care Act 2001 and Foundation Trusts also have a duty to engage with local communities. A plethora of initiatives have been introduced to guarantee service user involvement in service delivery (see Chapter 6 on participation, involvement and engagement).

Need versus rationing

- How can the idea of universal needs that deserve to be met be reconciled with the reality of a limited budget and rationing of services?

One strategy is to define core services and aspects of such service provision as universal, implying universal needs that deserve to be met in a similar way throughout the country. Examples of such policies are the National Service Frameworks which outline what service users can expect of services for different conditions (such as coronary heart disease) or population groups (such as older people). However, in reality funding is always limited and hard decisions have to be taken about which services to fund and which to withhold. One casualty of rationing is infertility and reproductive services, which have been rationed and withdrawn in various areas at different times as a result of funding constraints. This dilemma is likely to become more problematic due to the ageing population, as it is generally accepted that an ageing population will have a greater level of health and social care needs. Already there have been instances of ageist policies and practices when service providers have been accused of failing to meet elderly clients' needs solely on account of their age. Chapter 6 discusses how public involvement has been extended to priority setting for healthcare services.

Managerialism versus professionalism

- Should services be controlled by management or professionals?
- Which form of authority is most transparent and trustworthy?

The modernization agenda in the UK has prioritized managerialism over professionalism. Strategies such as performance targets and quality audits are intended to make practice transparent and accountable. While these aims are laudable, it is questionable whether the increasing use of numerical data actually provides the relevant information. Professionals complain that such monitoring leads to a 'tick box' mentality where quantity is valued over quality. This shift has been widely interpreted as an attack on professional autonomy.

 Box 4.24 **Activity**

Within your workplace, do managers or professions wield the most power? Is the balance of power static or a constantly shifting battleground?

Centralized versus devolved services

- Should health and social care services be nationally run?
- Or should the planning and delivery of services be locally organized?

There is a tension between providing centralized services that are the same for everyone, and providing locally sensitive services which may then vary nationwide. Equity underpins the NHS and is part of its perennial popularity – the same service for everyone, according to need, not social or geographical status. Yet local services which are responsive to local circumstances are also popular and a politically sensitive issue. At least one local election has been fought and won on the issue of retaining a local hospital threatened with closure. The existence of pressures to both centralize decision making and devolve services may make it difficult for practitioners to work in a way that supports both strategies. Practitioners may end up feeling torn between contradictory demands and as a consequence become demoralized and disillusioned.

Conclusion

The policy context is one of the most important factors affecting practitioners' focus, priorities and workload. Although the policy process may appear to be remote from everyday work, this chapter has sought to demonstrate that practitioners are a key stakeholder group (alongside service users). Practitioners can have an impact on policy through networking, professional and local lobbying groups, and research evidence. Policy is often presented as a rational result of weighing up the evidence, but this chapter has underlined the importance of values and ideology in the policy process. Practitioners who reflect on their own values and ideological position will be able to locate policies in terms of underpinning values, and also to identify stakeholders' views and positions. This understanding will enable practitioners to maximize their input through effective lobbying with like-minded partners.

Policies may set the overall context and direction, but there is ample scope for local and individual flexibility in the frontline implementation of policies. An understanding of the power relationships of key partners enables practitioners to reflect on their own and others' contribution to policy implementation. For the reflective practitioner, an understanding of how the policy process works and impacts on day-to-day work is fundamental for enhancing effectiveness. Policy, alongside theory, research and evidence, is a key driver for public health and health promotion practice. While there are links between all these elements, policy may also act as an independent and value-based driver for practice.

Further discussion

- In what ways, both positive and negative, does policy affect your practice?
- Policy is a preferred driver for practice when compared to:
  a. economic cost-effectiveness criteria
  b. professional experience and knowledge.

Critically discuss this statement.

- Consider an organization with which you are familiar. How, if at all, is policy resisted or transformed on the 'front line'?

Recommended reading

- Baggott R: *Understanding health policy*, Bristol, 2007, The Policy Press.

  A user-friendly text that examines the processes associated with policy making, and the role of different stakeholders in the policy process. The focus is on the

UK, although the role of European and international organizations is also discussed.

- Blakemore K, Griggs E: *Social policy: an introduction*, edn 3, Maidenhead, 2007, Open University Press.

  An excellent introduction to the field of social policy, written in an accessible and user-friendly manner. Chapter 9 focuses on health policy and health professionals.

- Buse K, Mays N, Walt G: *Making health policy*, Maidenhead, 2005, Open University Press.

  A very useful introduction to the policy process that explains how and why issues get onto agendas, and the policy-making and implementation processes.

- Hunter D: Public health policy. Chapter 2. In Orme J, Powell J, Taylor P, Grey, M: *Public health for the 21st century: New perspectives on policy, participation and practice*, edn 2, Maidenhead, 2007, Open University Press/McGraw Hill.

  A critical review of the current government's approach to public health policy. The distinction between policy directed towards public health and policy focused on health services is examined, and various tensions between the two are identified and discussed.

- Pitt B, Lloyd L: Social policy and health. Chapter 7. In Naidoo J, Wills J, editors: *Health studies: An introduction*, edn 2, Basingstoke, 2008, Palgrave Macmillan.

  A clear and readable account of the history of social policy and the policy process, focusing on how social policy affects health. The chapter adopts a critical stance, examining critiques of social policy, as well as acknowledging its positive effects.

References

Action on Smoking and Health (ASH): Submission to the comprehensive spending review 2007, 2007. available from http://www.ash.org.uk/files/documents/ASH_502/ASH_502htm.

Baggott R: *Public health: policy and politics*, London, 2000, Macmillan.
Baggott R: *Understanding health policy*, Bristol, 2007, The Policy Press.

Baum F: Health, equity, justice and globalization: some lessons from the People's Health Assembly, *J Epidemiol Community Health* 55:613–616, 2001.

Blakemore K: *Social policy: an introduction*, edn 2, Maidenhead, 2003, Open University Press.

Buse K, Mays N, Walt G: *Making health policy*, Maidenhead, 2005, Open University Press.

Cabinet Office—Strategic Policy Making Team: *Professional policy making for the twentyfirst century*, London, 1999, Cabinet Office.

Cm 4310: White Paper: modernizing government, presented to parliament by the prime minister and the minister for the Cabinet Office by command of Her Majesty, London, 1999, The Stationery Office.

Colebatch HK: *Policy*, Maidenhead, 1998, Open University Press.

Department for Education and Skills (DfES): *Every child matters: Green Paper (Cmd 5860)*, London, 2004, HMSO.

Department of Health (DH): *Review of the Mental Health Act 1983*, London, 2000, The Stationery Office.

Department of Health (DH): *Choosing health: making healthy choices easier*, London, 2004, DH.

Department of Health (DH): *Healthy weight, healthy lives: a cross government strategy for England*, London, 2008, DH.

Dickinson A: Implementing the single assessment process: opportunities and challenges, *J Interprof Care* 20(4):365–379, 2006.

Dunsire A: *Control in a bureaucracy: the execution process, vol 2*, Oxford, 1978, Martin Robertson.

George V, Wilding P: *Ideology and social welfare*, London, 1985, Routledge.

Giddens A: *The third way: the renewal of social democracy*, Cambridge, 1998, Polity Press.

Hill M, Hupe P: *Implementing public policy*, London, 2002, Sage.

HM Treasury: *Every child matters: change for children*, Cm. 5860, London, 2004, The Stationery Office, Foresight Report on Obesity 2008.

Jarvis MJ, Wardle J: *Social patterning of health behaviours: the case of cigarette smoking*. In Marmot M, Wilkinson R, editors: *Social determinants of health*, edn 2, Oxford, 2005, Oxford University Press.

Lipsky M: *Street-level bureaucracy: dilemmas of the individual in public services*, New York, 1980, Russell Sage Foundation.

Macintyre S, Chalmers I, Horton R, et al: Using evidence to inform health policy: case study, *Br Med J* 322: 222–225, 2001.

Malin N, Wilmot S, Manthorpe J: *Key concepts and debates in health and social policy*, Maidenhead, 2002, Open University Press.

Meier P, Brennan A, Purshore R, et al: Independent review of the effects of alcohol pricing and promotion, University of Sheffield, School of health and related research, 2008.

Milward L, Kelly M, Nutbeam D: *Public health intervention research: the evidence*, London, 2001, Health Development Agency.

Mokdad AH, Ford ES, Bowman BA, et al: Prevalence of obesity, diabetes, and obesity-related health risk factors, 2001, *J Am Med Assoc* 289:76–79, 2003.

Naidoo J, Wills J: *Foundations for health promotion*, edn 3, London, 2009, Baillière Tindall.

Rokeach M: *Understanding human values*, New York, 1973, The Free Press.

Simon H: The role of expectations in an adaptive or behavioristic model. In Bowman MJ, editor: *Expectations, uncertainty and business behavior*, New York, 1958, Social Science Council.

Sutton R: *The policy process: an overview*, working paper 118, London, 1999, Overseas Development Institute.

The Victoria Climbie Inquiry: Report of an Inquiry Lord Laming, London, 2003, Department of Health, Home Office.

Titmuss RM: *Social policy*, London, 1974, Allen & Unwin.

United Nations: The Kyoto protocol to the United Nations Framework Convention on Climate Change (UNFCCC), 1997.

Walker L, Gilson L: We are bitter, but we are satisfied: nurses as street level bureaucrats in South Africa, *Soc Sci Med* 59(6):1251–1261, 2004.

Walt G: *Health policy: an introduction to process and power*, London, 1994, Zed Books.

Wanless D: *Securing our future health: taking a long-term view, Final report*, London, 2002, HM Treasury.

World Health Organization (WHO): *Second International Conference on health promotion*, Adelaide, 1988, South Australia.

World Health Organization (WHO): *Framework convention on tobacco control*, A56/8, Geneva, 2003, WHO.

Yeatman HR: Food and nutrition policy at the local level: key factors that influence the policy development process, *Crit Public Health* 13(2):125–138, 2003.

Part Two
Strategies for public health and health promotion practice

Introduction

Part 1 has explored the drivers for public health and health promotion practice, including theoretical frameworks, research and the growing evidence base, and the policy context and underlying values that inform policies. Part 2 goes on to explore core strategies that are used in health promotion and public health. Strategy is defined as a plan of action that specifies how targets and goals are to be achieved. Health promotion and public health goals are varied and include maximizing the potential for health and well-being, the appropriate provision and use of services, and reducing mortality and ill health. Part 2 identifies four key strategies that contribute towards the achievement of these goals: tackling health inequalities, the participation and involvement of patients, users and the public, partnership working, and empowerment. These strategies (amongst others) have been identified in many international and national health policy documents (e.g. DH 2001a,b; WHO 1986) as the means whereby health promotion and public health goals can be translated into practice. As such, they embody core values identified as equity, empowerment and collaboration.

Equity, defined as equal opportunity and social justice for all, was cited as a fundamental prerequisite for health by the World Health Organization (WHO 1985). Tackling health inequalities, defined as avoidable and unjust health differences, is identified as a key goal for governments internationally (e.g. DH 2001a,b; Howden-Chapman and Tobias 2000 and www.health-inequalities.org for examples of EU countries tackling socio-economic determinants of health). The aim is to improve health by focusing on the most disadvantaged and deprived groups in society, including indigenous peoples in Canada, Australia and New Zealand. Whilst many practitioners may feel sympathetic towards the underlying ethical value – equity – the required focus on the most disadvantaged groups is challenging and may sit uneasily alongside training in the provision of universal services. Chapter 5 seeks to demonstrate how practitioners can tackle inequalities in health effectively and why tackling inequalities is a central strategy at the level of personal service delivery as well as at the central government policy level.

The World Health Organization has defined health as:

the extent to which an individual or group is able, on the one hand, to realize aspirations and satisfy needs; and, on the other hand, to change or cope with the environment. Health is, therefore, seen as a resource for everyday life, not an object of living; it is a positive concept emphasizing social and personal resources, as well as physical capacities.

WHO (1984)

Implicit within this statement is the need for information and participation in order to achieve health. Information and participation are also necessary to achieve empowerment, defined as the central goal and principle of health promotion (Tones 2001). Public participation and involvement is a key strategy for service delivery in any democracy. Robust strategies for participation and involvement ensure that services are appropriate, accessible and meet needs. Public participation and involvement also facilitates the accountability of health professionals and managers. Participation and involvement of service users, members of the public and communities have been recognized in many government policies and documents (e.g. DH 2001a,b). Chapter 6 seeks to demonstrate the relevance and feasibility of participation strategies for everyone. Being aware of this issue, and having the skills to achieve participation, is fast becoming part of every health practitioner's repertoire.

Collaboration or partnership working is recognized as a key strategy to effectively address the multidisciplinary nature of health and the multi-agency nature of relevant service providers. In the UK, the historical separation of health from other social care services has had negative effects in terms of duplication of work and service providers focusing on compartmentalized aspects of health instead of addressing health in holistic terms. The separation of responsibilities and functions can also make it hard for clients to access appropriate services. Partnership working has been identified as the solution to these problems, facilitating seamless services that meet people's needs effectively and efficiently. Working in partnerships is often assumed to be an unproblematic aspect of practice, but research and experience show it requires dedicated resources and specific skills. Working in partnerships is becoming a recognized part of the core training and education for health and social care practitioners. Chapter 7 discusses how partnership working can be facilitated and supported and identifies the resulting benefits.

Empowerment is the fourth key strategy to be identified and discussed in Part 2. Empowerment is an elusive concept incorporating many elements, including self-esteem, control and decision making. Enhancing individual and collective assets and capabilities is key to strategic development. Access to appropriate information is a crucial aspect of health promotion and public health. People can only take advantage of opportunities, access services and make voluntary informed choices, and thus exert power and self-efficacy, if they have the information to do so. The explosion of information networking and availability via the Internet has demonstrated that people want information and want to be able to make informed choices. Health messages may include public information campaigns, commercial product marketing and entertainment. Such information varies widely in its accuracy, scope and persuasiveness. Information dissemination does not stop with the written word and includes storytelling, festivals and theatre. Health practitioners remain trusted and valued sources of information, and they have a responsibility to inform clients of relevant, up-to-date findings and knowledge on matters of interest. Chapter 8 discusses how practitioners can communicate effectively with clients and provide accessible and appropriate information and education.

Together, the four chapters in Part 2 discuss core strategies for health promotion and public health and explore how practitioners can most effectively use and contribute to such strategies. Policies may specify strategies and place duties on practitioners to adopt such strategies; but the degree to which this is acted upon varies widely. Part 2 aims to encourage practitioners to use strategies proactively for public health and health promotion. Each chapter discusses the strategy in the context of public health and health promotion policy and includes examples of good practice. We hope the chapters in Part 2 will stimulate practitioners to reflect on their potential to use the four key strategies, and to incorporate them into their everyday practice.

References

Department of Health (DH): *The expert patient: a new approach to chronic disease management for the 21st century*, London, 2001a, DH.

Department of Health (DH): *Tackling health inequalities: consultation on a plan for delivery*, London, 2001b, The Stationery Office.

Howden-Chapman P, Tobias M: *Social inequalities in health: New Zealand 1999*, Wellington, 2000, Ministry of Health.

Tones K: Health promotion: the empowerment imperative. In Scriven A, Orme J, editors: *Health promotion: professional perspectives*, Basingstoke, 2001, Palgrave.

World Health Organization (WHO): *Health promotion: a discussion document on the concept and principles*, Copenhagen, 1984, WHO Regional Office for Europe.

World Health Organization (WHO): *Targets for health for all*, Copenhagen, 1985, WHO.

World Health Organization (WHO): *Ottawa charter for health promotion: an international conference on health promotion*, November 17–21, Copenhagen, 1986, WHO.

Chapter Five

Tackling health inequalities

Key points

- Definition and scope of inequalities
- The link between social and health inequalities
- Tackling inequalities: policies and strategies
- Tackling inequalities: the practitioner's perspective
- Evaluating what works to reduce inequalities

OVERVIEW

'Health inequalities' is the phrase used to refer to patterned socio-economic differences in the health status of populations. People with a lower level of education, lower occupational class or lower level of income tend to die at a younger age and have a higher prevalence of all kinds of health problems. Whilst differences in people's health are unavoidable and natural, structured differences that are related to socio-economic factors are deemed to be unjust and inequitable. Despite high levels of prosperity and developed health and social care systems, inequalities have increased in the last 20 years in many countries. Inequalities in social circumstances are linked to inequalities in health via a variety of mechanisms. Whilst there is debate concerning the magnitude of effect of different factors, material disadvantages, such as low income, are generally viewed as central. Other key factors are environmental, such as poor housing and low levels of social support; psychosocial, such as low self-esteem and chronic stress; and accumulated disadvantages experienced during the life-course or concentrated into particular geographical areas (Brunner and Marmot 1999; Wilkinson 1996). Factors other than social class (such as gender and ethnicity) that show patterned associations with health status are generally perceived to be linked to health via material circumstances and income, although cultural norms and lifestyles are also involved.

The documented rise in social inequalities in the UK since the 1970s and 1980s has been mirrored by a growth in health inequalities (Acheson 1998; Shaw et al 1999). The UK Labour government recognized inequalities in health as a major public health issue. In 2001, two targets to reduce inequalities in infant mortality and life expectancy were set, and there has also been ongoing consultation and debate around strategies and policies to tackle inequalities and how these should be evaluated (DH 2001, 2004, 2005, 2008a).

This chapter reviews the evidence of widening social and health inequalities and then goes on to look at the mechanisms which link social and health inequalities. The current policy context is briefly reviewed, demonstrating a supportive environment for tackling inequalities. Strategies to enable practitioners to tackle health inequalities are discussed, using several examples of innovative work in this area.

Introduction

For those working to promote health, recognition and understanding of the social structural factors that underpin health experiences and health status are fundamental. Practitioners work with individuals and communities, but underpinning the experience of clients are basic social structures such as income distribution, education provision, employment prospects, and housing access and affordability. These basic social determinants of health are discussed in detail in Chapter 9. One of the key characteristics of these social structural factors is their non-egalitarian and inequitable distribution both worldwide and within different countries. For health practitioners, the link between social and health inequalities is central. Whilst it may appear at first sight to be impossible to address such structural causes of health inequality, this chapter argues that practitioners do have the potential to intervene successfully to address inequalities in health. Practitioners may feel that addressing poverty or unemployment is potentially stigmatizing and victim-blaming and therefore avoid such topics. The good practice examples in this chapter demonstrate how tackling inequalities can be

undertaken in a constructive, empowering and health promoting manner.

Defining health inequality

Inequalities refer to differences in circumstances, or the state of being unequal. The current usage of this term in public health includes the additional element of inequity, or being unjust or unfair:

> The term inequity has a moral and ethical dimension. It refers to differences which are unnecessary and avoidable but, in addition, are also considered unfair and unjust ... Our aim is not to eliminate all health differences, for that would be impossible, but rather to reduce or eliminate those that result from factors which are avoidable and unfair ... Equity in health implies that ideally everyone should have a fair opportunity to attain their full health potential and, more pragmatically, that no-one should be disadvantaged from achieving this potential if it can be avoided.
>
> Whitehead (1990, p. 1)

'Inequalities' is the common term used in the UK, but other countries use the terms 'inequities' or 'disparities' to refer to the same phenomenon. There are different types of inequalities in health, including:
- socially patterned differences in life expectancy
- socially patterned differences in health and ill health (both acute and chronic) status
- inequalities in access to, and use of, services
- geographic or regional differences
- differences in treatment outcomes.

 Box 5.1 **Practitioner talking**

My case-load spans a deprived inner city area and a more affluent adjacent area. There's more health problems in the inner city area, granted, but there's also health problems in the affluent area, and there are plenty of

perfectly healthy people living in both areas. Everyone's health is different, you can't expect it to be otherwise. We need to make sure that everyone can get the services they need but that's about all we can do.

Box 5.1 **Practitioner talking—cont'd**

Commentary

It is unrealistic to expect everyone to have equal income or health. Some factors (e.g. gender, ethnicity, age) are clearly unalterable and may include a biological dimension that impacts on health. Some practitioners may argue that other factors such as education or employment include an element of individual choice, although this is debatable. Being unemployed may be a result of a lack of training and employment prospects, determined in turn by wider economic factors such as recession. Even where it appears that

there is an element of individual choice (as in behaviours such as smoking), social norms and networks will, to a large degree, determine lifestyle choices. As Dr. Chan (2008) put it: 'Lifestyles are important determinants of health. But it is factors in the social environment that determine access to health services and influence lifestyle choices in the first place'. This is why such factors are socially patterned rather than randomly distributed. There are variations in health but their social patterning rather than random distribution makes them unjust.

Equity, or social fairness and justice, is an acknowledged goal of many health services and interventions. Equity is not the same as equality, or everyone being equal, which is clearly unrealistic in relation to people's health status. People have varying degrees of health, but the goal of health equity is the absence of unfair and avoidable or remediable differences in health among social groups (Solar and Irwin 2007). Public health and health promotion strategies may improve health overall but at the same time actually increase inequalities as the better off are more likely to access services or adopt health messages (Kelly et al 2006). In 2002, the NHS foregrounded equity by adopting tackling health inequalities as a key priority area (DH 2002).

The scale of inequalities

Inequalities in health are apparent worldwide as well as being manifest within countries. Today the life expectancy for a child born in Japan or Sweden is more than 80 years; for a child born in Brazil it is 72 years, for a child born in India it is 63 years, and in several African countries it is less than 50 years (CSDH 2008). The following example demonstrates how globalization may reinforce and magnify inequalities rather than tackle and reduce them. Globalization may also impact on inequalities through factors associated with economic growth and development, such as the loss of diverse natural habitats,

the risk of pollution, and the vulnerability of single crop economies to infestation or disease.

 Box 5.2 **Example**

Global inequalities in health

In Britain, 1 child in every 150 dies before the age of 5. Average per capita spent on health is £927. In Ghana, 1 child in 10 dies before the age of 5. Average per capita spent on health is £6. In addition, Britain has saved £65 million in training costs by recruiting Ghanaian doctors since 1998, whilst Ghana has lost £35 million of its training investment in health professionals (Ray 2005).

Within many countries, including the UK, the USA, the Netherlands and India, there is a wealth of evidence documenting the continued existence of health inequalities (Acheson 1998; DH 2005; Dorling 2006; Groffen et al 2008; Lantz et al 2001; ONS 2004; Subramanian et al 2006). Box 5.3 gives a summary of this evidence for the UK, most of which focuses on social class or socio-economic status, as measured by the Registrar-General's occupational classification system, as the key variable. In 2001, the old classification of 5 categories was replaced by the NS-SEC (National Statistics Socio-economic Classification). The NS-SEC has 8 categories, including a new category (8) for 'never worked and long-term unemployed'. This issue is discussed in more detail in

Chapter 2 in our companion volume *Foundations for Health Promotion* (Naidoo and Wills 2009). Other forms of inequality linked to factors such as geographical area, gender and ethnicity, and the ways in which inequalities accumulate over the life-course, are also the focus of considerable research (Graham 2000).

Box 5.3 **Health inequalities in the UK in the twenty-first century**

- The social class difference in life expectancy is around 9 years for men and 5 years for women (ONS 2007).
- In 2001–2003, the infant mortality rate (IMR) for the 'routine and manual' group was 19% higher than for the total population, which was an increase compared to the 13% difference between the two groups in 1997–1999 (DH 2005).
- Babies of unskilled manual workers are almost three times more likely to die than babies with fathers in professional occupations. In England and Wales in 2002 the estimated IMR among children whose fathers were in higher managerial and professional occupations was 3.1 per 1000 live births compared to 9.2 for children whose fathers were in routine and semi-routine occupations (ONS 2004).
- The IMR for babies of mothers born in Pakistan is almost double the overall IMR (DH 2006)
- Material disadvantage is an independent risk factor for disability in older adults. The most disadvantaged groups are 2.5 times more likely to report severe disability than the reference group (Adamson et al 2006).
- Death rates from circulatory disease are over 25% higher in the North West than in the South West of England (DH 2006).
- The life expectancy for men in Blackpool is 8 years less than for men in Kensington and Chelsea (DH 2006).

In the UK, socio-economic differences in life expectancy have proved to be a persistent trend, with people in social class group 1 enjoying longer life expectancy than those in lower social class groups. These socio-economic differences increased from the 1970s to the mid 1990s, when the difference peaked at 9.5 years for men and 6.5 years for women (see Figure 5.1). Since then socio-economic differences have declined slightly, but remain very significant.

There is a noticeable stepwise gradient of health outcomes across all socio-economic groups. Higher socio-economic status is linked to increased longevity, reduced incidence of premature mortality at all ages, and reduced incidence of ill health and disease. There are a few exceptions to this rule (e.g. some cancers, hypertension, type 1 diabetes mellitus, inflammatory bowel disease and rheumatoid arthritis), but the overall pattern is consistent and marked (Asthana and Halliday 2006).

Socio-economic differences in mortality are most marked amongst children, young people and younger adults, although they persist into older age groups as well. The infant mortality rate (IMR) is also patterned by socio-economic status. Morbidity is also affected by socio-economic status. Whilst it may be no surprise that social class group 8 (never worked and long-term unemployed) experience five times as much long-term illness as social class group 1, long-term illness is also twice as common in social class group 7 (routine occupations) compared to social class group 1 (ONS 2001). Many other illnesses (although not all) are more common amongst lower socio-economic groups (Asthana and Halliday 2006).

Whilst the link between socio-economic status and health is strongly documented, there is also evidence that geographical area, gender and ethnicity are also linked to health status. In the UK, there is a big North–South divide with higher rates of poor health found in Wales, the North East and North West regions of England than elsewhere. The widest health gap between social classes, however, is in Scotland and London, illustrating some of the complexities of area-based strategies and resource funding (Doran et al 2004).

Gender differences and inequalities, especially in relation to income, may result in inequalities in health status and access to health care. In terms of gender differences in health status, women tend to live longer

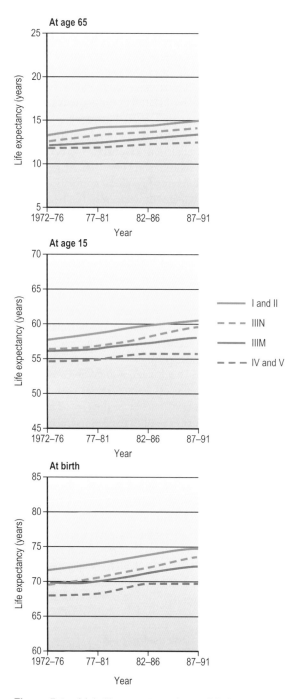

Figure 5.1 ● Male life expectancy by social class, England and Wales. Source: Drever and Whitehead (1997).

than men, but experience more ill health and make more use of health services such as GPs than do men. Commentators (Daykin 2001; Doyal 1995) suggest no single cause but a combination of factors including continued gendered inequalities in society (e.g. the fact that women bear most of the burden of caring and domestic work and are discriminated against in the paid employment sector) and cultural stereotyping (e.g. doctors' readiness to interpret women's symptoms as evidence of mental illness).

The links between ethnicity and health are complex, with some evidence of better than average health status (e.g. low mortality from cancers amongst people from the Caribbean and the Indian subcontinent) but a general pattern of poorer than average health status. There is excess mortality among migrant ethnic minority groups with higher rates of infant mortality, especially among babies of Pakistan-born mothers (Davey Smith et al 2002), and a more common perception of poor health among minority ethnic groups. Material factors, including poorer living circumstances and institutional racism and discrimination, make a central contribution to these findings (Bhopal 2007). Public services may be more punitive to people from Black, Asian and minority ethnic groups (BAME). For example, rates of compulsory detention under Part 11 of the Mental Health Act 1983 for BAME people are six times the rate for white people (Audini and Lelliott 2002). Chapter 12 discusses the benefits and challenges of targeting sections of the population who experience health inequalities, such as women and BAME.

 Box 5.4 **Discussion point**

Despite increased overall prosperity and population longevity, socially patterned health inequalities persist. How can this be explained?

Explaining health inequalities

There are five main theories proposed to explain socio-economic inequalities in health (Davey Smith 2003; Kelly and Bonnefoy 2007):

- Materialist/structuralist theory suggests that low income leads to a lack of resources which in turn leads to ill health.
- Social production of health model suggests that capitalist processes of wealth accumulation are achieved at the cost of the disadvantaged, who become socially excluded.
- Psychosocial model suggests that social discrimination based on one's position in the social hierarchy leads to a biological response in the neuroendocrine system that in turn leads to disease.
- Ecosocial theory brings together the psychosocial and social production of health models and suggests that social and physical environments interact with individual biological systems.
- Life-course model proposes that the accumulated disadvantages experienced throughout the life-course or through generations has an impact on health.

 Box 5.5 **Activity**

Smoking is the biggest single cause of the differences in death rates between rich and poor people, and accounts for half the difference in death rates between men in the top and bottom social classes (Jha et al 2006). Which of the following views comes closest to your own?

- 'Poor people bring illness upon themselves. They don't care about their health, they smoke and drink too much and eat junk food. They could spend the money on healthy activities if they really wanted.'
- 'People's use of tobacco and alcohol is to a large extent determined by their social relations and social networks, which in turn affect their self-esteem and levels of stress. When social support is poor, tobacco and alcohol offer a prop of sorts.'

Adverse socio-economic circumstances and the unequal distribution of income are the key contributors to inequality. Poverty and its links with health and illness are discussed in more detail in the section on poverty

and income in Chapter 9. Poverty may be defined in different ways. Objectively poor people are defined as those living in households with incomes below 60% of the median income level of that year, taking housing costs into account. Poverty may lead to an inability to access the essentials for healthy living (e.g. a warm and safe living environment, adequate nutrition).

But poverty may also be defined relatively, in terms of social expectations, resources and activities. There is a strong relationship between being poor, being unemployed, having few social contacts or support, and having little say in decisions affecting one's life. The term 'social exclusion' has been defined as the state of being unable, because of low income, to participate in many of the activities which society regards as normal or appropriate (Social Exclusion Unit 1997). Social contacts are reduced, the pursuit of individual interests is likely to be impossible, and choices are severely constrained. In a sense, poor people become socially excluded second class citizens, without the resources to enjoy what constitutes everyday life for most people.

Social exclusion is not synonymous with poverty and includes a number of characteristics that are not always included in the concept of poverty. The concept of social exclusion implies exclusion *from* something – typically 'normal society'. As we have seen in Chapter 4, policy interventions are underpinned by clear moral values. Those not working, for example, are seen not only as excluded but also dependent, irrespective of whether or not employment is desired (as may be the case for mothers in two-parent households). Voluntary self exclusion (as in some rough sleepers) may be seen as undesirable and demanding intervention. The ways in which socially excluded groups are targeted for specific interventions are discussed in Chapter 12.

 Box 5.6 **Discussion point**

Why do you think that it is not the richest countries that have the best health, but those that have the smallest income differences between the rich and the poor?

Affluent countries with unequally distributed resources have populations with poorer health status than countries with equal distribution of resources (Wilkinson 1996). Conversely, poor countries or areas with egalitarian resource distribution mechanisms and policies experience better than expected health status. This is illustrated by the example of Kerala in South India. Mortality rates in Kerala are close to those of much wealthier, industrialized countries, and very different from other states in India. Kerala has redistributive policies and many years of investing in human resources, particularly promoting women's access to education (Lynch et al 2000). Wealthy countries with redistributive policies, for example Nordic countries, Belgium and Japan, have the healthiest populations.

The psychosocial model proposes that the perception of inequality and disadvantage is mediated by biological processes that lead to poorer health outcomes. It is not so much the stark lack of resources, as the perception of something lacking that other people have, that is responsible for this process, producing a stress response:

> The power of psycho-social factors to affect health makes biological sense. The human body has evolved to respond automatically to emergencies. This stress response activates a cascade of stress hormones which affect the cardio-vascular and immune systems. The rapid reaction of our hormones and nervous system prepares the individual to deal with a brief physical threat. But if the biological stress response is activated too often and for too long, there may be multiple health costs. These include depression, increased susceptibility to infection, diabetes, high blood pressure and accumulation of cholesterol in blood vessel walls, with the attendant risks of heart attack and stroke.
>
> Brunner and Marmot (1999, p. 41)

The ecosocial model states that it is the interdependent action and effect of many different determinants of health (including environmental, social and physical) that leads to health inequalities. This model flags up the need to address these different domains simultaneously in order to reap the most rewards. What is needed is joined-up thinking and action across the different domains.

The life-course model proposes that the clustering of advantages and disadvantages across the life-course and through generations is the key to health inequalities. This model shares many features with the ecosocial model, but includes a timeline. Deprivation experienced in utero or as a child has a biological effect (e.g. on height, weight, lung function) that impacts on a person's health in later years: 'Human bodies in different social locations become crystallized reflections of the social experiences within which they have developed' (Davey Smith 2003, p. xlvii).

It appears that a number of factors are responsible for these patterned inequalities in health, including poverty, social exclusion, cultural stereotypes, and professional and institutional inflexibility. Poverty is not the only explanation for observed socio-economic, gender and ethnic inequalities, but it plays a central role.

Tackling inequalities

It is clear that inequalities in health are not just a consequence of health service delivery but have complex origins in socio-economic conditions, living and working conditions, and people's lifestyles. The implications of this are that tackling health inequalities involves all sectors of society:

> the high burden of illness responsible for appalling premature loss of life arises in large part because of the conditions in which people are born, grow, live, work, and age. In their turn, poor and unequal living conditions are the consequence of poor social policies and programmes, unfair economic arrangements, and bad politics. Action on the social determinants of health must involve the whole of government, civil society and local communities, business, global fora, and international agencies. Policies

and programmes must embrace all the key sectors of society not just the health sector.
CSDH (2008, p. 1)

Strategies for tackling health inequalities focus on four main areas:

1. Macro-economic social policies (such as reducing unemployment levels).
2. Living and working conditions (including the use of community development approaches).
3. Behavioural risk factors (particularly where focused on disadvantaged groups).
4. Healthcare systems (improving access, particularly for marginalized groups).

Most public policies impact on health and can contribute to or reduce inequalities, hence the importance of 'joined-up government' – a cross-cutting approach that examines all policies for their impact. As we have seen, income is a major determinant of health status. Improving material conditions for the worst off is therefore an important step towards health improvement.

 Box 5.7 **Discussion point**

Should governments focus on closing the gap between the rich and the poor or raising the floor, that is, bringing more people out of poverty?

Traditionally, social democracy has responded to inequality with a simple solution of taking from the rich and giving to the poor. But most governments have pulled back from using redistributive policies that use taxation for fear of alienating the better-off sections of the electorate. Instead, low income has been tackled through increased targeted benefits and the establishment of a minimum wage. The catch-phrase of American democrats is that welfare should offer a hand-up not a hand-out and this is reflected in the emphasis on job creation, education for employability and flexible working.

The Acheson (1998) Report into inequalities in health made 39 policy recommendations, only 3 of which related to the NHS. The report also recommended that priority should be given to improving the health of women of childbearing age, expectant mothers and young children. This reflects a focus in many developed countries struggling with welfare reform to shift redistribution forward in the life-course and concentrate on the young. Attention has also been focused on the working population and the economic case to be made for tackling ill health in a more proactive and integrated fashion. Each year sickness absence and worklessness costs the UK over £100 billion. Mental ill health is a major contributor to the absence of sickness, with over 200,000 people moving onto incapacity benefit due to mental ill health over the last decade (Black 2008). The review 'Working for a Healthier Tomorrow' (Black 2008) advocated the establishment of a new integrated, multi-disciplinary 'Fit for Work' service to manage ill health at the early stages of absence due to sickness and to encourage staff back to work.

In the past decade attention has also focused on area-based strategies to regenerate and revitalize disadvantaged localities. This is in part due to recognition of the interlinked environmental, social and physical factors that affect health, as proposed in the eco-social model of health inequalities.

A raft of interlinked policies and interventions to tackle inequalities has been launched by the UK government. Key policies are outlined in Box 5.8.

If progress is to be made towards tackling inequalities, agencies need to be able to measure local inequalities. Traditionally, data on health status and outcomes, such as standardized mortality rates (SMRs) for diseases or indicators such as the percentage of low birthweight babies, would be used. This chapter shows the complexity of health inequalities and that tackling the wider determinants of health inequalities requires action across a range of factors. Health equity audits (HEAs) were introduced to ensure local health and development plans prioritize those with the greatest need (DH 2003). A HEA aims to systematically review inequities in causes and outcomes of ill health and access to preventive and treatment services within a specific population.

Box 5.8 **Policies that tackle health inequalities**

Tackling low income

- In 1999, a minimum wage was established, which in 2008 was £5.73 per hour for an adult (aged 22 plus). Low income workers and their families also benefited from the introduction of the Working Tax Credit and the Child Tax Credit, the introduction of a lower income tax rate and reform of the national insurance system. Benefits levels for families with children and pensioners have increased.

Tackling child poverty and ill health

- Sure Start is a national programme in England to support children, families and communities to achieve the best outcomes. Sure Start is involved in many interventions, for example an £18 million national programme to loan home safety equipment to disadvantaged families to be run by ROSPA (Royal Society for the Prevention of Accidents).
- Every Child Matters: Change for Children works to improve the well-being of children and young people from birth to age 19. Key outcomes for children that should guide all policies and children's services are: be healthy, stay safe, enjoy and achieve, make a positive contribution, and achieve economic well-being.

Tackling health in the workplace

- Establishing a new 'Fit for Work' service to provide an integrated, multi-disciplinary service for people in the early stages of sickness absence. Such a service will provide health support (including mental health support) and employment and skills programmes.
- The Department of Health will adopt the Single Equality Scheme 2009–2012 which will commit to a plan of action across the six equality strands of ethnicity, gender, disability, age, sexual orientation, and religion or belief. The SES also incorporates the Human Rights Programme.

Tackling area-based inequalities

- Joint Strategic Needs Assessment (JSNA) was introduced in 2008. Local authorities and primary care teams (PCTs) have a statutory duty to produce a JSNA for their area, which feeds into Local Area Agreements and the sustainable communities strategy. The JSNA focuses on the health and well-being needs of a population and involves a range of statutory and non-statutory partners.
- Local Area Agreements (LAAs) are 3-year agreements developed by local councils with their partners in a Local Strategic Partnership (LSP). The aim is to identify local priorities that will improve the quality of life for inhabitants, and to channel resources (including mainstream funding and the new Area-Based Grant) accordingly. LAAs were introduced in 2004/5 in England, and by 2008 were in place for all 150 upper-tier local authority areas. LAAs are normally drawn from the Sustainable Community Strategy (SCS) for the area. The SCS is a longer term vision based on evidence and forecasts as well as extensive local consultation.
- Healthy Living Centres (HLCs) were established as a UK-wide initiative in 1999. The aim of HLCs is to influence the wider determinants of health such as social exclusion, poor access to services, mental health, diet and fitness. HLCs are targeted at the most disadvantaged 20% of the population. Projects are flexible to meet local needs and local community involvement is encouraged. Examples of projects include smoking cessation, dietary advice, training and skills schemes, arts programmes and complementary therapy. HLCs were funded with lottery money and managed by the New Opportunities Fund. HLCs have been recognized as providing value for money and tackling health inequalities in an effective manner. Following the end of lottery funding,

Box 5.8 Policies that tackle health inequalities—cont'd

the Scottish parliament made available up to £70,000 per centre for 2009–2010 in order to allow them to continue to function and to set up sustainable funding arrangements for the future.

- Neighbourhood Renewal Unit (NRU) oversees and supports local strategic partnerships in the 86 most deprived districts in England.

The aim is to respond to local circumstances. The NRU runs a number of programmes including New Deal for Communities partnerships which tackle five key themes: poor job prospects, high levels of crime, educational under-achievement, poor health, and problems with housing and the physical environment.

Box 5.9 Activity

In your practice you may need to show that you are tackling health inequalities. What methods of monitoring would you use to show progress?

Box 5.10 Example

Health equity audit

A HEA is designed to answer the following questions in a local area:

- What are the known health inequalities for a particular population group or area?
- What are the significant equity issues in relation to provision/access to services, facilities and the determinants of good health?
- Which of these are priorities for action?
- What programmes already exist which might help reduce the inequities?
- Are there any relevant national targets?
- Should a local target be set?
- What further action can be taken by existing public services or through more targeted action with key groups and areas?
- Have resources been reallocated to take the most effective action?
- Has there been any impact on the inequities targets?

Source: Hamer et al 2003

Although many interventions and services are provided on a universal basis for all people within a defined population (e.g. within an age group or diagnosed with a certain condition), in practice service uptake is often poorer amongst more disadvantaged social groups. This phenomenon – the inverse care law – was first described by Tudor Hart (1971) and applies to screening and preventive services as well as for acute services. Equity audit provides a potentially powerful tool to try to tackle unequal uptake of services, and it is encouraging that equity audit has been highlighted as a required strategy in England.

Another kind of strategy involves identifying indicators that are monitored in order to assess whether or not reductions in inequalities are occurring. This could be undertaken as part of a local area needs assessment.

Two 'headline' inequalities targets are used in England (DH 2001):

1. Starting with IMRs, by 2010 to reduce by at least 10% the gap in mortality between manual groups and the population as a whole.

2. Starting with health authorities, by 2010 to reduce by at least 10% the gap between the fifth of areas with the lowest life expectancy at birth and the population as a whole.

Box 5.11 Discussion point

Why were these chosen as the targets for reducing inequalities?

These inequalities targets were seen to be achievable yet challenging. The first target focuses on children and the next generation, an important priority group for breaking the generational transmission of poverty and disadvantage. The targets can be measured using data that are already routinely collected and available.

Since then health inequalities targets have been included in Department of Health Public Service Agreement (PSA) targets. For example, DH PSA for 2004 (http://www.hm-treasury.gov.uk/media/70320/sr04_psa_ch3.pdf) included the following targets:

- Reduce mortality rates from heart disease and stroke and related diseases by the year 2010 by at least 40% in people under 75, with at least a 40% reduction in the inequalities gap between the fifth of areas with the worst health and deprivation indicators and in the population as a whole.
- Reduce mortality rates from cancer by 2010 by at least 20% in people under 75, with at least a 6% reduction in the inequalities gap between the fifth of areas with the worst health and deprivation indicators and the population as a whole.
- Reduce adult smoking rates to 21% or less by 2010, with a reduction in prevalence among routine and manual groups to 26% or less.

The White Paper 'Choosing Health – making healthier choices easier' (DH 2004) led to the adoption of a Public Health Service Agreement target to address geographical inequalities in life expectancy and cancer, heart disease, stroke, and related disease rates. The targets aimed for faster than average progress in the fifth of areas with the worst health and deprivation indicators – the Spearhead Group comprising 70 Local Authorities and 88 Primary Care Trusts (PCTs) – by 2010. The targets require concerted and coordinated action by local authorities and PCTs working together in Local Strategic Partnerships in order to address the determinants of health – income, employment, healthy local environments and transport systems, housing, education and health, and social care services.

Evidence on whether or not these targets to reduce health inequalities are being met is mixed. To date, 41% Spearheads are on track to meet their target of a 10% reduction in the life expectancy gap between themselves and England as a whole (DH 2008a). However, the socio-economic gap in life expectancy is increasing rather than reducing (2% wider for men; 11% wider for women in 2004–2006 compared to the baseline 1997–1999), even though life expectancy for everyone is increasing (DH 2008a). The infant mortality health inequalities gap is narrowing, but is still wider than the 13% gap that existed in the baseline period of 1997–1999 (DH 2008a).

 Box 5.12 **Example**

Area-based Initiatives

The establishment of the Healthy Towns initiative is an example of the focus on physical area (DH 2008b). Nine areas in England have been awarded a total of £30 million in order to support initiatives for a healthier population. Each council will match this funding and develop its own schemes and initiatives. The driving force has been the alarming increase in obesity, and initiatives include encouraging walking and cycling as the means of transport, and promoting healthier diets through, for example, the establishment of breakfast clubs and subsidized fruit and vegetables.

Smoking provides a good example of how what are viewed as individual lifestyle choices are in fact the result of continuing health inequalities. There is a strong association between smoking and lower socio-economic status. The contribution of smoking to persistent inequalities in health has been widely acknowledged and attempts to tackle health inequalities often focus on this issue (Jarvis and Wardle 1999). A recent cohort study found that smoking was a greater source of health inequality than social position, and suggested that the priority should be on getting smokers in lower social positions to stop smoking (Gruer et al 2009). However, even if smoking-related diseases and premature deaths decline, other competing mortality risks will rapidly increase in prevalence, resulting in the maintenance of long-term social class inequalities in mortality (albeit at higher levels of overall life expectancy) (Scott Samuel 2009).

Addressing living and working conditions is evident in the Mayor of London's draft strategy below. Key aims of the strategy included encouraging physical activity and supporting individuals to make healthier choices and promoting well-being in the workplace.

 Box 5.13 **Example**

The Mayor's Draft Health Inequalities Strategy for London

- To increase people's opportunities to benefit from employment and other meaningful activities by supporting equality in the workplace, providing ongoing opportunities for skill development, and raising the profile of unpaid work opportunities
- To empower individuals and communities by building capacity and skills, supporting cultural activities and community work, and increasing community and individual involvement in public services
- To develop London as a healthy place for all by providing affordable housing and local facilities, safe, accessible local environments that facilitate social cohesion, and working towards a sustainable environment and stable climate

(Mayor of London, 2008)

 Box 5.14 **Discussion point**

A local partnership is tasked with reducing health inequalities. What factors can you identify that would assist you in this task?

There is now a concern to learn from experience and to look beyond 2010 and set on-going and challenging targets and goals to reduce health inequalities. One of the key challenges is to translate national goals into effective local action. In many ways tackling health inequalities should be a mainstreamed aspect of all public health work. The following list, compiled by the National Support Team for Health Inequalities and based on their experience, identifies what works locally (DH 2008a):

- A strategic evidence-based approach.
- Scaling action to the size of the problem locally.
- Leading from the top.
- Ensuring the quality and quantity of primary care.
- Actively seeking out people who already have a disease or are at high risk but are not accessing services early enough.
- Capitalizing on community infrastructures to engage individuals, families and communities.
- Ensuring that partnerships are effective.
- Considering and addressing workforce implication.
- Innovating.

Tackling inequalities aims to raise the level of the less well off. This strategy ignores the fact that widening inequalities are driven not just by an increase in the poorest and most disadvantaged groups, but also by a rise in the income and wealth of the richest groups in society. As Professor Dorling put it on the BBC news in 2005, 'without tackling wealth inequalities, which are widening, it is not going to be able to tackle health inequalities'. The current approach is to try to break the cycle of inequalities rather than close the gap. Health promotion strategies such as those suggested to tackle coronary heart disease and cancer focus on individualized risk management and health education and are less widely taken up by disadvantaged groups. Such interventions may therefore actually increase inequalities despite improving the overall health of the population. Chapter 11 on lifestyles discusses the approaches used to change behaviours and some of the resulting dilemmas.

The performance of agencies tackling inequalities is to be monitored against targets. Whilst the setting of national inequalities targets is important in directing strategies and funding, targets are fairly blunt instruments with which to measure change and improvement. The development and use of local targets is problematic, especially when partnership working is required. It is likely that different agencies and professional groups will have different priorities that will in turn hinder the identification of shared targets. Partnership working and community development approaches are rightly seen as the means towards achieving a reduction in inequalities. However, in order to achieve these aims, these strategies need to be resourced adequately. This is not always recognized or accounted for in funding arrangements. The challenges for practitioners of working with communities and across agencies are discussed in Chapters 6 and 7.

Box 5.15 **Activity**

To what extent do you feel able to address health inequalities in your practice?

Tackling inequalities: the practitioner's perspective

Many of the policies and strategies designed to reduce inequalities appear to be beyond the scope of individual practitioners, unless they are specifically employed as project workers. However, there are examples of how practitioners can routinely include tackling inequalities in their work practice.

Box 5.16 **Examples**

Practitioners tackling health inequalities

1. Community nurses tackling health inequalities

A community nurse-led health shop in a disadvantaged area of London reports that 'Community nurses can play a significant part in helping marginalized groups access healthcare services and health promotion initiatives more effectively. Key to this success is the contextualization of health issues, messages and initiatives in the local culture, making it easier for people to participate …'. One of the stories cited concerned a middle-aged Bengali woman who attended the health shop to express her dismay at being told she had cancer and to find out more about it. She described how she received a letter, which her friend interpreted for her, saying that she had 'low cancer'. The letter actually said that she had had a normal cervical smear result and therefore a 'low' probability of developing cervical cancer. The report argues that using an interpreter would not change or alter the power relations of the Bengali population, nor lessen their alienation. Community nurses can provide community members with the strategies and knowledge necessary to be informed users of services rather than remaining passive recipients, and thereby embed significant changes and improvements within communities.

(Forbes 2000)

2. Tackling inequalities through the Healthy Living Centre programme

A research study exploring practitioners' perspectives on tackling health inequalities through their involvement in the Healthy Living Centre programme (which targets services at the most deprived local communities) identified several challenges. These included positioning services to appeal to and reach the target groups, and the difficulties in evaluating the impact of their work on reducing health inequalities. Practitioners identified several key processes, for example gaining acceptance and overcoming barriers to engaging with disadvantaged communities, allowing sufficient time to achieve such engagement, the proximity of service providers to service users, and adaptable services to address evolving needs.

(Rankin et al 2009)

Compared to many other public health and health promotion interventions, welfare benefits screening and advice services appear to be of proven effectiveness using a variety of criteria:

- The service avoids victim blaming by focusing on benefit entitlement not unhealthy lifestyles.
- Services may be accessed by many of the most marginalized and 'hard to reach' groups.
- Quantitative positive outcomes are apparent, both in terms of numbers of users, and in terms of additional income flowing into the area.
- Qualitative outcomes are provided in the form of individual case studies where increased income leads to health benefits.

A recent review of delivering welfare rights advice in healthcare settings concluded that there was evidence that such interventions resulted in increased financial benefits (Adams et al 2006). There are sound theoretical reasons to suppose that this would in turn lead to improved health, but there is currently a lack of good quality evidence to this effect.

Box 5.17 Discussion point

As a health practitioner working with a disadvantaged population in a deprived inner city area how might you go about reducing health inequalities?

For practitioners with case-loads, tackling inequalities may seem beyond their remit and there are enormous challenges. However, local practitioners and services have the potential in their day-to-day work to address the more immediate health needs of the most disadvantaged. Examples include ensuring that people are receiving their full benefits income entitlement, supporting and facilitating community initiatives and resources, signposting clients to appropriate community networks, and providing individually tailored information and advice about healthy lifestyles. Practitioners can also reflect on how they deliver services to ensure that they have maximum impact on inequalities and provide accessible and empowering services. Table 5.1

Table 5.1 Providing supportive and empowering services: helpful and unhelpful strategies

Helpful	Unhelpful
An integrated approach	Services that treat financial, health and social problems as unrelated
A coordinated response	Individual agencies working on separate sets of problems
Services which offer realistic advice and recognize the limitations that poverty places on people	Providing help only when families are in crisis Interventions which individualize problems
Partnerships between families and workers where families' contributions are valued	Services based on what professionals think that families want rather than what families say they want Failure to recognize what families do achieve in adversity Blaming families for their poverty
Services that are permanent	Temporary or short-term projects
Services that are relevant	Forcing families to define financial problems as emotional problems or personal inadequacy before help is given
Services that are easy to use	Only providing help when families are labelled as a problem

Source: Laughlin and Black (1995).

above illustrates some guiding principles to help review service delivery.

Evaluating policies to reduce inequalities

Despite the interest in inequalities there is very little evidence of the impact of policy interventions. A recent report of the House of Commons Health Committee on health inequalities was highly critical of the neglect of evaluation and the manner in which policy has been implemented, which has made rigorous evaluation impossible (House of Commons 2009). Kevin Barron MP, Chair of the Health Committee, said: '… while our Committee commends the Government on its commitment to reducing the health gap, we were shocked by the lack of meaningful evidence and evaluation available on this subject'.

The debate about evaluation is made more complex because of the diverse goals that different interventions have. Whilst some interventions target the most deprived in an attempt to reduce their poverty and social exclusion, other interventions are targeted at the whole population in an attempt to reduce the health inequalities gradient.

The Dutch strategy for tackling inequalities recommends a combination of 'upstream' measures targeting the socio-economic factors that are pushing people into the river and 'downstream' measures that target the accessibility and quality of services (that might help to pull people out of the river) (Mackenbach and Stronks 2002). Upstream measures include improving the physical and psychosocial work environment, reducing smoking in lower socio-economic groups, improving nutrition (preferably through universal measures such as healthier school meals), and reducing childhood poverty. Downstream policies include healthcare policies that improve accessibility for lower socio-economic groups.

Whilst there is a solid theoretical base that suggests 'upstream' interventions would be the most effective, most policy in practice is more 'downstream', where there is a dearth of either theoretical or research evidence of effectiveness. In particular,

local initiatives, although very popular with government, frequently have no solid evidence base of effectiveness (see Box 5.18).

> Box 5.18 **Interventions to reduce health inequalities that have a good evidence base**
>
> - Area-wide traffic calming schemes reduce traffic injuries
> - Smoke detectors and child-resistant containers reduce injury in the home
> - Drunken driving legislation and enforcement (via breath testing) reduces alcohol-related accidents, deaths and injuries
> - Increasing the price of cigarettes reduces tobacco use amongst adolescents and young adults
> - School-based sex education programmes linked to community contraceptive services reduces the incidence of STIs (sexually transmitted infections)
> - Dietary and vitamin supplementation improves foetal growth and reduces pre-term births and the incidence of low birth weight
> - Multi-faceted interventions increase breastfeeding initiation and duration
> - Home visiting and parenting programmes improve mothers' health and children's behavioural development
> - The provision of early years child care improves children's development and school achievement, and mothers' education, employment and interaction with children
>
> Source: Asthana and Halliday 2006.

Policy evaluation is very difficult because of the complexities of the policy process and the pathways linking social policy interventions to individual outcomes. Experimental methodologies are usually impossible due to the broad impact of policy interventions, and the difficulty of finding comparable population groups who have not been subject to the policy in question, or one that is similar in intent. However, other rigorous methodologies, including international comparative studies and theory-based evaluation, exist and should be used when appropriate (Mackenbach and Bakker 2002).

Whitehead et al (2000) describe a framework which is intended for researching policy impact on health inequalities (see Figure 5.2). This framework seeks to evaluate the different pathways that link individuals and policies, including the impact of policies on social position (including educational policies and policies which affect social networks and social inclusion), specific exposure to risks and hazards (e.g. housing, occupational, and food policies), and the impact of being ill (e.g. healthcare and disability policies).

Conclusion

Social and health inequalities remain a significant and preventable cause of much ill health and prema-

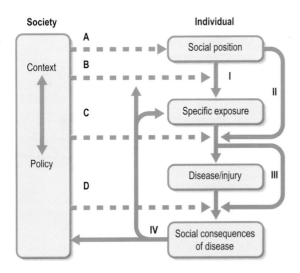

Figure 5.2 ● Framework for researching policy impact on health inequalities. Source: Whitehead et al: In Graham H, editor: *Understanding health inequalities*, 2000. Reproduced by permission of Open University Press.

ture death. The impact of such inequalities on health is apparent both between countries worldwide and within countries. The health inequalities agenda is now firmly established on the health agendas of many developed countries. However, the gap from policy to practitioner level can appear daunting and practitioners may feel tackling inequalities is beyond their remit and that they do not have the necessary knowledge, skills and resources to do so effectively. This chapter has sought to demonstrate that practitioner interventions to address inequalities are feasible and effective, and has argued that the extent of health problems related to inequalities makes such action a priority.

Inequalities due to socio-economic position, gender, ethnicity and geography impact on health via complex pathways involving material resources, the physical and social environment, behaviour and lifestyles, and physiological responses. Inequalities often cluster and accumulate over the course of a lifetime or may become concentrated within small geographical areas. Tackling inequalities requires policy initiatives aimed at reducing the gap between the wealthiest and the poorest sections of society. This is generally interpreted as raising the income and improving the circumstances of the poorest groups, but equally it could involve reducing the incomes of the wealthiest through redistributive taxation policies. Many countries (e.g. the UK, The Netherlands and Sweden) have adopted targeted interventions aimed at disadvantaged groups. Some commentators argue for a simpler intervention aimed at raising incomes of people living in poverty, and argue that international comparisons suggest this simpler strategy is more effective in reducing inequalities with all the benefits this brings to individuals and society in general (Whitehead et al 2000). The UK has followed the route of raising people out of poverty rather than reducing the health gap, and has achieved some success with this approach. Practitioners can support such activity by being aware of the current policy context, supporting individual clients to claim their full benefits entitlement, and working with communities to address inequalities in the local environment.

Being aware of the constraints of poverty and social inequalities on lifestyles and behaviours can enable practitioners' health promotion work with individuals and families to be sensitive, appropriate, enabling, and ultimately more effective.

Further discussion

- With reference to your own practice, identify how (if at all) social inequalities result in health inequalities.

- What 'downstream' initiatives might help improve the accessibility and quality of services for disadvantaged clients?

- The life-course perspective shows how health disadvantage accumulates throughout life. How can practitioners help to make a difference?

- Should priority be given towards 'upstream' or 'downstream' interventions to tackle inequalities? Why?

Recommended reading

- Asthana S, Halliday J: *What works in tackling health inequalities? Pathways, policies and practice through the lifecourse*, Bristol, 2006, Policy Press.

   This text examines the research basis for interventions at different stages in the life-course, and the efficacy of policies directed at reducing health inequalities. The role of theory, research and policy in identifying and tackling health inequalities is debated.

- Davey Smith G, editor: *Health inequalities: lifecourse approaches*, Bristol, 2003, Policy Press.

   An edited collection of articles supporting the life-course theory of health inequalities.

- Dowler E, Spencer NJ, editors: *Challenging health inequalities: from Acheson to 'Choosing Health'*, Bristol, 2007, Policy Press.

   Nearly 10 years after New Labour's election commitment to tackle inequalities, this book examines and evaluates the impact of different policy areas that are drivers of health inequalities (e.g. education, employment, poverty, and income distribution). A multidisciplinary perspective is adopted and determinants of health, factors impacting on health, and health strategies are all examined.

- Graham H, Kelly MP: Health inequalities: Concepts, frameworks and policy Health Development Agency Briefing Paper, 2004.

   A useful 'unpacking' of the different concepts used in health inequalities research and literature. The links between different concepts and policies is explored.

- Kelly MP, Bonnefoy J: The social determinants of health: Developing an evidence base for political action. Final Report to World Health Organization Commission on the Social Determinants of Health from Measurement and Evidence Knowledge Network Universidad del Desarrollo, Chile and NICE, UK, 2007.

   This report looks in detail at the challenges of developing and using evidence of health inequalities in policy and practice. Illustrative case studies from around the world help to demonstrate the variety of challenges and strategies.

- Marmot, M: Fair society, healthy lives: The Marmot Review of Health Inequalities in England post-2010 www.ucl.ac.uk/ marmotreview, 2010.

   This strategic review of the government's actions to reduce health inequalities concludes that what is required is a comprehensive and participatory approach to tackling social inequalities - what it terms 'proportionate universalism'. Such action will have economic and environmental benefits. Six policy objectives are identified, embracing action directed at children and young people, employment, economic status, sustainability and the prevention of ill health.

- Shaw M, Galobardes B, Lawlor DA, et al: *The handbook of inequality and socioeconomic positions*, Bristol, 2007, Policy Press.

  This book provides a valuable resource or 'toolbox' for anyone interested in socio-economic inequalities. Key concepts and measurements are described, and the complexities of the methodologies used to measure inequalities explained.

- Wilkinson R, Pickett K: *The Spirit Level: Why more equal societies almost always do better*, London, 2009, Allen Lane.

This book makes a robust case for arguing that among rich countries, more unequal countries fare worst on virtually all quality of life indicators, including physical and mental health and wellbeing, criminality and educational attainment. The UK ranks amongst the more unequal societies (with the USA ranked the most unequal), and thus stands to make very significant gains if social and economic inequality is tackled effectively.

References

Acheson D: *Independent inquiry into inequalities in health*, London, 1998, The Stationery Office.

Adams J, White M, Moffatt S, et al: A systematic review of the health, social and financial impacts of welfare rights advice delivered in healthcare settings. *BioMed Central Public Health* 6:81, 2006.

Adamson JA, Ebrahim S, Hunt K: The psychosocial versus material hypothesis to explain observed inequality in disability among older adults: data from the West of Scotland Twenty-07 Study, *J Epidemiol Community Health* 60:974–980, 2006.

Asthana S, Halliday J: *What works in tackling health inequalities? Pathways, policies and practice through the lifecourse*, Bristol, 2006, Policy Press.

Audini B, Lelliott P: Age, gender and ethnicity of those detained under Part 11 of the Mental Health Act 1983, *Br J Psychiatry* 180:222–226, 2002.

Bhopal RS: *Ethnicity race and health in multicultural societies: foundations for better epidemiology, public health, and health care*, Oxford, 2007, Oxford University Press.

Black DC: *Working for a healthier tomorrow. Dame Carol Black's Review of the Health of Britain's Working Age Population*, London, 2008, The Stationery Office.

Brunner E, Marmot MG: Social organization, stress and health. In Marmot MG, Wilkinson RG, editors: *The social determinants of health*, Oxford, 1999, Oxford University Press.

Chan Dr. M: Director General of World Health Organization's speech at the launch of the Commission for Social Determinants of Health Final Report, Geneva 28/8/2008, 2008.

Commission on Social Determinants of Health: *Closing the gap in a generation: health equity through action on the social determinants of health*, Final Report of the Commission on Social Determinants of Health, Geneva, 2008, World Health Organization.

Davey Smith G, Chaturvedi N, Harding S, et al: Ethnic inequalities in health: a review of UK epidemiological evidence. In Nettleton S, Gustaffson U, editors: *The sociology of health and illness: a reader*, Cambridge, 2002, Polity Press.

Davey Smith G, editor: *Health inequalities: lifecourse approaches*, Bristol, 2003, Policy Press.

Daykin N: Sociology. In Naidoo J, Wills J, editors: *Health studies*, Basingstoke, 2001, Palgrave.

Department of Health (DH): *Tackling health inequalities: consultation on a plan for delivery*, London, 2001, DH.

Department of Health (DH): *Improvement expansion and reform: the next three years' priorities and planning framework 2003–2006*, London, 2002, DH.

Department of Health (DH): *Health equity audit: a guide for the NHS*, London, 2003, DH.

Department of Health (DH): *Choosing health: making healthy choices easier*, London, 2004, DH.

Department of Health (DH): *Tackling health inequalities – Status Report on Programme for Action*, London, 2005, DH.

Department of Health (DH): *Fact sheet on health inequalities*, London, 2006, DH.

Department of Health (DH): *Health inequalities: progress and next steps*, London, 2008a, DH.

Department of Health (DH): *Healthy weight, healthy lives: a cross government strategy for England*, London, 2008b, DH.

Doran T, Drever F, Whitehead M: Is there a north-south divide in social class inequalities in health in Great Britain? Cross sectional study using data from the 2001 census, *BMJ* 328:1043–1045, 2004.

Dorling D: Commentary: the fading of the dream: widening inequalities in life expectancy in America, *Int J Epidemiol* 35(4):979–980, 2006.

Doyal L: *What makes women sick? Gender and the political economy of health*, Basingstoke, 1995, Macmillan.

Drever F, Whitehead M, editors: *Health inequalities*, London, 1997, The Stationery Office.

Forbes A: A community nurse-led project to tackle health inequalities, *Br J Community Nurs* 5(12):610–618, 2000.

Graham H: *Understanding health inequalities*, Maidenhead, 2000, Open University Press.

Groffen DAI, Bosma H, van den Akker M, et al: Material deprivation and health-related dysfunction in older Dutch people: findings from the SMILE study, *Eur J Public Health* 18(3):258–263, 2008.

Gruer L, Hart CL, Gordon DS, et al: Effect of tobacco smoking on survival of men and women by social position: a 28 year cohort study, *Br Med J* 338:b480, 2009.

Hamer L, Jacobson B, Flowers J, et al: *Health equity audit made simple: a briefing for primary care trusts and local strategic partnerships*, London, 2003, Health Development Agency and Public Health Observatories.

House of Commons: Health committee health inequalities. Third Report of Session 2008–9 vol.1, 15 March 2009, http://www.publications.parliament.uk/pa/cm/cmhealth.htm.

Jarvis M, Wardle J: Social patterning of individual health behaviours: the case of cigarette smoking. In Marmot M, Wilkinson R, editors: *Social determinants of health*, Oxford, 1999, Oxford University Press.

Jha P, Peto R, Zatonski W, et al: Social inequalities in male mortality, and in male mortality from smoking: indirect estimation from national death rates in England and Wales, Poland and North America, *Lancet* 368(9533):367–370, 2006.

Kelly MP, Bonnefoy J, Morgan A, et al: *The development of the evidence base about the social determinants of health*, London/Chile, 2006, WHO Commission on Social Determinants of Health Measurement and Evidence Knowledge Network, NICE /UDD.

Lantz P, Lynch J, House J, et al: Socio-economic disparities in health change in a longitudinal study of US adults: the role of health-risk behaviours, *Soc Sci Med* 29–40, 2001.

Laughlin S, Black D: *Poverty and health: tools for change*, Birmingham, 1995, Public Health Alliance.

Lynch J, Davey Smith G, Kaplan G, et al: Income inequality and mortality: importance to health of individual income, psychosocial environment or material conditions, *Br Med J* 320:1200–1204, 2000.

Mackenbach JP, Bakker M: *Reducing inequalities in health: a European perspective*, London, 2002, Routledge.

Mackenbach JP, Stronks K: A strategy for tackling health inequalities in The Netherlands, *Br Med J* 325:1029–1032, 2002.

Mayor of London: *Living well in London: the mayor's draft health inequalities strategy for London*, London, 2008, Greater London Authority.

Office of National Statistics (ONS): *Census: longitudinal study*, 2001, available online at www.statistics.gov.uk.

Office of National Statistics (ONS): *Mortality statistics: childhood, infant and perinatal*, Review of the Registrar General on deaths in England and Wales 2002, Series DH3 No. 35, London, 2004, ONS.

Office of National Statistics (ONS): *Health statistics quarterly No. 33*, London, 2007, ONS.

Rankin D, Backett-Milburn K, Platt S: Practitioner perspectives on tackling health inequalities: findings from an evaluation of healthy living centres in Scotland, *Soc Sci Med* 68(5):925–932, 2009.

Ray S: The NHS as part of global health. In *Politics of health group UK health watch 2005: the experience of health in an unequal society*, 2005.

Scott Samuel A: What the Renfrew/Paisley data really tell us about tackling health inequalities: the need to refocus upstream, *BMJ* 338:b480, 2009.

Shaw M, Dorling D, Gordon D, et al: *The widening gap: health inequalities and policy in Britain*, Bristol, 1999, The Policy Press.

Social Exclusion Unit: *Purpose, work priorities and working methods*, London, 1997, HMSO.

Solar O, Irwin A: *A conceptual framework for action on the social determinants of health*, 2007. http://minority-health.pitt.edu/archive/00000757/accessed 26/03/09.

Subramanian SV, Nandy S, Irving M, et al: The mortality divide in India: the differential contributions of gender, caste, and standard of living across the life course, *Am J Public Health* 96(5):818–825, 2006.

Tudor Hart J: The inverse care law, *Lancet* 1:405–412, 1971.

Whitehead M: *The concepts and principles of equity in health*, Copenhagen, 1990, World Health Organization.

Whitehead M, Burström B, Diderichsen: Social policies and the pathways to inequalities in health: a comparative analysis of lone mothers in Britain and Sweden, *Soc Sci Med* 50(2):255–270, 2000.

Wilkinson RG: *Unhealthy societies: the afflictions of inequality*, London, 1996, Routledge.

Chapter Six

Participation, involvement and engagement

Key points

- The context for public and patient involvement
- The context for community engagement
- Typologies of participation
- Patient and user involvement
- Participation in needs assessment and priority setting
- Community development, community engagement and capacity building
- Evaluating public involvement and community engagement

OVERVIEW

This chapter examines the growth of participation and involvement as key strategies in public health and health promotion. The concept of public involvement is not new, and international and national bodies have advocated participation since the 1980s. However, public participation is now increasingly being seen as relevant to improvements in service delivery, monitoring and management. The NHS Plan (DH 2000) envisaged a service which is shaped around the convenience and concerns of patients. Patient and public involvement (PPI) is carried out at the level of the individual, involving patients in decisions about care and treatment, and at the collective level, involving patients and the public in decisions concerning the planning and delivery of services. PPI therefore covers a broad range of activities from providing information to gathering feedback to involvement in decision making. Community engagement, especially with marginalized and seldom heard groups, is a key feature of public policy to reduce health inequalities. This chapter discusses some of the strategies which may be used to engage the public and service users. Finally, the chapter discusses the difficulties of evaluating participation and involvement strategies and concludes with a discussion of public involvement from the perspective of a health practitioner.

Introduction

There is no simple explanation of why public participation has become so significant in governmental discourse and practice in many countries in recent years. This paradigm shift, whereby the public are seen as co-producers of health, draws from social and patient rights movements (Brown and Zavestoski 2005). The Department of Health reflects this in naming its involvement section 'Patient and Public Empowerment'. Popular neoliberal ideology (see Chapter 4) has recast the public as active consumers rather than passive recipients of services with new forms of governance of public services (Newman and Clarke 2009).

There is a broad spectrum of attitude and purpose in relation to 'involvement'. The emphasis is now on participatory and bottom-up approaches (rather than control by experts) reflected in a range of actions including:

- User participation in decisions about treatment and care.
- User involvement in service development.
- User evaluation of service provision and a shift to public accountability.
- User involvement in teaching and training of practitioners.
- User involvement in research.

A commitment to a community-oriented health approach informs the UK government health and care programmes (see Chapter 4). NICE, the standard-setting body for the NHS, has set out guidelines for patient and public involvement (PPI) (see http://www.nice.org.uk/getinvolved/patientandpublicinvolvement/), and for commissioning organizations' work with partners to engage communities in identifying their health needs and aspirations when developing strategic plans. This includes making sure community perspectives – people's preferences, felt needs and expectations – are built into the Joint Strategic Needs Assessment (JSNA) and health needs assessments undertaken with particular communities, moving beyond a solely data-driven approach to needs assessment to one that is complemented by the views of those in the community. For example, Competency Three of the requirements for World Class Commissioning, the means by which the government aims to deliver high-quality services (DH 2007), states: 'PCTs are responsible through the commissioning process for investing public funds on behalf of their patients and communities. In order to make commissioning decisions that reflect the needs, priorities and aspirations of the local population, PCTs will have to engage the public in a variety of ways, openly and honestly. They will need to be proactive in seeking out the views and experience of the public, patients, their carers and other stakeholders, especially those least able to advocate for themselves'.

'Involvement' is a principle across all health and social care sectors but is central to health improvement, and there are specific reasons why public health and health promotion practitioners may lead on this issue. *Foundations for Health Promotion* (Naidoo and Wills 2009) highlighted how the role of communities in health improvement has been signalled in key international agreements:

- Equity and participation were central concepts of the World Health Organization Health for All 2000 strategy.
- The Ottawa Charter (WHO 1986) made community participation and strengthening communities a central principle and level of action for health promotion.
- The Jakarta conference on Health Promotion into the Twenty-First Century (WHO 1997) highlighted the need to increase community capacity and empower the individual as one of five priorities for health promotion.

PPI, empowerment and community engagement pose real challenges for practitioners. Although there have been moves to client-centredness in care, a professional service culture continues to be reluctant to let communities or users lead. The need to meet centrally imposed targets (see Chapter 4) means that the organizational ethos is very task-focused. To increase involvement means consciously reaching out and being proactive in enabling communities to play a real role in planning services and programmes. It means discovering a community's health needs and priorities and then supporting and enabling them to improve their health. This involves uncertainty and giving up some aspects of power.

This chapter explores some of the challenges of PPI and community engagement:

- How users and communities can be involved in decision making about services and generating knowledge and evidence.
- How communities can be supported to deliver health improvement.
- How the professional service culture can be changed to acknowledge the importance of users and communities as partners in health improvement.

The context for PPI

A dictionary definition of 'involvement' is 'to include' or 'to be part of'. The definition of participation is simply 'taking part in' and the definition of 'empowerment' is 'to take control of'. Obviously encompassed within these definitions is the possibility of a variety of activities and outcomes ranging from someone merely being present at a decision-making forum to a form of empowerment whereby people have a real say in decisions and issues that affect their lives.

 Box 6.1 **Activity**

Why is involving people seen as a 'good thing'?

Involving people:
- enables organizations to get a clearer idea of what is important to local communities
- identifies unmet needs
- enables resources to be targeted effectively and to prioritize future spending
- ensures that services will be used and are relevant for the local context
- improves quality through measuring satisfaction
- encourages people to feel a greater ownership and commitment to services and projects that they have been involved in designing and may help to restore confidence in public services
- contributes to greater openness and accountability.

The growth of participation can be traced through several parallel developments:

- *The growth of the power of the consumer* There is increasing attention given to service users in all public sectors. This can be traced back to a desire to reduce the role of the state and roll back paternalistic government. The construction of league tables of performance and charters have introduced the concept of minimum entitlement that indicates what users have a right to expect, and is used by government to make services more accountable.

- *The growth of citizenship* The World Health Organization identified the basic right of any citizen to participate in their health care and a 'duty' or 'obligation' to exercise that right in the Alma Ata Declaration (WHO 1978). As citizens, people have been encouraged to have a legitimate expectation to participate in decisions that affect them. Alongside rights come responsibilities. There is also therefore an expectation that citizens will use services appropriately and contribute to their own health improvement. This is reflected in the NHS Constitution for England (DH 2009, p. 7) which states: 'You have the right to be involved, directly or through representatives, in the planning of healthcare services, the development and consideration of proposals for changes in the way those services are provided, and in decisions to be made affecting the operation of those services'.

- *The lay voice* In recent years, there has been a questioning of professional and policy assumptions about the best way of delivering services. There is an increasing recognition that the lay perspective gives insight into patterns of behaviour and lifestyles and subjective experiences. This understanding can help to 'unpack' global concepts such as health inequalities, and enable the development of appropriate and accessible services. There is a commitment to involving patients in the management of chronic conditions and valuing individual expertise developed through experience in the 'Expert Patient' initiative (DoH 2001a).

- *Legislation* The importance of listening to the public has been reinforced by several inquiries including the Kennedy report on the Bristol Royal Infirmary Inquiry (DH 2001b), which recommended that the perspectives of patients and of the public must be heard, be taken into account and permeate all aspects of health care.

Box 6.2 **Discussion point**

What differences are implied in the different terms used to refer to public involvement – that is, consumers, users, citizens, lay people?

These different terms, although sometimes used interchangeably, denote different levels of power. Consumers and users have limited power to affect services. Their ultimate sanction is to refuse to use services, and take their custom elsewhere. The terms originate in an economic model of relationships within capitalism, and the relevance of such terms to universal state service provision has been questioned. Most people cannot afford the alternative of private sector services, although the UK government has encouraged the notion of competition and 'shopping around' within the state sector for services. The concept of citizenship implies a more active engagement and use of power to determine the kinds of services offered. Citizens hold power, even if at several removes, through the democratic process, and services need to be accountable to citizens. The term 'lay people' suggests an intermediate level of power between consumers and citizens. Lay people hold local lay knowledge, but lack expert professional knowledge. Lay people are therefore vital partners if services are to develop in appropriate and accessible ways.

Internationally, public health planning has tended to be a top-down process based on expert identification of priorities and strategies and donor agencies financing piecemeal health projects. People living in low-income/developing countries often consult an array of practitioners and there are few safeguards and little monitoring of providers. Households may also make substantial contributions to health activities in cash and in kind. Many governments have tried different forms of decentralization such as district management boards and local health committees. Such structures can provide a means whereby local voices, particularly those of poor people and women, can be represented. However, Greenhalgh (2009) uses the example of patient activism in South Africa to point out the naivete of narrow views of participation. Obtaining AIDS treatment at all has been a political struggle of far greater importance than patient involvement and self-management.

Box 6.3 **Example**

Participation in healthcare planning

In a remote rural area of China, the maternal mortality rate and infant mortality rate were much higher than the national average. A loan from the World Bank intended to improve maternal and child services stipulated that the poorest families should be allocated money from the loan to enable them to access ante- and postnatal care, hospital deliveries for emergency or high-risk pregnancies, and treatment for infant pneumonia and diarrhoea. But 99% of women continued to deliver at home attended by an untrained person, some counties did not spend the money, and some used it only for obstetric emergency care. A participatory planning workshop was attended by all the major stakeholders (service providers at province, district, county, township and village levels; health officials and managers; township leaders). The priorities for the loan were identified and concerns shared about its administration – that it should not be used all at once; the inability to encourage the poor to access the fund; that the limited money should be used on emergencies only; that the limited money should be used on infant disease treatment rather than maternity care. As a result of the workshop, the project was able to 'correct' the misuse and underuse of the funding and ensure that the project became sustainable.

Source: Institute of Development Studies briefing papers www.ids.ac.uk

The context for community engagement

The discourse of community is pivotal to the policy agenda of the past decade and a plethora of policies.

Box 6.4 **Discussion point**

How do examples of public policy reflect different concepts of community?

The 'community' is seen as the site where needs are both defined and met. The public health White Paper 'Choosing health: Making healthy choices easier' refers to how 'the environment we live in, our social networks, our sense of security, socio-economic circumstances, families and resources in our local neighbourhood can affect individual health' (DH 2004, Ch. 4). Policy initiatives have attempted to address many of the characteristics of the community: There has been a raft of regeneration initiatives intended to transform the country's most deprived and excluded areas. There is recognition in policy that the sense people have of community is also forged through everyday societal interactions and networks of friends, families and neighbours. Health inequalities are now clearly linked with the concept of social exclusion, the latter being defined as:

'What happens when individuals or areas suffer from a combination of linked problems such as unemployment, low incomes, poor housing, a high crime environment, poor health and family breakdown' (www.socialexclusion.gov.uk). The concept of social inclusion in which everyone, whatever their circumstances, is encouraged to make use of opportunities to participate in society, has permeated policy. The English government Department for Communities and Local Government (www.communitiesgov.uk) is responsible for, among other things, building sustainable communities, neighbourhood renewal, and tackling anti-social behaviour (see, for example the White Paper 'Stronger and prosperous communities' (Department for Communities

and Local Government 2006); and recent public service agreement targets outlined in 'Building more cohesive, empowered and active communities' (HM Treasury 2007)). Working with and for communities through community development has now ceased to be seen as experimental and radical but much more mainstream in policy and service delivery and a vital public health function.

Box 6.5 **Discussion point**

Why has the driver for community engagement become such a central feature of governmental discourse?

In part, community engagement means people have opportunities for participation in all sorts of decisions in their lives, whether it is their choice of treatment or place of schooling, and it is assumed that by being involved, people are more likely to get the services they want and need. A more cynical view might see this as a strategy of governance of the public that seeks to encourage self-dependent responsible citizens who take care of their own welfare. By seeking to engage marginalized groups, individuals are connected with a plurality of networks which it is assumed will help overcome social fragmentation and the alleged breakdown of parenting and families. People will therefore rely on each other rather than the state.

Understanding involvement and participation

Recent guidance on the evidence supporting community engagement (NICE 2008a) proposes a theoretical framework (see Figure 6.1) that outlines why different levels of community engagement could directly and indirectly affect health in both the intermediate and longer terms. The framework proposes that those community engagement approaches used to inform (or consult with) the public may have an impact on the appropriateness, accessibility and uptake of services. Approaches that help communities

Figure 6.1 ● Community engagement for health. Source: NICE (Popay J in press).

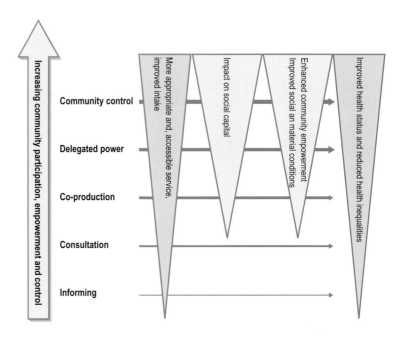

to work as equal partners (co-production), or which delegate power to them may lead to more positive health outcomes which may also include enhancing their identity as a community.

 Box 6.6 **Discussion point**

In what ways can involvement and participation promote health?

The guidance suggests this may arise because these approaches:

• utilize local people's experiential knowledge to design or improve services, leading to more appropriate, effective, cost-effective and sustainable services

• empower people by, for example, giving them the chance to co-produce services: participation can increase confidence, self-esteem and self-efficacy (i.e. a person's belief in their own ability to succeed). It can also give them an increased sense of control over decisions affecting their lives

• build more trust in government bodies by improving accountability and democratic renewal

• contribute to developing and sustaining social capital (social support networks)

• encourage health-enhancing attitudes and behaviour.

(Attree and French 2007 cited in NICE 2008a).

The NICE guidance reflects the struggle to bridge the conflicting paradigms of evidence-based practice and values-based practice (see Chapter 3). NICE recognizes that evidence of the effectiveness of community engagement strategies may simply not be possible as 'research in this area has often been the result of haphazard and unrelated decisions by both funders and researchers' (p. 12) and 'community-based activities are difficult to evaluate because of their complexity, size, the speed of rollout, their (usually) limited duration and the multiple problems they try to address' (p. 12). Yet the NICE guidance asserts that community engagement is desirable practice.

The framework described above suggests that there are levels of participation. Several writers have developed typologies of participation (e.g. Arnstein 1969; Wilcox 1994). These models make a hierarchical distinction between approaches to involvement according to the amount of power sharing involved and the degree of influence over decisions. Arnstein's (1969) model, shown in Figure 6.2, is presented as a ladder where the lower rungs are participation activities designed to give people a voice as a way of making them involved but they remain recipients of services and there is little commitment to them having real influence. The next rungs are about consultation activities that seek to identify with communities and find out what is needed and listen to views before decisions are made. The higher rungs of the ladder identify forms of participatory activity in which the community has greater power and influence and there is a commitment to integrating their views in wider processes. The top rung is user-led activities in which agencies step back from the identification of priorities or the definition of solutions and help communities to do what they want.

Arnstein's model has been criticized as a simplistic rationalization, but it has enjoyed considerable currency as it was the first to put forward the idea of establishing a structured framework of engaging a community and using consultation within the planning/participatory framework of decision making. Models of participation that are presented as hierarchies imply that projects should aspire to the highest level; yet participation needs to be appropriate to its context and take account of the issues involved.

A further major challenge for organizations and practitioners is to create opportunities for people to be involved. In some situations it may be sufficient to inform or consult while in others the principle of partnership and working with communities is important.

 Box 6.7 **Discussion point**

What criticisms might be made of this model of involvement?

In Figure 6.3, the main dimensions of involvement are seen at the level of the individual, involving patients in decisions about care and treatment, and at the collective level, involving patients and the public in decisions concerning the planning and delivery of services. Possible aims and objectives for local PPI may be to:

- get feedback on the quality of services
- learn more about patients' experiences of care
- identify unmet needs
- gain ideas about priorities.

 Box 6.8 **Practitioner talking**

We carried out a consultation exercise with the local community about whether to set up a new health centre that would act as a local resource for advice, exercise and complementary therapies.

We held a public meeting that we advertised in the local press, community centres and libraries and in shops. About 200 people came. We then met with 23 local groups and held 6 focus groups of local people. We carried out a street survey. We also took comments in writing, on a website and in telephone calls and there were about 2000 of these. There was no problem getting a response and enormous efforts were made with the modes of communication and language.

If I were being cynical I would say that despite the number of responses, we had to be seen to be consulting. I think it was just a

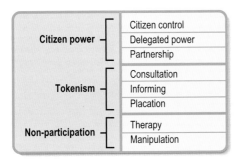

Figure 6.2 ● Ladder of participation. Source: Arnstein 1969.

Box 6.8 **Practitioner talking—cont'd**

means of getting an existing decision across and getting public support made the case more powerful. Lots of people in the focus groups seemed to think the decision had already been made and there would not be a response to their concerns.

Commentary

Involvement in decision making is part of a new thrust to enable patient and public to engage with health services. Frequently such efforts are tokenistic and the scope for responding to views is limited. Harrison and Mort (1998) argue that involvement is frequently used as a way of legitimizing corporate decisions or 'placation' on Arnstein's ladder. There may be a lack of openness about any decisions to be taken and the professional expectations from any consultation. Users and carers may then become cynical about the value placed on any consultation.

As much as the challenges of transferring power, public involvement also poses the challenge of ensuring that decisions are representative of a public view. The current drive for 'involvement' refers to 'patients' and 'public'. These terms have been criticized. Those who use services may not identify themselves as patients or users and view their involvement as time-limited and condition-specific. The term 'user' implies independence, but as Ovreteit (1996) states, 'it gives the impression of someone exploiting the practitioner and does not advance the idea of partnership'.

Box 6.9 **Discussion point**

The national Teenage Pregnancy Strategy contains a commitment to involving stakeholders in the development of local responses. Who would you regard as stakeholders in relation to this issue?

'Stakeholders' is the term frequently used to signify those who have a personal interest in an issue. The question of who to involve in a 'community' is complicated. Early attempts to increase participation focused on a strategy of involving those who were most accessible, who tended to be local leaders. For example, attempts to reach ethnic minority groups frequently employed strategies of contacting faith leaders or using existing groups that met at religious

Figure 6.3 ● Levels of involvement (from DH 2003).

Public Involvement Continuum				
Minimum involvement ←				→ Maximum involvement
Giving information	**Getting information**	**Forums for debate**	**Participation**	**Partnership**
• Exhibitions • Leaflets and written documents • The press	• Citizens' panels • Open surgeries • Patient diaries • Radio or live phone-ins • Self-completed questionnaires • Semi-structured one-to-one interviews including discovery interviews • Structured one-to-one interviews	• Focus groups • Meetings with patients and carer groups • Public meetings • Seminars • Target interested people including the voluntary sector	• Citizens' Juries • Expert Patients • Health panels • Shadowing • Story telling	• Community development • Large group processes

buildings. Identifying 'activists' and those used to participating in groups – those in tenant groups or parents' associations – were also seen as ways of increasing involvement and getting a 'lay voice'. Where there is no clear constituency these representatives tend to be drawn from voluntary sector agencies. Jewkes and Murcott argue that in seeking representatives pragmatic considerations often become paramount: 'These constraints result in the community representatives being drawn from one small part of the voluntary sector, the larger funded organizations' (Jewkes and Murcott 1998, p. 855). Organizations such as Age Concern or Mind have broad memberships but nevertheless may not enable access to try harder to reach groups such as ethnic minority elders or mentally disordered offenders.

The Kennedy Report (DH 2001c) states that the public should be represented by a wide range of individuals and groups and not by particular 'patient groups', valuing the voices of individuals and communities whose views are seldom heard. Asylum seekers, the homeless, drug users and people with a disability are examples of groups that are hard to reach, may not have a strong voice and yet have significant health needs that may not be directly addressed by the services. Some groups have traditionally not had a voice although their right to do so is increasingly enshrined in statute. For example, in many countries it is assumed that children and young people are unable to take decisions despite the UN Convention of the Rights of the Child which states that a child who is capable of forming his or her own views has the right to express these views freely and to have his or her views given due weight in accordance with his or her age and maturity (Article 12 of the UN Convention of the Rights of the Child 1989). The White Paper 'Every child matters' (DfES 2004) aimed to ensure that every child, whatever his or her background or circumstances, has the support he or she needs to:

- be healthy
- stay safe
- enjoy and achieve
- make a positive contribution
- Achieve economic well-being.

Successful involvement of young people in decision making may require specific strategies (DH 2002):

- interesting and fun activities to hold their interest
- incentives and rewards
- ways of demonstrating respect and the value of their views
- structured activities to elicit views
- feedback about what will happen as a result of their contribution.

Types of involvement

Involvement in primary care is a broad concept. It may range from individual patient experience to the social and economic regeneration of communities. Opportunities exist for patient and public participation in:

- individual decisions about treatment
- user views on service provision
- health needs assessments to determine community priorities and views on an issue in order to inform service or programme development
- public consultation exercises about service provision or development
- citizen involvement in public policy panels
- strategic planning groups
- community development and neighbourhood regeneration.

 Box 6.10 **Activity**

Think of an example where you have sought the views of clients/service users. What prompted you to undertake this activity? How did you do this and what methods did you use? What did you do with the information generated?

Patient and user involvement

As we have seen in this chapter, there has been a significant change in emphasis in public service reform from service providers to service users. There has been a corresponding shift from matters of service provision – such as choice among providers and performance against targets – to a more explicit concern with the needs of the people who use public services. Patient and service user involvement at an individual level involves patients in discussions and decisions about their own care and treatment or at a collective level in decisions regarding the planning, delivery and monitoring of services. The involvement may range from a one-off consultation to long-term representation on a steering group.

A fundamental shift in care has taken place that recognizes that people are partners in their own care and treatment. Many people now suffer from long-term conditions and experience physical and psychological difficulties, social and economic problems, and social exclusion due to restricted work and leisure opportunities. Yet it is widely recognized that patients do not feel involved in decisions, do not feel they have anyone to talk to about their anxieties and may feel unclear about tests and treatments, and there may be insufficient information for family and friends (Coulter 2002). Many users and carers have not been active participants in their own care planning.

 Box 6.11 **Discussion point**

What factors are likely to promote patient participation in decision making?

Patient self-management programmes were first advocated in *Saving Lives: Our Healthier Nation* (DH 1999). *The Expert Patient: a new approach to chronic disease management for the 21st century* (DH 2001b) is based on the Chronic Disease Self Management Programme, a 6-week education course developed at Stanford University in the USA that covers relaxation, symptom management, fatigue,

exercise, nutrition, problem solving and communication. It has been widely adopted in Australasia, the USA, Europe and China. Structured self-management programmes are said to be successful in contributing to:

- reduction in the severity of symptoms
- decrease in pain
- improved life control and activity
- improved resourcefulness and life satisfaction
- improved doctor–patient communication.

These initiatives are not about instructing or educating patients about their condition but about developing the confidence and motivation of patients to use their skills and knowledge to take control over living with a chronic illness. This applies to both the management of their own condition and helping others in education programmes. In the UK, such programmes have been developed with the support of voluntary agencies to help in the management of many conditions including arthritis, bipolar disorder and multiple sclerosis.

 Box 6.12 **Discussion point**

How do patient management groups differ from the self-help groups that have mushroomed since the 1970s?

The ideological tension between responsibility and involvement discussed earlier in this chapter and in Chapter 8 on empowerment strategies is evident in these moves to patient involvement. There is an expectation that people want to be involved and yet this can move from empowerment to moral coercion – that with the rights to treatment and care come responsibilities. As Small and Rhodes (2000) put it: 'Problems arise where opportunity turns into obligation and user involvement comes to be seen as a condition of receipt of services and more widely of responsible citizenship'.

The 'Expert Patient' document recognizes that practitioners may have concerns and asserts that the Expert Patient programme is not an 'anti-professional initiative but one based on partnership.

The expertise of professionals is no less essential in treating chronic disease when patients are involved in self-management' (DH 2001b, p. 6). What does change with the Expert Patient programme is that the relationship between the patient and the professional is enhanced through a recognition that the patient holds expert knowledge too, of how his or her condition impacts on his or her life and how it may best be managed. The relationship thus becomes one between equal partners or co-producers who each have a valuable expertise and perspective.

Patients as service users may also be involved in an advisory or management capacity as part of quality

Box 6.13 **Activity**

What challenges would be posed to your practice by greater patient involvement?

standards monitoring or strategic planning. Patient Advisory and Liaison Committees (PALS) act as a point of contact and information for patient concerns, whilst scrutiny of health services is undertaken by local authorities. Ensuring that such processes are productive and not tokenistic conduits for involvement is a major challenge.

Box 6.14 **Practitioner talking**

I was part of a multi-agency group carrying out a review of mental health services. We hired an independent researcher to lead focus groups of users and carers, health professionals and the general public. The members of the public and users were paid and this ensured good attendance. But those who didn't use the services found they had little to contribute and those who did had plenty to say about their experience but very little about how the services could be better organized or delivered. Some of the health professionals didn't listen when the users were talking and dismissed what they said as 'just their opinion'. The carers were worried about saying anything that could be seen as critical. The health professionals did not attend regularly and were not a cohesive group but had different responsibilities and roles. The process was valuable but I think that overall people were disappointed.

Commentary

The level of involvement expected here was not great and the exercise was a consultation with little opportunity to develop plans from the views expressed. Health professionals may see any views expressed as a challenge to their expertise and users may not feel they are taken seriously, or fear their care might be affected. It is important that

users do not feel they are merely commenting on issues, but that they can be consultants. Some users have begun to develop research skills in order to find out about issues in a 'scientific way'. In other situations, Anderson et al (2002) describe how the 'outsider voices' may be strong enough to have input because they are seen as representative of a wider community. The legitimacy of views can be called into question when the organizational culture is predominantly professional.

In order to avoid accusations of tokenism, organizations need to be clear about why they are seeking participation, what they want it to achieve and what level of involvement is appropriate. There needs to be transparency about which decisions are open to change so expectations aren't raised or organizations presented with a long list of actions that they are unable to deliver on. Preparatory work before any consultation is therefore vital to ensure a commitment to the process and so that everybody is clear about what is achievable and why the process is being undertaken. Clear mechanisms for feeding back information and decisions are also needed. As Brooks and Gillam (2002, p. 55) found in their case studies of PPI in primary care, 'the single biggest criticism made of public involvement work by professionals and lay people alike is that it fails to bring about change. It simply doesn't make any difference'.

Box 6.15 **Activity**

What guidelines for user involvement would you propose?

Participation should be a mainstream part of health and social care, not a marginal activity or one left to a few 'experts' such as advocates or 'champions'. It is not easy to manage effectively and many organizations have guidelines on how best to achieve better participation by users:

- asking more than one user to attend
- using language that is free from jargon
- ensuring specialized support is available if necessary (e.g. translators, interpreters)
- meeting all expenses for travel, time, child care, and being aware of the effect of payment on benefits (e.g. payment in vouchers)
- explaining the structure of meetings to the attendees beforehand
- providing training, for example assertiveness skills, chairing meetings, confidentiality
- offering appropriate settings that are comfortable and accessible
- ensuring that there is feedback about the ways in which user views have influenced decisions.

Participation in needs assessment and priority setting

Comprehensive health and social needs assessment is the starting point for the development of any intervention strategy, service development or health improvement programme. National priority areas demand local strategies based on local knowledge of local needs. In Chapter 17 of *Foundations of Health Promotion* (Naidoo and Wills 2009), we discussed the question of what needs are and different ways of assessing needs. A health needs assessment is a systematic review of the health issues of a population leading to agreed priorities that will improve health and reduce inequalities.

Needs assessment uses quantitative and qualitative methods to investigate and understand:

- demographic and social characteristics of the population (its structure, socio-economic environment, lifestyles, history, culture and religion, its social institutions and interaction patterns)
- what medical conditions have the most impact: extent and scale of the issue (incidence and prevalence) and the burden and impact on those affected, their families and society
- current services and their utilization, unmet needs or excessive levels of service provision
- people's perception of what services and interventions should be developed and how they should be delivered
- views of professionals, managers and policy makers about the type and prevalence of problems and the best means to deliver services
- views of policy makers on resource feasibility.

All too often in health needs assessments, health professionals take the lead and define 'health needs and services' from their perspective, which usually means adopting what the epidemiological data suggest as the main priorities and what they are able to provide. Techniques that prioritize the involvement of communities and members of the public in the process include rapid appraisal.

Box 6.16 **Example**

Rapid Appraisal as a method of needs assessment

Rapid Appraisal is a professionally led research approach that aims to provide policy makers with an understanding of communities. Rapid Appraisal gathers information about the health situation of a particular community in a short period of time and without large expense and is based on a community's own priorities (see Ong 1996). Rapid Appraisal typically involves interviewing a range of key local informants, collecting existing records and making observations in the neighbourhood. This information is then collected into an information 'pyramid' that describes the neighbourhood's issues and priorities. The validity of the approach depends on triangulation – data from one source is cross-checked against data from at least two other sources or methods of collection.

Box 6.17 **Discussion point**

What criticisms could be made of these methods of community needs assessment?

Participatory needs assessment (PNA) emphasizes participatory processes which enable community members to set the agenda, analyse their situation and identify their own plans for action. This approach provides a useful starting point for engagement with a community and provides policy makers with quick and accurate assessments of the implications and impact of policies and services. PNA utilizes various methods including problem solving, community walks, force field analysis and ranking exercises that are highly visual. The use of several different methods increases the likelihood of engaging different groups within the community, including people who might be excluded by formal paper exercises. The collected data form the basis for dialogue and can be discussed and modified.

One way in which individuals or groups may be involved in service planning is through deciding the priorities of different services or the allocation of resources. Governments, as a consequence of service modernization, have sought new ways to encourage active citizenship, including using information technology, for example blogs and online discussions. One mechanism used by many Local Authorities is the Citizens' Panel or Citizens' Jury, which typically comprises 100–1000 local residents who are presented with information and asked to help in decision making. An early exercise in community priority setting was the one started in 1982 by Oregon Health Council to decide health service priorities and which services should be part of the local health plan. This eventually developed into an independent civic organization that has focused on access to health care, allocation of resources, and which services should be included as part of Medicaid (Ham 1998; Hogg 1999).

In Canada, day-long dialogue sessions with representative groups of ordinary 'unorganized' citizens have been used to draft the healthcare policy. This process involves complex value judgements about

responsibilities and choices and begins to redefine the role of a citizen from a passive consumer to an active participant in the governance of the healthcare system (Maxwell et al 2003).

In England, the JSNA (see Chapter 5) is the key means of identifying priorities for action to improve health and well-being. In addition to the core data set, community and user engagement is emphasized, giving people a chance to voice their needs.

Box 6.18 **Discussion point**

What factors are likely to influence the decisions made by citizens' groups?

Depending on which professional discourses have entered the public domain, public decision making through consultation often leads to a majority view predominating. Decision making favours services that have impacted on participants' own families. Conversely, marginal or specifically targeted services and the needs of the most excluded get selected out.

Box 6.19 **Example**

Visioning as a strategy for community engagement

The 'imagine' project on participative democracy run by the New Economics Foundation encourages communities to identify what works by getting them to tell stories about the good things in their community. The method is familiar, fun and flexible enough to be used in public areas. It is then used to create a shared vision and future priorities.

Involving the many different sections of a widely spread rural community in a visioning process provided a real challenge for Ryedale District Council's Community Strategy team. The New Economics Foundation facilitated a core group of 12 community and voluntary-sector workers using the Imagine method. They developed and used Imagine questions

Box 6.19 **Example—cont'd**

in conversations and in workshops out and about, gathering stories and images of what people value about the region in order to shape a shared vision for Ryedale's future. These stories became the raw material for the vision upon which the 10-Year Community Plan is now based. Ryedale District Council is taking this visioning process forward through its website: www.imagine-ryedale.org.uk

(Source: New Economics 2003)

Community engagement

The terms community development and community engagement are often used synonymously. Community development involves active engagement with a defined group of people over an extended period of time in order to identify and tackle some of the social, economic, environmental and political issues that determine their health and quality of life. In addition to leading to desirable outcomes, the process itself is important because its aim is to encourage participation and involvement and this is in itself beneficial to health. Chapter 10 in *Foundations for Health Promotion* (Naidoo and Wills 2009) discusses some of the issues associated with working with communities and the range of strategies and methods involved. Increasingly, the focus is on asset-based work that involves the nurturing and release of talents, skills and capabilities. This requires time and trust in order to develop relationships, networks and effective ways of working. Goals may be initially unclear but become clarified and change over time. The process of community development therefore sits uneasily with the pressure on many practitioners to meet predetermined targets and objectives. Much of this work is resourced by short-term funded projects which do not recognize the time required to work successfully in this way. Experienced practitioners report that typically the time needed to establish relationships is underestimated but vital.

Community engagement is the involvement of the public, either as individuals or as a community, in policy and service decisions which affect them. Barriers to health services exist for many people and those barriers are often rooted in the failure of agencies to recognize adequately the complex social, cultural, religious, economic and generational experiences of some distinct communities. According to the NHS Pacesetters programme on community engagement, 'the complete body of knowledge required to identify the needs of all people, raise awareness on a range of health and social care issues, educate and disseminate information does not lie wholly with the community or with the agencies. Hence, creating an environment where communities and agencies can share that knowledge will fill the gaps' (Scott 2008, p. 6).

Box 6.20 **Discussion point**

Why might it be difficult to engage communities?

There may be longstanding feelings of disaffection, suspicion or powerlessness or a lack of structures to enable people to become involved. Freire (1972) argued that liberation requires people to develop a critical awareness of the world in which they live (conscientization) and to define problems as well as being involved in decision making to resolve problems. Communities cannot become active if people are not willing or able to give time or energy, where there are high levels of distrust or where people do not know each other and there are no networks that link people together.

Box 6.21 **Example**

Engaging with the gypsy and traveller community

The gypsy and traveller communities are typically tight-knit and separate from other local residents. This is partly due to their nomadic traditions, but is also the result of their distinctive culture and exclusion from local communities.

Box 6.21 **Example—cont'd**

- Low literacy levels reinforce the need for audio/audiovisual communication materials distributed via outreach activity.
- This is a close-knit community. As such, the use of intermediaries (via outreach) is key to engaging the community and engendering trust.
- There has been a rise in Evangelical Christianity among the Romany Gypsy community in recent years. The religious rallies that they hold are a useful opportunity to meet people from the community.
- Issues concerning children are generally the province of mothers, so messages should be targeted at them in the first instance.

Source: Scott (2008) A dialogue of equals
The Pacesetters programme Community Engagement
Guide p. 28

Evidence of effectiveness

In this chapter, we have explored the current drivers towards PPI and community engagement and some of the health outcomes expected from greater participation by individuals and communities:

- increased access to information
- greater ability to identify and articulate health needs
- increased self-esteem and confidence in individuals
- more responsive services
- better relationships and greater understanding between stakeholders
- stronger community networks, relationships and support.

The evaluation of such processes is still in its infancy. Inspection bodies for public services are developing frameworks to investigate the extent to which services are user-driven and to use local intelligence to evaluate service performance.

Greater participation and involvement is likely to lead to empowered individuals and communities (See Chapter 8). Evaluating each of these outcomes poses difficulties because they refer mainly to qualitative changes in people's perceptions rather than quantitative factors which can be counted. However, it is important that such outcomes are not ignored or devalued simply because they are hard to evaluate.

Box 6.22 **Discussion point**

Why might it be difficult to evaluate community engagement initiatives?

The methodological challenges of evaluating community development initiatives are common to many health promotion interventions (see Naidoo and Wills *Foundations for Health Promotion* 2009, Chapter 19, and Chapter 3 in this volume). Community development typically involves different partners, each with their own agenda, criteria for success and preferred method of evaluation. Deciding what to measure, when, and what threshold to accept as evidence of success are current dilemmas for many community development projects. This may be crudely stated as a preference for outcomes (e.g. How many people became involved? In what ways did their behaviour change?) versus impact (e.g. What did people gain as a result of participating? How do people feel the project has affected their health and that of the community'), although the reality is more complex than this. There are frameworks for evaluating community development approaches to improving health and well-being. For example, the Achieving Better Community Development (ABCD) framework (Barr and Hashagen 2000a) and the Learning Evaluation and Planning Model (LEAP) (Barr 2002) both provide a structure within which community development work to promote health may be measured and evaluated.

Box 6.23 **Discussion point**

Indicator 4 of the Public Service Agreement 21 to build sustainable and empowered communities (Treasury 2007) is the percentage of people who feel they can influence decisions in their locality. How could this be measured?

Increasing involvement: The practitioner perspective

Community development and engagement are key competences for health promotion and public health practitioners. The Faculty of Public Health in England identifies the following learning outcomes for public health specialists in relation to community development (http://www.fph.org.uk/training/curriculum/learning_outcomes_framework/default.asp):

- 5.2 Debate the theory of community development and action.
- 5.7 Influence a community development project or action showing understanding of relationships with the community and the community development staff, including issues of power and politics.
- 5.10 Play an active role in engaging the public in solving their own health problems.

The overriding principle of community development approaches is social justice. This is reflected in part by the reference to power and politics in 5.7 above, but there is no reference to the necessity of practice being imbued by values or an awareness of the political context. The focus of these competences is on doing – through projects – rather than through education for

learning as envisaged in the radical community work of Freire (1972). Chapter 8 on empowerment distinguishes between practice that simply ameliorates and that which is intended to transform.

Many of the barriers to public involvement are linked to the culture of healthcare professionals and their employing agencies. This culture fosters a belief in professional expertise and often reinforces the dependent status of patients and service users. The shift required to move from this position to one where members of the public are valued as equal experts is significant. In many instances, public involvement is regarded as a 'time-consuming indulgence' – desirable and helpful but not necessary. Public and patient involvement is not yet mainstreamed into all areas of service delivery.

 Box 6.24 **Activity**

What arguments could you put forward to colleagues to support greater public or user involvement in your work?

For the individual practitioner working in primary care, for example, there are considerable disincentives to work in this way. It is time-consuming and challenging to professional authority.

 Box 6.25 **Practitioner talking**

Staff attitudes to patient and public involvement

Ironically, staff at the coalface who interact every day with patients and public see the concept of involvement as an additional task. Managers and commissioners of services also have a dilemma in prioritizing the views of local service users when bound by their own professional judgement, targets, planning constraints and finite resources. To make public involvement their business, staff have to see it as part of the organizational culture and they need to have some decision-making power to

improve services for patients. Opportunities need to be taken to involve the public within working and development groups, team meetings and larger conferences and events. Rich patient stories about patient experience, outcomes of care, environment and the organization of care are everyday bread and butter for community staff. They may need to tweak their listening skills, but at the individual level, patient involvement can be easily facilitated. A more difficult area is how staff involve patients in their own care and treatment. It may feel a bit messy and out of control for the

Box 6.25 **Practitioner talking—cont'd**

clinician to give the patient more responsibility, but patient involvement and increased self-management will shift the balance of power. Staff should see this opportunity as another string to their bow, not the straw that ... well you know the rest ...

Commentary

Greater public involvement can be supported on many grounds – professional, ethical and practical. From a health practitioner perspective, greater public involvement will ensure that services provided are accessible and appropriate, and are therefore used more effectively by patients. The new public health and health promotion are characterized by a concern to start with people's self-defined health needs and issues, which means taking a broad social perspective on health. Integral to this is the need to foster public involvement, both as a means of establishing public priorities and as a means of increasing public health and well-being through the participatory process. From an ethical perspective, greater involvement fosters autonomy and helps reduce inequalities associated with socio-economic factors as well as bringing additional benefits to service users. From a practical point of view, greater involvement will mean that resources are used efficiently and not wasted or duplicated, because services will be more closely tailored to needs. Public involvement may pose challenges, but this is part and parcel of the quest to broaden and develop practitioner expertise. As public involvement appears to be a permanent fixture on the public health agenda, developing expertise in this area will enhance professional and career development.

Practitioners may adopt a variety of different roles in relation to user-led services, all of which demand a change in ethos away from simply being providers (House of Commons 2007):

- Advisers or advocates: helping users to assess their needs and forge plans for their future care.
- Navigators or link workers: helping users find their way to the services they want.
- Brokers: helping users to put together a package of services that meets their needs where services might come from different sources.

Conclusion

Public involvement is a diverse phenomenon that refers to different models of 'the public', including patient, consumer, user, citizen and lay person. The implications of these different ideal types in terms of the kind of relationship and activities envisaged in public involvement have been discussed. Three particular strategies for public involvement – patient and user involvement, PNA and priority setting, and community development and engagement – have been explored in more detail. Particular challenges facing practitioners who wish to support greater public involvement have been identified and discussed throughout the chapter. The rationale for public involvement includes enhanced efficiency, effectiveness and quality as well as a moral and political ideal (House of Commons 2007). A key challenge, which has been discussed in more depth, is the need to evaluate public involvement activities in ways which are appropriate and meaningful.

This chapter has discussed 'co-production' in public services – the notion that service users work with service practitioners and professionals to 'co-produce' desired outcomes such as good health or safe communities. In user-directed services, service users are able to control or direct (often by financial means) the services they receive, for example through holding personalized budget accounts for care or learning. User-driven services include all the different ways in which users are consulted or involved in design and delivery. The core underpinning idea is the same, however, that successful public services will enable and engage the public.

Public involvement is a relatively new concept within the health services, and health professionals are unlikely to have received training to support efforts in this field. In addition to being an unfamiliar field for many practitioners, public involvement may also be viewed as a threat to professional expertise and autonomy, and a waste of time and resources. However, this chapter argues that public health and health promotion are inseparable from public involvement and participation. This is because the content of efforts to improve public health must relate to public perceptions and priorities and also because the process of participation is a key factor in health and well-being. Reliance solely on the medical model of health and professional expertise ignores many fundamental socio-economic determinants of health and fosters an unhealthy dependency and passivity amongst patients. An understanding of the benefits of public involvement and skills in supporting public involvement are vital aspects of the role of the public health and health promotion practitioner today.

Further discussion

- Do you think public involvement knowledge and skills should be part of every health practitioner's training? Why?

- What strategies and techniques can be used to increase the involvement of the poorest and most marginalized groups in your community?

- What opportunities are there to encourage participation in your organization? Where

are these on the Arnstein's ladder of participation?

Recommended reading

- Orme J, Powell J, Taylor P, et al, editors: *Public health for the 21st century: new perspectives on policy, participation and practice*, edn 2, Maidenhead, 2007, Open University Press/McGraw-Hill Education.

   A useful text that explores participation and partnership as part of contemporary public health practice.

- Rifkin SB, Lewando-Hundt G, Draper AK: *Participatory approaches in health promotion and planning: a literature review*, London, 2000, Health Development Agency; available at http://www.nice.org.uk/niceMedia/documents/partapproach_hp2.pdf

   A useful review of definitions and theory of community participation with case study examples from practice.

- Wallerstein N: *What is the evidence on effectiveness of empowerment to improve health?* Copenhagen, 2006, WHO Regional Office for Europe (Health Evidence Network report; http://www.euro.who.int/Document/E88086.pdf

- The Healthy Communities web pages can be found at www.idea.gov.uk/health

References

Anderson W, Florin D, Gillam S, et al: *Every voice counts. Primary care organization and public involvement*, London, 2002, King's Fund.

Arnstein S: A ladder of citizen participation, *J Am Inst Plann* 35(4):216–224, 1969.

Attree P, French B: *Testing theories of change associated with community engagement in health improvement and health inequalities reduction*, Report prepared for NICE Guidance PH009, 2007.

Barr A: *Learning evaluation and planning*, London, 2002, Community Development Foundation.

Barr A, Hashagen S: *ABCD handbook: a framework for evaluating community development*, London, 2000a, CDF Publications.

Brooks F, Gillam S: *New beginnings: why patient and public involvement in primary care?*, London, 2001, King's Fund.

Brown P, Zavestoski S (eds): Social movements in health: an introduction, *Sociol Health Illn*, 26(6):679–694, Oxford, 2005, Blackwell.

Coulter A: After Bristol: putting patients at the centre, *Br Med J* 324:648–651, 2002.

Department for Communities and Local Government: *Stronger and prosperous communities – the local government white paper*, London, 2006, Department for Communities and Local Government.

Department for Education and Skills: Every Child Matters: *Change for Children*, London, 2004, HMSO.

Department of Health: Saving Lives: *Our Healthier Nation*, London, 1999, The Stationery Office.

Department of Health: *The NHS Plan: a plan for investment, a plan for reform*, London, 2000, DH.

Department of Health (DH): *The Health and Social Care Act (Section 11 Public involvement and consultation)*, London, 2001a, The Stationery Office.

Department of Health (DH): *The expert patient: a new approach to chronic disease management for the 21st century*, London, 2001b, DH.

Department of Health: *Learning from Bristol: the report of the public inquiry into children's heart surgery at the Bristol Royal Infimary (Kennedy Report) 1984–1984*, London, 2001c, DH. www.bristol-inquiry.org.uk

Department of Health: Listening, hearing and responding: Department of Health action plan: core principles for the involvement of children and young people, 2002, http://www.dh.gov.uk/assetRoot/04/06/62/14/04066214.pdf

Department of Health (DH): *Strengthening accountability: involving patients and the public policy guidance*, London, 2003, DH.

Department of Health: *Choosing health: making healthy choices easier*, London, 2004, Department of Health.

Department of Health: *World class commissioning. Competencies*, London, 2007, Department of Health.

Department of Health: *NHS Constitution for England*, London, 2009, TSO.

Freire P: *Pedagogy of the oppressed*, Harmondsworth, 1972, Penguin.

Greenhalgh T: Patient and public involvement in chronic illness: beyond the expert patient, *BMJ* 338:b49, 2009.

Ham C: Retracing the Oregon trail: the experience of rationing and the Oregon Health Plan, *Br Med J* 316:1965–1969, 1998.

Harrison S, Mort M: Which champions, which people? Public and user involvement in health care as a technology of legitimation, *Soc Policy Adm* 32(1):60–70, 1998.

Hogg C: *Patients, power and politics: from patients to citizens*, London, 1999, Sage.

House of Commons: Public administration select committee: user involvement in public services, 2007, http://www.publications.parliament.uk/pa/cm200708/cmselect/cmpubadm/410/410.pdf

Jewkes R, Murcott A: Community representatives: representing the 'community', *Soc Sci Med* 46(7): 843–858, 1998.

Maxwell J, Rosell S, Forest PG: Giving citizens a voice in health care policy in Canada, *Br Med J* 326:1031–1033, 2003.

Naidoo J, Wills J: *Foundations for health promotion*, edn 3, London, 2009, Baillière Tindall.

National Institute of Health and Clinical Excellence (NICE): *Community engagement to improve health PH009*, London, 2008a, NICE.

National Institute of Health and Clinical Excellence (NICE): Patient and public involvement programme, 2008b, http://www.nice.org.uk/getinvolved/patientandpublicinvolvement/

New Economics Foundation: *Participation works! 21 methods of community participation for the 21st century*, London, 2003, NEF.

Newman J, Clarke J: *Publics, politics and power*, London, 2009, Sage.

Ong BN: *Rapid appraisal and health policy*, London, 1996, Chapman Hall.

Ovreteit J: How patient power and client participation affects relations between professions. In Ovreteit J, Mathias P, Thompson R, editors: *Interprofessional working for health and social care*, Basingstoke, 1996, Macmillan.

Popay J: Community empowerment and health improvement. In: Morgan A, Ziglio E, Davies M, editors: *International health and development: investing in assets of individuals, communities and organisations*, New York, in press, Springer.

Scott S: *A dialogue of equals: the pacesetters programme community engagement guide*, London, 2008, Department of Health, available at http://www.dh.gov.uk/en/Publicationsandstatistics/Publications/PublicationsPolicyAndGuidance/DH_082382.

Small N, Rhodes P: *Too ill to talk. User involvement and palliative care*, London, 2000, Routledge.

Treasury HM: *PBR CSR public service agreements. PSA delivery agreement 21: build more cohesive, empowered and active communities*, London, 2007, HM Government.

Wilcox D: *A guide to effective participation*, Brighton, 1994, Pavilion.

World Health Organization (WHO): *Alma Ata 1978 primary health care*, Copenhagen, 1978, WHO.

World Health Organization (WHO): *Ottawa charter for health promotion: an international conference on health promotion*, Geneva, 1986, WHO.

World Health Organization (WHO): New players for a new era: leading health promotion into the 21st century. 4th International Conference on Health Promotion, Jakarta, Indonesia. Conference Report. Geneva, 1997, WHO.

Chapter Seven

Partnership working

- Defining partnership working
- Types of partnerships
- The impetus for collaboration
- Understanding effective partnership working

OVERVIEW

Partnership working or collaboration is based on the understanding that individual and community well-being is determined as much by social, environmental and economic systems as by healthcare provision. It follows then that the promotion and maintenance of health does not belong to one professional group or sector. Partnership working has been a central feature of health promotion and a cornerstone in the development of healthy public policy. National health strategies also support the concept of partnerships as the key way to deliver health improvement, better integrated services and reduce health inequalities. This chapter looks at the context in which this current emphasis on collaboration has arisen and explores the tensions underpinning current practice. It outlines how an understanding of organizational theory and group-work theory can help to identify key themes in successful partnership working.

Introduction

 Box 7.1 **Activity**

How many partnerships are you aware of in your area? What is their purpose? Who do they involve?

Policy and practice in health and social care is full of references to the need for agencies to 'work together' and 'collaborate' and for multidisciplinary working to blur professional boundaries. The term 'partnership' has become a catch-all phrase for a range of different concepts in relation to joint working. The Department of Health initially used the term 'healthy alliance' to define the way agencies can work together to promote health, emphasizing cooperation and partnership: 'A healthy alliance is in effect a partnership of individuals and organizations formed to enable people to increase their influence over the factors that affect their health and well-being' (DH 1993, p. 22). WHO used the term 'Intersectoral Collaboration' to emphasize that collaboration should take place across public sectors and involve a wide range of agencies. The Alma Ata declaration (WHO 1978) stated that health could only be attained by action in spheres additional to the health sector, in particular: agriculture, animal husbandry, food industry, education, housing, public works and communications. Accepting the impact on people's health of a variety of policies and programmes outside the health service sector requires the development of mechanisms so that policy makers are aware of the consequences of their actions on health. The WHO Health for All strategy stressed the need for intersectoral collaboration for just this reason (WHO 1985). The revisited Health for All strategy, 'Health 21, p. 21 targets for the 21st century', contains a specific target (number 20) on mobilizing partners for health: 'By the year 2005, implementation of policies for health for all should engage individuals, groups and organizations throughout the public and private sectors and civil society, in alliances and partnerships for health' (WHO 1998, p. 200).

By the late 1990s, a new partnership culture had emerged and partnerships were defined by WHO as 'a recognized relationship between part or parts of different sectors of society which has been formed to take action on an issue to achieve health outcomes or intermediate health outcomes in a way which is more effective, efficient or sustainable than might be achieved by the health sector acting alone' (WHO 1998, p. 14–15). The Jakarta Declaration (1997) and Bangkok Charter for Health Promotion (2005) both emphasize the importance of partnerships to development. National strategies also place partnership working as the cornerstone of health improvement strategy, for example the White Papers *Working Together for a Healthier Scotland* (Scottish Office 1998) and *Well Being in Wales* (Welsh Assembly 2002).

Box 7.2 **Activity**

Identify a partnership that develops and/ or delivers policies and strategies related to population health and well-being. Is there any 'added value' due to partnership working? If so, how can this 'added value' be defined?

Partnership working has come to represent a new means of governance – it has been at the heart of public service reform in England since the 1990s and the demand for health and social care to work together and for service providers to work with service users (see Chapter 8). The last decade has seen Local Strategic Partnerships (LSPs) between primary care and local authorities, Children's Trusts, Sure Start, and education, employment, health action and regeneration zones. Boydell and Rugkasa (2007) highlight concerns over whether the growing commitment to public governance through partnership adds value and suggest that there is little evidence that collaboration has improved health status, quoting Davies (2002, p. 175), who comments that 'it is easy to assume partnerships generate added value in a politico-ideological culture that assumes they will'. Partnership working is not necessarily straightforward and this chapter discusses some of its challenges. It requires different organizational structures, budgetary control and working practices. Instead of hierarchies or competition, the dominant mode of organization is networks. Networks are based on trust. Yet to expect this to happen automatically is unrealistic. Indeed, many practitioners' experience of collaborative working is of intense competition and rivalry and a reluctance to share information or 'give up' areas of work. Many professional training and education programmes stress the unique perspective and skills of the profession, which may lead to 'protectionism' when professionals feel threatened by rapid organizational change. In such uncertain situations, instead of recognizing the potential for partnership working, professionals may retreat within their own professional role and identity.

There are also the differing perspectives that organizations have on what exactly constitutes promoting health. There is little identifiable theory of collaboration which can help to illuminate this. There are a few empirical studies in the UK of intersectoral collaboration in the health promotion field which attempt to develop a theory of collaboration (Davies et al 1993; Delaney 1994a; Springett 1995). There are only a small number of studies which focus on collaborative activity for public health. Barnes and others (2005) conducted an evaluation of Health Action Zones (HAZ). These established partnership structures, albeit dominated by NHS Primary Care Trusts (PCTs), failed to move into the mainstream of working across sectors or change to pooled budgets, joint posts, joint performance management or planning. Similar challenges in working across boundaries and aligning planning were highlighted by Hamer and Smithies (2002) in their review of community strategies and health improvement. Other conclusions about the features of successful collaboration draw mainly on the experience of practitioners (see, e.g. Balloch and Taylor 2001). These accounts tend to be enthusiastic about the prospects but pessimistic about the actual outcomes of partnerships.

Working in partnership is a core competence for public health practice. The knowledge required to do so is identified as (www.skillsforhealth.org.uk):

- Knowledge of the range of organizations, teams and individuals that contribute to developing and delivering policies and strategies related to population health and well-being.
- Awareness of the ways in which organizations, teams and individuals work in partnership to improve and protect population health and well-being.
- Knowledge of the principles of effective partnership working and how to apply these in one's own work.

 Box 7.3 **Activity**

Has your professional training included partnership skills? What would these be?

Key to understanding partnership working is an understanding of the process. This chapter draws on organizational studies and groupwork theory to explore why collaboration is a difficult principle to put into practice.

Defining partnership and collaboration

As discussed in the introduction, there is uncertainty and overlap in the definitions of concepts such as partnership, collaboration, alliance, network and coalition. Table 7.1 shows the distinctions made by Leathard (1994) between:

- concept-based terms
- process-based terms
- agency-based terms.

The underlying assumption of partnerships is that agencies work together. In Table 7.1, there are many process-based terms to describe working together, most of which involve sharing, trust, and a willingness to work towards a common purpose.

 Box 7.4 **Discussion point**

What is the difference between networking, coordinating, cooperating, collaborating?

Plampling et al (2000) make a distinction between coordinating partnerships, where the partners agree about the nature of the problem and its solution, and corporate partnerships, in which partners pursue their own goals most effectively by working with others. In a coordinating partnership the underlying assumption is that all the partners agree about the nature of a problem, the nature of its solution, and how it is to be achieved. Every organization has to do its own part of the work in a manner that allows the whole project to be completed. This usually means appointing someone to manage the joint work, chase everyone up, and hold everyone to account. Cooperative partnerships enable partners to pursue

Table 7.1 Alternative terms used variously for inter-professional work denoting learning together and working together

Concept-based	Process-based	Agency-based
Interdisciplinary	Joint planning	Interagency
Multidisciplinary	Joint training	Intersectoral
Multiprofessional	Shared learning	Trans-sectoral
Transprofessional	Teamwork	Cross-agency
Transdisciplinary	Partnership	Consortium
Holistic	Merger	Commission
Generic	Groupwork	Healthy
	Collaboration	alliances
	Integration	Forum
	Cooperation	Alliance
	Liaison	Centre
	Synergy	Federation
	Bonding	Confederation
	Common core	Inter-institutional
	Interlinked	Locality groups
	Interrelated	
	Joint project	
	Collaborative care	
	planning	
	Locality planning	
	Unification	
	Coordination	
	Multilateral	
	Joint learning	
	Joint management	
	Joint budgets	
	Working interface	
	Participation	
	Collaborative	
	working	
	Involvement	
	Joint working	
	Jointness	

Source: Leathard (1994).

their own goals most effectively by cooperating with others using enlightened self-interest. 'Cooperative' partnerships use mechanisms that facilitate the completion of individual goals and targets: 'you scratch my back and I'll scratch yours'.

 Box 7.5 **Discussion point**

'The general pattern of collaboration would seem to be one of the health service eliciting support of other sectors for the implementation of NHS initiated policies' (Farrant 1986).

Do you agree with the above statement? Can you identify any changes in collaborative working since 1986?

Concept-based terms include those most commonly used in the health sector: 'interdisciplinary' or 'multidisciplinary' working. Both these terms refer to a team of individuals from different professional backgrounds (e.g. nursing, education, social work) who contribute a distinctive perspective and skills to the team. Interdisciplinary working usually means within the same professional group, for example community nurses and acute sector nurses, whereas the term multidisciplinary is normally taken to refer to a wider group which includes members from different professions. Multidisciplinary public health is a term used to describe the many different practitioner groups and associated bodies of knowledge that are involved in promoting public health.

Types of partnership

The agency-based terms in Table 7.1 illustrate the different forms partnership can take:

- linking individuals, informal networks of agencies and organizations
- loose networks or informal arrangements about clients or service delivery
- single issue, usually around a specific project or broad-based
- having a fixed timescale, usually with limited funding or an on-going remit

- neighbourhood, community, nationally or internationally based
- concerned with a client group, a health issue, or broader issues such as environmental responsibility
- strategic, facilitative or implementing, such as the arrangements that exist to commission services or coordinate policy across organizations.

Partnerships for public health can cover a variety of arrangements, ranging from parallel working with some informal contact through to integrated working on many different levels. In the UK, the following types of partnerships can be found:

- Service delivery partnerships – these are frontline staff networks aimed at improving on the ground service delivery through coordination of the work of two or more agencies or professional groups (such as groups set up to discuss improved maternity care).
- Learning and best practice partnerships – these are groups of similar agencies working in a town, city or region, who come together to share best practice and to provide peer support and learning (such as Drug Action teams).
- Influencing and strategic partnerships – these are partnerships with organizations with funding, strategic or statutory responsibilities.
- Consortia – groups of organizations approaching public sector agencies to lobby or deliver contracted-out services.

Partnerships are not natural for organizations or professions. They tend to emerge when there is a financial advantage of obtaining extra resources, especially financial resources and staff, or where there is an instruction to do so. Other partnerships exist to commission services that cross service boundaries such as substance misuse. There has been a proliferation of strategic partnerships in the UK in the past decade. Some of these partnerships are a statutory requirement or there is a strong policy expectation from the central government, for example a Joint Strategic Needs Assessment (JSNA) of an area's needs will be carried out by the Primary Care organization and Local Authority; Local Involvement Networks (LINKS) encourage involvement of the public in the design and delivery of services (see Chapter 6). Others focus around the achievement of shared goals and targets, for example reducing teenage pregnancy. Partnerships are therefore a fact of life for many practitioners. Understanding how they work and how to ensure they are productive and facilitate one's own goals is therefore an important area of expertise.

 Box 7.6 **Discussion point**

What makes a partnership strategic?

LSPs coordinate improvements in public services to achieve sustainable economic, social and physical regeneration and to narrow the gap between the quality of life in deprived areas and the rest of the country. LSPs are strategic because they address agreed social priority areas and operate from the higher echelons of the involved organizations.

LSPs may oversee other partnerships, for example:
- Economic and Local Employment
- Children and Young People through a Children's Trust
- Sustainable Neighbourhoods
- Crime and Disorder Partnership or Safer City Partnership
- Health Inequalities
- Transport
- Culture Contact.

Understanding effective partnership working

Much of the literature on partnership working in health and social care is concerned with analyses of practice – what partnerships do and how they can be more effective (e.g. Audit Commission 1998; Hardy et al 2000; HDA 2003). Recent policy reforms have encouraged different professional groups to break down barriers and work together, and there has been some analysis of how the governance of welfare has driven this (Balloch and Taylor 2001; Glendinning et al 2002).

Increasingly, there have been attempts to theorize partnerships and the literature discussing definitions and concepts is plentiful (Carnwell and Carson 2005; Peckham 2003; Plampling and Pratt 1999; Plampling et al 2000; Pratt et al 1998a,b). However, understanding how to facilitate partnership working remains limited (Whitelaw and Wimbush 1998) even where services have been brought together into single organizations as in, for example, PCTs. Partnerships appear to be a rational response to service delivery and professional working. They expand the budget available to tackle an issue, they may help to achieve better coordination and through the pooling of ideas and resources may achieve 'added value'.

Partnerships are seen as important tools for improving public health because:
- Complex problems require complex solutions – no one agency can resolve these issues alone.
- Shared intelligence – of both 'soft' and 'hard' information – improves understanding of the needs and wants of local communities.
- Shared resources – pooling people and funds – is a rational way of dealing with issues that cut across organizational boundaries.
- Partnerships have complex governance which leads to greater challenge and scrutiny.
- Avoidance of gaps and duplication of effort.
- Opportunities for shared learning across organizations.
- Supports the development of good relationships across organizations that can have on-going benefits (e.g. when partnership has finished).

Yet there is an increasing acceptance that partnership working is neither easy nor a panacea for tackling big issues. That organizations will find issues of commonality is unrealistic given that they all recognize that they each have a legitimate 'core business' – what Braito et al (1972) have described as 'domain consensus'. The legitimacy of their 'core business' rests partly on perceived expertise, on funding streams, on governance arrangements and partly on statutory responsibilities. As a Health Education Board for Scotland report comments (HEBS 2000, p. 7), 'many writers stress the inevitability of conflict and

the need to accept it and work with it' and the need to identify the collaborative advantage (Huxham 2003; Huxham and Vangen 2005).

Much of the guidance about partnership working is about improving process; building a shared vision and trust; brokering power, information and resources; and monitoring progress (Audit Commission 1998; HDA 2003). The public health competences for practitioners and specialists (www.skillsforhealth.org.uk) reflect this in their focus on the development of negotiation, influencing and interpersonal skills. An awareness of how different organizational cultures can influence outcomes of collaborative work and of the roles different organizations, agencies, individuals and professionals play is also key to partnership working.

 Box 7.7 **Discussion point**

What features or characteristics would lead you to the conclusion that a partnership was unsuccessful?
- *Leadership and vision*: Lack of agreed vision; competing targets; divergent organizational priorities; differing perspectives such as medical versus social models of health
- *Organization and involvement*: Key agencies missing from the table; lack of clarity about relative roles of partners; unrealistic expectations of partners' capabilities and capacity (e.g. voluntary sector)
- *Development and coordination*: Lack of agreement in relation to needs; no clear agreed plans; no sense of coordinated joint endeavour
- *Learning and development*: Unwilling to share knowledge and skills; organizational or professional defensiveness; unwilling to take risks and innovate
- *Resources*: Unwilling to share human, financial, technical and information resources
- *Evaluation and review*: No clarity or consensus about the criteria defining a 'good' output or outcome; no process review; no agreed success measures

Box 7.8 **Activity**

Interagency partnerships reflect many of the characteristics that contribute to successful personal partnerships. What do you think these are?

Plampling et al (2000) identified a series of steps that are important when establishing a partnership:

1. Find a shared goal.
2. Build trust gradually.
3. Find a common currency/fair exchange.
4. Clarify vision and objectives.
5. Include a wide range of stakeholders.
6. Have good communication, visibility, and transparency of working.
7. Develop human resources.

These seven stages will now be discussed in greater depth.

The attributes of partnerships

Find a shared goal

For participants to believe that the partnership is beneficial, there needs to be a clear, shared vision of what it intends to achieve (Delaney 1994a; DH 1993; Nutbeam 1994; Powell 1992). When partnerships to promote health try to identify their goals, a lack of agreement often comes to the fore with competing rationales. Taking the time to identify shared values and a common starting point through workshops and open discussions is deemed to be the first task of a partnership.

Build trust gradually

It cannot be assumed that a partnership will fall into place because there are structures and processes supporting it. Building trust is an important ingredient in successful partnerships. Trust includes recognizing the purpose and value of partners' work, and knowing

that others value one's own contribution, skills and knowledge. To be effective, partners need to discover how each other's organizations are structured; how decisions are taken and by whom; their financial and planning processes; and the ways in which information is communicated. This vital stage may be overlooked when partnerships see their priority as getting things done.

Box 7.9 **Practitioner talking**

We have an obesity strategy group whose purpose is to identify the goals and actions we need to take. The group has a wide range of members including managers from dietetics, health promotion, leisure services, schools and children's services, pharmacy and planning. The chief planner rarely attends and obviously doesn't want to be there although we think it is clear that the environment has an impact on health and on rising trends in obesity. We have discussed the importance of green spaces for exercise opportunities and how to build in more cycle routes. We are also going to discuss food access and security and we want to get more food in the area to be locally grown which will mean limiting the number of large-scale supermarket outlets.

We asked him to explain his priorities and how he understood the statutory requirements for spatial planning and sustainability. It became obvious that we had similar objectives but used different language and had different imperatives. Once we indicated that we understood his political drivers and working culture and made a conscious effort to ask for his views on every matter, he became a committed and active proponent of planning for health.

Commentary

Although urban planning has a long tradition of improving public health in relation to housing and sanitation, embedding public health priorities in

Box 7.9 Practitioner talking—cont'd

the planning process is a challenge. The different cultures, language and priorities make it difficult for planners and health professionals to work together. There are numerous contemporary drivers for considering health, well-being and inequalities within land-use plans and Local Development Frameworks. Increasingly, Health Impact Assessments are used for planning development. These use a variety of methods and tools to systematically judge the potential effects of a policy or project on the health of a population and the distribution of those effects within the population. The Healthy Urban Development Unit (www.healthyurbandevelopment.nhs.uk) has produced a tool kit to enable engagement between planners and health professionals. Its guidance includes having arrangements for good communication: agreeing a simple protocol for managing communication, making sure of mutual consultation in statutory requirements such as the Local Development Framework, and agreeing arrangements for the monitoring of all policies that impact on health.

The fragmentation and compartmentalizing of practitioners and services which is typical of the role culture of the NHS can make collaboration difficult. Guidance on partnership working (DETR 2001) recommends that individuals clarify what they bring to a partnership as representatives of their community, as a service provider and as a partner. Those working in the NHS may be particularly bound by their roles and hierarchical structures. Participants may lack the status to take decisions or commit money or may be unclear about the roles of other departments within the organization. Representatives who are committed to the partnership and who share the same values as the other members may not be representative of their organization. Glover describes a workplace project in which 'building on an individual's enthusiasm without getting the agreement of the organization they represented created a problem. Consequently, when there were changes of personnel, commitment

to the project was lost and support had to be renegotiated with the individual's successor' (Glover 2001, p. 213). Where partnerships have a strategic role, partners need to have enough influence within their own organization to secure a commitment to the policy.

Box 7.10 Example

Organizational cultures

Recognition of different organizational cultures is an important element in the understanding of the partners in an alliance. Handy (1976) has identified organizations like tribes and families, with their own ways of doing things. He uses the symbolism of four gods to describe the varying types of management that can be discerned in organizations:

- The club culture symbolized by Zeus. This organization is characteristic of small family-type companies. Control is exercised from the centre with little bureaucracy.
- The role culture symbolized by Apollo. This a typical bureaucracy with different departments for different functions such as finance, purchasing, marketing, etc. These are coordinated by a hierarchy of managers.
- The task culture symbolized by Athena. This is a matrix organization with a team culture. Expertise rather than position is important and management is flat and low key.
- The existential culture symbolized by Dionysus. This organization is a cluster of individuals, each of whom is fairly autonomous.

Find a common currency/fair exchange

The concept of exchange is seen as the key to understanding collaboration. Regardless of the overt purpose of an organization (e.g. to provide services or meet client needs), most organizations are also concerned about preserving their interests – to ensure adequate resources, their autonomy, status and authority. Working with other agencies results in some loss of independence and control and necessitates the investment of scarce resources into building partnerships, the outcomes of which are by no means clear. Consequently, organizations only enter into collaborative working if they can see that the needs of their organization are being met and they will benefit in some way.

One of the key factors in effective collaboration is achieving an interagency equilibrium where power is balanced among the participating agencies. A sense of equality among partners is important in generating commitment. This can be problematic when partner organizations vary widely in terms of size, status and funding, and span across the statutory and voluntary sectors. The role of service user partners, who may not have the backing or resources of any agency or organization behind them, is particularly fragile.

The source of power for an organization varies. Local authorities are controlled by elected politicians; voluntary organizations are accountable to management committees and their client group; health authorities have a duty to develop mechanisms for consultation but have no direct local accountability. The different bases of local and health authorities' membership can create different priorities. Local authority officers who have to work from election to election can find longer-term strategic planning difficult. Health services' accountability is governed by the Patient's Charter and various statutory responsibilities and the recently embraced principle of participation and the need for consultation and involvement (see Chapter 7).

work and contribution of partners not being equally valued. The exchange theory of organizational relations suggests that for partnerships to develop, there needs to be some brokerage and matchmaking, recognizing what each brings to the task and negotiating on points of conflict. Financial clout is at the heart of power relations. Organizations may be wary of joint working if they are concerned about their partner's commitment but may equally embrace it if they believe it will increase access to other pots of money.

Clarify vision and objectives

Partnerships often emerge as strategies to bid for specific funding streams. This can lead to conflict. In a resource-starved environment, different imperatives become clear. The pots of money that are available for new initiatives such as Sure Start or Neighbourhood Renewal can lead to competition rather than developmental commissioning. Differential budget growth, a reluctance to share resources, and different budget cycles may all be barriers to successful public sector partnerships. Partnerships where time has been taken to allow a common shared vision and objectives to be defined are much stronger, more stable, and stand a better chance of survival. It may be difficult to take time out at the outset of partnerships to establish a shared vision, but experience suggests this is time well spent.

 Box 7.11 **Discussion point**

What factors might constitute 'power' for an organization in a partnership?

Power might include information, access to important networks or groups the organization is intended to serve, and, crucially, sources of funding. Power also manifests itself in partnerships through the way participating organizations negotiate the remit of the partnership and whether they are 'invited' to join a partnership by a lead agency. This can lead to the

 Box 7.12 **Practitioner talking**

This isn't a very successful partnership as we seem rather peripheral. There isn't a stable and linked structure for the Sure Start programme so we don't link in with people as well as we should. Where we do, it's because I go round chasing and go out to meet people. But I am not sure we know who the key partners are. Certainly I don't think I know much about what is happening. There's supposed to be a system of communication and feeding back but it doesn't filter through

Box 7.12 **Practitioner talking—cont'd**

to the ground and there isn't a good uptake of people at the meetings. We just don't have time and it doesn't get prioritized.

This partnership includes a major agency from the voluntary sector. What they seem to be doing is trying to promote themselves. They want an active role like having their facilities used even when it isn't necessarily the most effective or cheapest option. It's like they are competing for resources and leadership. I know it's important within such a tight geographic boundary to include all the organizations but everybody needs to be considered and acknowledged equally.

Commentary

A shared set of values is deemed the most important prerequisite for a partnership (DETR 2001). In this Sure Start partnership there appear to be different priorities. Large-scale programmes such as this have major funding attached that provides an incentive to organizations to work together. This seems to have supported innovative projects but has not had much impact on the departmental ways of working. Existing power relationships remain and practitioners (and service users) are at the margins of the partnership process. The partnership 'table' takes people away from 'the frontline' and their constituency. Those left delivering the service can become resentful as they get stretched and may feel that they have been neglected for more attractive work. Along with the cultural challenge, there are structural and managerial challenges as well requiring ways of sharing and disseminating information.

Include a wide range of stakeholders

Many issues involve a wide range of stakeholders and it is important to identify gaps and duplication in service provision. Stakeholder mapping is a term used in project management to describe a process where all the individuals or groups that are likely to be affected by the activities of a project or involved in an issue are identified and may then be sorted according to how much they can affect the issue and how much the issue can affect them. This information is used to assess how the interests of those stakeholders should be addressed in any strategic or project plan.

Some partnerships tend to focus on statutory agencies only. Although there may be professional barriers, there are also commonalities – a professional work role, a service sector employer, and bureaucratic work cultures – which make it relatively easy to work together. To embrace voluntary agencies and service users as equal stakeholders represents a much greater challenge. Voluntary sector organizations sometimes find it difficult to be active partners. They are unable to commit funds to joint working and their organizational culture is different from the statutory and private sectors. Although they are not bound by the roles of the statutory sector, they may be perceived as amateurish and as not accountable and unable to deliver. Voluntary groups may not only feel compelled to be part of partnerships because of access to extra funding but also feel that their lobbying role is thereby compromised. What voluntary organizations do bring is the understanding of the perceptions, attitudes and values of service users which will ultimately determine how acceptable and effective service provision is. Understanding this different, but equal, basis for stakeholders is one important aspect of successful partnerships.

Box 7.13 **Activity**

Think of a partnership where you have been a partner. Were there any partners who questioned their participation? What did each of the partners bring to the alliance?

Have good communication, visibility and transparency of working

Good communication, including the transparency of decision making, is a central factor underpinning effective partnerships. Communication includes face-to-face contact such as in meetings as well as written documentation, and increasingly, email networks. Every avenue of communication needs to be scrutinized to ensure that it is inclusive, accessible and understandable to all partners. For example, acronyms and abbreviations that may be obvious to practitioners may be unknown to other agencies or service users. Everyday words (e.g. assessment, scrutiny) may mean something quite specific in policy or programme terms. Good practice includes spelling out every acronym in full the first time it is mentioned, and including a glossary of terms in every report or document.

Develop human resources

Most studies on interagency working have concentrated on the structures of organizations and the context in which it takes place. Nevertheless, most partnerships attribute their success or failure to 'personalities' and individual members. Whilst the role of personalities can be overplayed, most studies suggest that 'networking' is at the heart of collaboration and that nurturing relationships is crucial. Group theory can help us understand how networking takes place, how groups can fail to achieve their task, and how conflict can arise.

Box 7.14 **Discussion point**

What reasons might there be for conflict in joint working?

As we saw in the previous section, organizations have partisan interests and want to hold on to their resources and autonomy. In addition, there are professional constraints on collaboration. Lack of role clarity is often cited as an explanation for conflict when members are not clear about their contribution or that of others. Sentiments such as these are commonplace:

- 'I don't know what I'm doing here or why I've been invited. I've got nothing to do with health'.

- 'The PCT (or any of the other participants) are just doing this to get more money for themselves'.
- 'This is just a talking shop. It's got nothing to do with our priorities'.

Davies et al (1993) identify a key role in alliances for the mediator, who can resolve conflicts through bargaining and exchange. They also identify a role for 'the reticulist' – someone who plays a bridging role, spanning organizational boundaries, and who can harness energies and skills. It is often necessary for a formally appointed coordinator to take on this bridging role.

Box 7.15 **Activity**

Belbin's research into the working of teams (Belbin 1981) has been extremely influential in understanding the particular problems which may arise in groups and how the contribution of individuals can be enhanced. Belbin identified eight roles which together create a balanced, high-performing group:
- leader (the coordinator)
- task leader (the shaper)
- ideas person (the plant)
- analyst (the monitor/evaluator)
- practical organizer (company worker)
- fix it (the resource investigator) mediator (the team worker)
- details person (the finisher).

Can you identify the role you normally play in groups?

Tuckman's model of group development (Tuckman 1965) has been influential in showing how groups have common characteristics in their development. Tuckman describes groups as moving through five identifiable stages:

1. *Forming* – in which a group first meets and works out the roles of members and tries to agree upon a task and some way of working.

2. *Storming* – in which the group becomes polarized and may form subgroups. There may be reactions to power distribution and some resistance to the task.

3. *Norming* – in which the group begins to establish some shared goals and to find a way of working. Members take on roles to support the group in its task or to help the group to work well together.

4. *Performing* – in which the group begins to work well. There is more trust and acceptance of the contribution of each member. Interpersonal issues get resolved. Members approach the task with energy.

5. *Mourning* – the group disbands, sometimes reluctantly, and there may be attempts to continue the life of the group.

In the initial stages of partnerships, there may be competition (the storming phase) as the balance of power within the group is worked out. For a group to move on, however, a safe enough environment has to be created.

 Box 7.16 **Activity**

Think of a partnership where you have been a partner. Can you identify stages in the 'life' of the partnership? What helped to move the group through the stages or did it get stuck?

Participants have to relinquish some control in joint working. For professions in health and social care which have been seeking to define their professional competence and difference such as nurses and health promotion specialists, crossing professional boundaries and finding ways to work together can be challenging. Beattie (1994) cites the following as common barriers to intersectoral working:

1. professional ambition and competition

2. territoriality and protectionism

3. information used as a major source of power and shared only reluctantly

4. different terminology and jargon.

In partnerships, participants often focus on the task for which they have come together. Difficulties arise over the nature of the task and the role of the participating agencies in the partnership. What often gets ignored in partnership working is the 'maintenance' of the partnership – those ways of being which help people to work together. Markwell (1998), for example, identifies the importance of making sure that participants are acquainted. The motivation of someone drafted in or someone who has little influence or knowledge of the echelons of their own agency may be limited. So effort in communicating about the work and keeping participants on board is vital. Having a task focus with equal opportunities for contribution and responsibility through, for example, the setting of the criteria for the alliance and chairing meetings can help to defuse power conflicts. Conventional ways of working, such as committees, steering groups and formal minute taking can hamper the development of ideas and inhibit the contribution of community representatives who may be unused to such ways of working.

Beattie argues that groups also need to develop the ability to give feedback on how the group is working and that there is a strong case for drawing on 'the theory and practice of psychodynamics of relationships within institutions to explore the significance of emotional processes and interpersonal defence mechanisms' (Beattie 1994, p. 119). Members need to spend time talking over differences and reviewing relationships within the partnership. The Health Education Board for Scotland (HEBS 2000) also identified 'transparency', 'mutual trust and confidence' and 'open and honest communication' as key indicators of successful partnerships.

This section has looked at organizational and interpersonal issues drawing on established theories from management and organizational studies and social psychology and psychodynamic work. These ideas help us to make sense of those factors, identified from empirical studies, which are the ingredients for successful collaboration. The insights gained from practice can also help us to 'test' these theories to see if they do offer explanations of what goes on in collaborative and alliance work.

Box 7.17 **Example**

Healthy schools partnership

Read the following information about a Healthy Schools Partnership and then answer the following questions.

The healthy schools partnership has existed for nearly 10 years. It has always been a small group of key people, chiefly from the council and the primary care organization. It has principally focused on the process issues associated with the implementation of the healthy schools programme in the borough. It has no links or reporting to wider strategic partnerships in the area such as Children's Board or LSP.

Its purpose is to
- oversee the implementation of the healthy schools programme in the area
- agree the allocation of resources to support the implementation of the programme.

The partners involved are
- Local authority Children's Services
- Health Promotion staff
- Primary School Head Teachers × 2
- Secondary School Deputy Head Teacher × 1 (a member, but in practice struggles to attend)
- There used to be a wider reference group involving a range of partners, but this has not met for a number of years.

So far, it has overseen a process which has exceeded the government targets for the area. All local schools are participating in the scheme and many have already achieved the standards required. There is good communication and dissemination of information, with a website dedicated to the programme in the borough and regular newsletters sharing good practice. There is a bi-annual health-related behaviour survey funded by the primary care organization. All schools are invited to participate in the survey to provide them with an up-to-date snapshot of the health behaviours of their pupils in order to help them plan in relation to need. Half of the eligible schools take up the offer.

The people directly involved in the partnership are at middle management level. They all feel that the programme does not have the profile it deserves across agencies. There have been tensions between the council and the Primary Care Organization about the use of resources throughout the period that the partnership has operated. The council physically holds the money, and ultimately takes the decisions. Whilst there is a nationally set target for local areas regarding healthy schools programmes, this is not included in the Vital Signs targets of the Primary Care Organization or the 198 National Indicator Set that councils are measured against. Healthy schools is not a target for the Local Area Agreement between primary care and local authority in this area.

- Does the partnership appear to have common agreed goals, shared targets, commitment and effort?
- Does there appear to be good participation of key stakeholders, agreement of relative roles and clarity of expectation? Are the right people and partner agencies involved?
- Is there evidence of needs assessment and appropriate policies, plans, objectives, targets, delivery mechanisms and funding?
- Is there evidence of the partnership enabling the sharing of knowledge and skills across boundaries and groups and supporting innovation?
- Is there evidence of the sharing of human, financial, technical and information resources?
- Is the partnership clear about what success looks like and whether it is achieving it?

Conclusion

The existing literature on partnerships is based on process evaluations, although there is an implicit assumption that partnership working is 'a priori' a good thing. However, theoretical frameworks and reported experiences of participants reveal a number of common themes concerning the difficulties and opportunities for successful collaboration. There are obvious costs and benefits involved. Partnership working is about compromise and entails some change in normal patterns of working. It may require additional and specific skills such as effective group working and management skills. Partnership means relinquishing control and the inclination to put one's own interests first and it entails crossing professional boundaries. Strategic partnerships are very expensive in time and resources with little evidence to date of effective outcomes.

On the other hand, at the level of a specific project or campaign, partnership working may lead to synergistic working with the achievement of more significant and long-term outcomes than would be achieved by agencies working in isolation. It may have a 'trickle down' effect whereby partner agencies become more committed to public health and health promotion and gain new insights into problem definitions and possible solutions. Where partnerships include voluntary organizations and members of the public, there may be additional benefits of empowerment and increased social capital. Partnership working offers the potential of more 'transparent' ways of working, with greater accountability to a variety of interest groups. Most fundamental of all, however, is that it can bring about a cultural change that recognizes health as a multidimensional concept that reaches far beyond the health services.

Further discussion

- Is partnership a consequence of joint working?
- Is the commitment to partnership working by government more rhetoric than reality?
- Do professional education and training courses equip people to work effectively in partnerships?

Recommended reading

- Balloch S, Taylor M: *Partnership working: policy and practice*, Bristol, 2001, Policy Press.

  A collection of case studies of partnerships in health, social care and regeneration. It examines the theoretical and practical reasons why partnerships do or do not work.

- Glasby J, Dickinson H: *Partnership working in health and social care*, Bristol, 2008, Policy Press.

  This book provides a very useful introduction to partnership working, summarizing current policy and research, and setting out useful frameworks and approaches. Others in this practice-based series include guides to effective team working (Jelphs K and Dickinson H) and managing and leading in interagency settings (Peck E and Dickinson H).

- Glendinning C, Powell M, Rummery K: *Partnerships, new labour and the governance of welfare*, Bristol, 2002, Policy Press.

  An edited collection examining the political drivers to partnership working as a means of 'joined up' government.

- Health Development Agency: *The working partnership*, London, 2003, HDA.

  http://www.nice.org.uk/nicemedia/documents/working_partnership_3.pdf

  A manual that examines the evidence from community involvement, business excellence and partnership dynamics for common features of successful partnership working. It includes assessment tools so that partnerships can identify their achievements and areas for improvement and capacity building.

- Health Education Board for Scotland: *Partnerships for health: a review*, HEBS working paper No. 3, Edinburgh, 2001, HEBS.

A paper that provides a useful overview of the published literature and a critical examination of the issues involved in successful partnership working.

- Peckham S: Partnership working for public health. In Orme J, Powell J, Taylor P, Harrison T, Grey M, editors: *Public health for the 21st century: new perspectives on policy, participation and practice*, edn 2, Maidenhead, 2007, Open University/McGraw Hill Education.

   This chapter examines different meanings and frameworks for partnerships, and focuses on the necessity of partnerships for public health.

- Watson J, Speller V, Markwell S, Platt S: The Verona Benchmark – applying evidence to improve the quality of partnership, *Promot Educ* VII(2):16–23, 2000.

   A benchmarking and assessment tool to enable participants to share good practice. The Verona Benchmark focuses on leadership, organization, strategy, learning, resources and programmes.

References

Audit Commission: *A fruitful partnership: effective partnership working*, London, 1998, Audit Commission.

Balloch S, Taylor M, editors: *Partnership working: policy and practice*, Bristol, 2001, Policy Press.

Barnes M, Benzeval M, Judge K, et al: *Health action zones: partnerships for health equality*, Routledge, 2005, Abingdon.

Beattie A: Healthy alliances or dangerous liaisons: the challenge of working together in health promotion. In Leathard A, editor: *Going interprofessional: working together for health and welfare*, London, 1994, Routledge.

Belbin RM: *Management teams: why they succeed or fail*, Oxford, 1981, Butterworth Heinemann.

Boydell LR, Rugkasa J: Benefits of working in partnership: a model, *Crit Public Health* 17(3):213–228, 2007.

Braito R, Paulson C, Klongon G: Domain consensus: a key variable in inter-organisational analysis. In Brinkerhoff M, Kunz P, editors: *Complex organisations and their environment*, *Dubuqu*, 1972; Wm C Brown cited in Hudson B, Hardy B: "What is a 'successful' partnership and how can it be measured?" In Glendinning C, Powell M, Rummery K, editors: Partnerships, new labour and the governance of welfare, Bristol, 2002, Policy Press, pp 51–67.

Carnwell R, Carson A: Understanding partnerships and collaboration. In Carnwell R, Buchanan J, editors: *Effective practice in health and social care: a partnership approach*, Maidenhead, 2005, Open University Press, pp 3–20.

Davies J: Regeneration partnerships under new Labour: a case of creeping centralization. In Glendinning C, Powell M, Rummery K, editors: *Partnerships, new labour and the governance of welfare*, Bristol, 2002, Policy Press.

Davies J, Dooris M, Russell J, Pettersson G: *Healthy alliances: a study of interagency collaboration in health promotion*, London, 1993, London Research Centre report for South West Thames Regional Health Authority.

Delaney F: Muddling through the middle ground: theoretical concerns in intersectoral collaboration and health promotion, *Health Promot Int* 9(3):217–225, 1994.

Department of Health (DH): *Working together for better health*, London, 1993, HMSO.

Department of Transport and the Regions (DETR): *Local strategic partnerships: government guidance*, London, 2001, DETR.

Farrant W: Health for all by the year 2000?, *Radical Community Medicine* Winter 1986/7 19–26, 1986.

Glover M: Alliances for health at work: a case study. In Scriven A, Orme J, editors: *Health promotion: professional perspectives*, ed 2, Maidenhead, 2001, Open University Press.

Hamer L, Smithies J: *Community strategies and health improvement: a review of policy and practice*, London, 2002, Health Development Agency.

Handy C: *Understanding organizations*, London, 1976, Penguin.

Hardy B, Hudson B, Waddington E: *What makes a good partnership: a performance assessment tool*, Leeds, 2000, Nuffield Institute of Health.

Health Development Agency (HDA): *The working partnership*, London, 2003, HDA.

Health Education Board for Scotland (HEBS): *Partnerships for health: a review*, HEBS working paper No. 3, Edinburgh, 2000, HEBS.

Huxham C, Vangen S: *Managing to collaborate: the theory and practice of collaborative advantage*, Oxon, 2005, Routledge.

Huxham C: Theorising collaboration practice, *Public Manage Rev* 9(3):401–425, 2003.

Leathard A, editor: *Going interprofessional: working together for health and welfare*, London, 1994, Routledge.

Markwell S: Exploration of conflict theory as it relates to healthy alliances. In Scriven A, editor: *Alliances in health promotion: theory and practice*, Basingstoke, 1998, Macmillan.

Nutbeam D: Intersectoral action for health: making it work, *Health Promot Int* 9(3):143–144, 1994.

Peckham S: Who are the partners in public health. In Orme J, Powell J, Taylor P, Harrison T, Grey M, editors: *Public health for the 21st century: new perspectives on policy, participation and practice*, Maidenhead, 2003, Open University/McGraw Hill.

Plampling D, Pratt J: *Partnership fit for purpose*, London, 1999, King's Fund.

Plampling D, Gordon P, Pratt J: Practical partnerships for health and local authorities, *Br Med J* 320:1723–1725, 2000.

Powell M: *Healthy alliances: report to the Health Gain Standing Conference*, London, 1992, Office of Public Management.

Pratt J, Plampling D, Gordon P: *Partnership: fit for purpose?*, London, 1998a, King's Fund.

Pratt J, Gordon P, Plampling D: *Working whole systems: putting theory into practice in organisations*, London, 1998b, King's Fund.

Scottish Office: *Working together for a healthier Scotland*, Edinburgh, 1998, Scottish Office.

Springett J: *Intersectoral collaboration: theory and practice*, Liverpool, 1995, Institute for Health, John Moores University.

Tuckman BW: Developmental sequence in small groups, *Psychol Bull* 63:384–399, 1965.

Welsh Assembly: *Well being in Wales*, Cardiff, 2002, Welsh Assembly Government.

Whitelaw S, Wimbush E: *Partnerships for health: a review*, (HEBS Working Paper No. 3), Edinburgh, 1998, Health Education Board for Scotland.

World Health Organization (WHO): *Alma Ata 1978 primary health care*, Copenhagen, 1978, WHO.

World Health Organization (WHO): *Health for all in Europe by the year 2000*, Copenhagen, 1985, WHO.

World Health Organization (WHO): *Health 21. 21 targets for the 21st century*, Copenhagen, 1998, WHO Europe.

Chapter Eight

Empowerment

Key points

- Empowerment as a cornerstone of health promotion
- Giving information
- Enhancing self-efficacy
- Developing skills
- Enabling change
- Empowerment dilemmas in practice:
  - Ethical concerns
  - Effectiveness

OVERVIEW

An integral part of the World Health Organization's definition of health promotion is empowerment – people's ability to increase control over their health. The Ottawa Charter (WHO 1986) uses the term 'enablement', and identifies enablement, mediation and advocacy as key health promotion processes. The concept of 'enablement' in the Charter is 'premised on the idea that in order to realize their freedom and assume greater responsibility for their health, individuals may require help in the form of know-how, resources and power to assume greater control' (Yeo 1993, p. 233). Empowerment therefore includes having access to information, possessing the skills to use such information in practice, and having the opportunity and power to use information to make desired

changes in one's life. Empowerment is closely linked to engagement and participation. When people feel they are able to take control over their lives, they will seek the opportunity to participate in factors affecting their lives, such as planning and developing services or programmes. Such involvement (as described in Chapter 6) can also generate a sense of empowerment and control.

This chapter explores the many ways in which individuals and communities can be empowered through the provision of education and skills training. Developing the health literacy of patients, users and the public, motivational interviewing and social marketing are all strategies that are currently in vogue and share a common objective of achieving behavioural change. These three strategies will be used to illustrate the different stages of empowerment throughout this chapter.

Empowerment is the process of people acquiring more power or control over their lives. Power is 'one of the more important determinants of people's health, whether regarded as the psychological experiences of control or analysed as the social organization of communities, societies and economies which creates and distributes risks and vulnerabilities amongst different population groups' (Labonte and Laverack 2008, p. 6). Empowerment can be defined as an approach which attempts to enhance health or prevent disease through the provision of information, the development of self-efficacy and skills to put knowledge into practice, and the opportunity to take control over one's life. Empowerment strategies seek to build capacity in individuals and communities, thereby enabling them to take control, via decision making and advocacy, over the determinants of their health. This chapter explores some of the challenges for practitioners in embedding empowerment within their work and ensuring that the planning and development of empowerment strategies are equitable, ethical, client-centred, participatory and sustainable. The question of whether empowerment strategies are effective is also debated.

Introduction

The Ottawa Charter (WHO 1986) identified enablement as a core health promotion strategy, and its definition of enablement includes: 'a secure foundation in a supportive environment, access to information, life skills and opportunities for making healthy choices'. This concept is more often referred to as empowerment, or the ability of people to affect their own lives in desired ways. The Health Promotion Glossary (Nutbeam 1998, p. 354) defines empowerment as a process through which people are able to 'express their needs, present their concerns, devise strategies for involvement in decision-making, and achieve political, social and cultural action to meet those needs'.

For people to be empowered, they need to not only feel strongly enough about their situation to want to change it but also feel capable of changing it by having the information, support and skills to do

so. Whilst health communication is an important element of empowering individuals and communities, it may also be criticized as a way of achieving support for compliance with predetermined objectives (Nutbeam 1998, p. 355). Education for empowerment means client-led learning, where people define for themselves their own needs and objectives, and the methods that are best suited to their needs. However, in practice much education in the health field is 'expert-led', with agendas and methods being predetermined by experts or practitioners.

Three separate elements may be identified as contributing towards the empowerment of individuals: information, attitudes and skills. In order to become empowered and to make decisions informed by knowledge, people need to have not just the correct knowledge, but also the attitude that endorses self-belief and efficacy, and the skills to put their knowledge into practice in diverse settings. Different groups will vary in their needs for each of these three components. For example, marginalized groups such as Black, Asian and minority ethnic groups (BAMEs) or people with disabilities may need more inputs around self-efficacy in order to combat their history of disenfranchisement (see Chapter 12). Young people may have the correct knowledge, but require inputs about how this knowledge can be put into practice. Older people may have the skills to effect change, but lack up-to-date knowledge about relevant issues.

 Box 8.1 **Discussion point**

How can individuals be empowered to take control over their health?

Many different strategies contribute towards the empowerment of individuals and communities. Health education, or as Tones (2002) suggests, its recent reincarnation as health literacy, is a central strategy, encompassing the possession of the correct and relevant information to enable informed decisions and actions to take place. Motivational interviewing is a potentially empowering strategy for those who wish to change their behviour by employing supportive attitudes. Social marketing is a strategy which borrows advertising and marketing techniques to encourage behaviour change. Social marketing might appear to be a variant of advertising, but its adherents argue that by packaging desired behaviour and goals as socially acceptable and desirable, it becomes much easier for people to make the changes they want. These three strategies are not exhaustive, but they do provide an illustration of the range of strategies used to empower people and communities, and are discussed in greater depth later on in this chapter.

The concept of empowerment applies not only to individuals but also to communities, societies and nations. Community engagement and involvement in decision making is discussed in Chapter 6. Our companion volume *Health Promotion: Foundations for Practice, edn 3* (Naidoo and Wills 2009) discusses community development as a health promotion strategy. This chapter focuses primarily on empowering individuals.

Empowerment is one tactic amongst many in the health promotion field. In order to make practical decisions about how prominent such an approach should be, and how well resourced, key questions concerning its ethical base and its effectiveness need to be answered. These two key issues are discussed in relation to specific strategies throughout the chapter.

Empowerment is the process of increasing people's capacity to make independent choices and being able to implement those choices in practice. Empowerment therefore depends not just on the person or people making the choices, but also on the environment offering appropriate choices. Traditionally empowerment has tended to focus on people rather than environments. The empowerment process is complex, and may conveniently be divided into four different stages: acquiring the correct and relevant information; having an attitude of self-belief and self-efficacy; having the necessary skills to be able to put choices into practice; and enabling opportunities to effect change. This chapter discusses one key strategy that underpins each stage: effective communication as a means of acquiring information; motivational interviewing as a means of acquiring self-efficacy; social marketing as a means of putting choices into practice; and health literacy as a means of enabling opportunities to effect change.

Giving and providing information

Giving health-related information to clients is a key task for most practitioners. This typically involves conveying a message about reducing risks, compliance or the effective use of services. To do this effectively, the practitioner needs to understand the audience, the best means of reaching them, and how this information will be received. There are many process models of communication, all of which adopt a mechanistic and linear orientation. The American Yale-Hovland model of communication which was designed to develop ways of influencing public attitudes and was later elaborated by McGuire (1978) is shown in Figure 8.1. It suggests that the process of mass communication entails five variables: source, message, channel, receiver and destination. The effectiveness of the communication depends on:

- the extent to which the source has credibility and trustworthiness
- the way the message is constructed and distributed

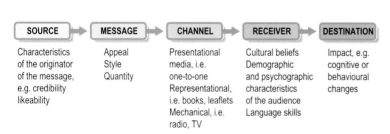

Figure 8.1 ● A model of communication.

- the receiver's receptiveness and readiness to accept the message.

Theories on behaviour change suggest that the adoption of healthy behaviour is a process in which individuals progress through various stages until the new behaviour is routinized. Behaviour models, such as the Health Belief model (Becker 1974) or the Theory of Reasoned Action (Ajzen and Fishbein 1980) or Ajzen's later Theory of Planned Behaviour (Ajzen 1988), which are discussed in *Foundations for health promotion*, edn 3 (Naidoo and Wills 2009), are based on a set of assumptions about the change process. These models show that the simple provision of information without some modification of attitudes and beliefs has little effect on behaviour. However, giving information is often the starting point for changing behaviour.

Information needs to be not just given but also received and correctly decoded. In most cases this means understanding the spoken language and/or being able to read the written language. Functional literacy (being able to read and write) is a key skill for living and learning, and there is a strong relationship between literacy and health (Parker 2000). Limited literacy has been identified as an independent risk factor for poor health, and increased health literacy is associated with improved health (Volandes and Paasche-Orlow 2007; von Wagner et al 2007). A significant percentage of the population, even in developed countries, is illiterate (estimates range from 7% to 47%; UN Development Program 2007).

 Box 8.2 **Discussion point**

What other methods can be used to provide health information in places where literacy levels are low?

Migrants and refugees may be literate in their own language, but lack literacy skills in the country they reside in. Translation and interpretation services are a necessary resource in such cases, in order to transmit and receive information. Such services are often poorly resourced and may be hard to access, particularly in areas that are not perceived as having a significant population of migrants. Using traditional channels of communication such as faith leaders or story telling and mass media such as radio or television, can also reach populations.

In any effective communication there are various stages to work through:

- Identify and understand your target audience – use knowledge about the target audience's demographic, social and psychographic variables to identify their priorities, values, beliefs and lifestyles. This will enable you to 'package' your information in ways that will appeal to them.
- Design the message – this needs to be 'packaged' in such a way that it will appeal to the target audience.
- Make it relevant – the information needs to be perceived as relevant to 'someone like me'.
- Make it credible – credibility may be enhanced by the use of people who are perceived to be experts, for example medical doctors; or conversely, by the use of 'people like me'.
- Make it motivational – there needs to be an appeal to desired values or attributes in order to convince people to act on the information. Commonly used motivating values are youth, energy and attractiveness.
- Make it seem possible – this might mean acknowledging that implementing changes to behaviour is not straightforward, and including information on negotiating barriers to change.
- Arouse emotional involvement – health promotion has a long history of using fear to increase the impact of messages. Whilst fear may be a powerful motivator in the short term (Montazeri 1998), repeated use of fear leads to denial and disassociation from the message. Appeals to positive emotions, for example self-confidence, may be more effective.

Box 8.3 **Example**

Communicating the risks about swine flu

In 2009, the UK government distributed a leaflet to every household providing information about swine flu, including:

- What swine flu is and how it could spread
- What has been done to prepare for a wider outbreak
- What people can do to protect themselves
- What to do if you develop symptoms

It employed a simple message: 'Catch it, bin it, kill it'.

To what extent does this information campaign meet the requirements for an effective behaviour change communication?

Enhancing self-efficacy

Self-efficacy is the belief in one's abilities and skills. In order to make behavioural changes to improve health, a person needs not just the correct information but also a mindset that believes such changes are possible. This belief in one's own abilities to make changes is fundamental to most health promotion programmes, especially in developed democratic countries where individual free will is highly valued. Rather than coercing or forcing people to adopt healthier behaviour, the overriding tactic in such countries is education and persuasion. Health promotion therefore competes with commercial advertising and promotion, all of which seek to persuade people to adopt certain behaviour. Peer-led strategies privilege the knowledge and experience of individuals themselves and use modelling to encourage change. Practitioner-led strategies seek to motivate change through empathic discussion.

 Box 8.4 **Example**

The Expert Patient Programme (EPP)

The EPP is a peer-led initiative for people living with long-term conditions. The aim of the programme is to increase people's confidence and improve their quality of life and their ability to self-manage their condition. The EPP is a 6-week course delivered locally by a network of trainers and volunteer tutors, and is also available online. The course enables people with chronic conditions to develop their communication skills, manage their emotions, engage with the health care system and find appropriate resources, plan for the future, and understand healthy lifestyles. The EPP has developed courses for a number of marginalized groups and communities, including young people and minority ethnic groups. Evaluation of the programme has been very positive, indicating that people who have undertaken the course feel they are less likely to let their symptoms interfere with their lives, report a lessening in the severity of their symptoms, feel better prepared for medical consultations, and make less use of health services.

Source: Department of Health (2007)

Motivational interviewing is a technique designed to assist people to make behavioural changes. It has its roots in clinical psychology and counselling (Miller and Rollnick 2002). Motivational interviewing has been used to help people change various types of behaviour, including alcohol and substance misuse and to achieve compliance with drug regimens. Motivational interviewing claims to be both client-centred and successful in achieving change. It seeks to help people understand the consequences and risks of adopting certain behaviour, and to become motivated to change such behaviour. Motivational interviewing is appropriate for people wherever they are in the behavioural cycle – whether they are in denial that there is a problem, or acknowledge that there is a problem but don't know where to start to change things. 'The strategies of motivational interviewing are more persuasive than coercive, more supportive than argumentative, and the overall goal is to increase the client's intrinsic motivation so that change arises from within rather than being imposed from without' (Rubak et al 2005, p. 305). These characteristics of motivational interviewing, especially its prioritizing of the principle of autonomy, ensure that it is an ethical approach.

There are five general principles underpinning motivational interviewing:

1. Express empathy – share clients' perspectives.

2. Develop discrepancy – help clients see the discrepancy between their actual lives and how they would like their lives to be.

3. Roll with resistance – understand and accept that clients' reluctance to change is natural.

4. Support self-efficacy – prioritize client autonomy (even if this means not accepting the need for change).

5. Avoid direct confrontation and arguments – argumentation creates resistance.

 Box 8.5 Activity

How easy or difficult would it be in practice to use this technique when encouraging a client to change his or her behaviour?

For many practitioners acknowledging a client's resistance to change can be challenging. If an issue is not accepted by the client as important despite its health risks (e.g. smoking in pregnancy) a practitioner may feel compelled, and even see it as their ethical duty, to point this out, often using fear to emphasize the risks. Such an approach is likely to lead to denial or resistance by the client.

 Box 8.6 Example

Effectiveness of motivational interviewing

There is a growing evidence base to support the use of motivational interviewing to achieve desired behavioural changes (Dunn et al 2001; Martins and McNeil 2009; Rubak et al 2005). Motivational interviewing has been shown to be an effective intervention for substance abuse although its effectiveness for other issues such as smoking and HIV risk has not been demonstrated (Dunn et al 2001). A more recent systematic review and meta-analysis of 72 randomized controlled trials that used motivational interviewing in relation to a variety of issues (including obesity, alcohol use and compliance with medication) showed that the use of motivational interviewing had a significant effect in approximately three quarters of the studies (Rubak et al 2005). Factors that increased the efficacy of motivational interviewing included its use by psychologists and physicians (rather than by other healthcare providers) and its use on more than one occasion. A review of 37 articles on the use of motivational interviewing to promote health behaviour in the areas of diet and exercise, diabetes and oral health concluded that this approach is effective (Martins and McNeil 2009).

Develop skills

Having information and a sense of self-efficacy are important but may not be sufficient to actually make changes in a person's life. In order to make changes a person also needs appropriate skills in decision making, such as evaluating information, negotiating change and being assertive. Health literacy is one of the many different activities that contribute to decision-making skills.

Health literacy is a term that encompasses many of the skills necessary to access, assess and use information in making life choices. Health literacy has been defined in many different ways, but a broad definition is provided by Zarcadoolas et al (2005): 'the wide range of skills and competencies that people develop to seek out, comprehend, evaluate, and use health information and concepts to make informed choices, reduce health risks, and increase quality of life'.

Box 8.7 **Discussion point**

In what ways might low literacy levels contribute to health inequalities?

Low literacy levels may mean that people

* struggle to understand health information such as leaflets or consent forms
* fail to fully understand healthcare procedures such as examinations or tests
* find signage confusing
* do not feel confident enough to take part in decision making.

Literacy has been identified as having a key role in health inequalities (CSDH 2008).

Pleasant and Kuruvilla (2008) identify two separate strands to health literacy. The clinical approach identifies health literacy narrowly as the ability to understand, analyse and use information to enable informed and effective use of healthcare services. This aspect of health literacy is to do with communication rather than skills development. In practice, this tends to mean complying with medical advice. Whilst this may mean service users are more knowledgeable about their diagnosis and treatment, whether or not this constitutes empowerment, or merely conformity and consent, is debatable.

Nutbeam (2000) argues that health literacy is a complex phenomenon, encompassing a variety of elements including functional, interactive and critical health literacy. Functional health literacy is being able to read and understand information about health risks and health services, which facilitates the appropriate and effective use of services. This is very similar to the general lay definition of literacy as the ability to read and write. Interactive health literacy includes the ability to develop skills in a supportive environment, leading to increased self-confidence and independent action to improve health. Critical health literacy includes the ability

to assess information on the wider socio-economic determinants of health, and to use this information to improve health and tackle health inequalities.

The public health approach is broader and encompasses the goal of empowerment. This broader view of health literacy is very similar to Freire's (1970) concept of education for critical consciousness, which proposed that education would illuminate the factors (including contradictory social and political factors) determining one's life chances, and also enable one to challenge such factors. Knowledge is defined more broadly within this approach, to include contradictions and awareness of different levels of knowledge and how knowledge is used in practice to both sustain and challenge the status quo.

Empowerment increases as one moves through the levels, from functional through interactive to critical health literacy. Literacy may therefore be seen as the foundation of health literacy, but in its more complex manifestations health literacy includes many other skills and abilities.

Box 8.8 **Example**

Schistosomiasis infection in China

Schistosomiasis is a serious endemic parasite infection in China. In the 1950s the Patriotic Health Campaign launched a programme against four devils – flies, mosquitoes, mice and sparrows – and people were instructed to clean their houses, which were regularly inspected. In the 1980s, health educators disseminated information through villages, complemented by a mass media campaign. None of these approaches has been successful. Evaluation of the campaigns showed that people expect the government to tackle the issue and lack motivation to plan waste disposal or individual and village hygiene systems, despite knowledge of the disease. Tackling the socio-economic determinants of health through education, policy and organizational change is more likely to be successful in addressing this issue.

Source: Wang (2000)

Enable change

Information by itself is often not enough to effect change; in order to have an impact, information will often need to be presented within a package that includes desired aims, goals, and images. Social marketing has arisen as a means of successfully marketing information and ideas in ways that prompt people to make changes. The term social marketing was first used in 1971 by Kotler and Zaltman (1971, p. 5) who described it as: 'the design, implementation and control of programs calculated to influence the acceptability of social ideas and involving considerations of product, planning, pricing, communication, distribution and marketing research'. They argued that just as there is a marketplace for products, there is a marketplace for ideas and the same techniques which are used to sell products can be used to sell an idea or cause or to persuade, influence or motivate people to change their behaviour or use a service. The process is based on the concept of a mutually beneficial exchange. In commercial terms, the consumer gets a product they want at a price they can afford and the producer gets a profit. In the marketing of health, the consumer gets the promise of improved health and quality of life (a benefit) at a possible cost, for example giving up a pleasure such as chocolate or cigarettes, or making some physical or psychological effort such as going to a gym.

According to Hastings and Haywood (1991) commercial marketing is 'essentially about getting the right product, at the right price, in the right place at the right time presented in such a way as to successfully satisfy the needs of the consumer'.

The marketing mix is thus said to be made up of:
- the product and its key characteristics
- the price and how important it is for the audience
- the place (where the message would be promoted)
- the promotion (how the message is to be presented).

Health promoters believe that social marketing can help them to use techniques to package 'health' to various target groups. Values which are seen as desirable to specific target groups, for example youth, attractiveness, control and self-discipline, and belonging would thus be used to motivate people or to 'sell' health. It is claimed that social marketing as a strategy provides a systematic approach to understanding behaviour and the key influences on it (DH 2008).

 Box 8.9 **Discussion point**

Consider the following messages which are used in health promotion campaigns. What is their appeal for their target audience?
- Break free (non smoking)
- Really Me (prevention of drug misuse)
- Vitality (healthy eating, physical activity)
- Slip Slap Slop (sun protection)

Branding plays a major part in selling commercial products. People buy things not just to satisfy a functional need but also to be seen to identify with a group. A very successful example of the development of a tangible product that indicates support of a cause is the Red Ribbon first used by a small charity in New York in 1991 as a symbol to unite the various groups working to get the AIDS epidemic acknowledged. The Red Ribbon was soon recognized by 50% of the population as 'something to do with AIDS' (Freeman 1995). Its success has led to the wearing of a coloured ribbon being adopted by other groups, for example those working for awareness of breast cancer use a pink ribbon.

The dilemma for health promotion if it adopts social marketing techniques is that it is most likely to be effective if it employs the images and values with which people are familiar. Those images are the ones produced by a consumer culture which attempts to sell products by associating them with desirable attributes – sex, power, wealth, success, escape, fantasy, glamour, energy, fitness and youth. Whilst marketers argue they are simply using a 'consumer orientation' to understand what influences behaviour, critics argue

Box 8.10 **Example**

VERB – It's what you do

VERB is a social marketing campaign designed to increase physical activity amongst 'tweens' – young people aged 9-13 years in the USA. Following extensive research conducted with young people and parents from all ethnic groups, the VERB brand was launched. Its key messages are about showing (not telling) young people that physical exercise is for people like them. The campaign used general and ethnic-specific advertising on television, radio, in print, the internet and through schools and communities. The following guidelines are used in the campaign:

- VERB is 'for tweens, by tweens', uses children's language, and focuses on having fun and being with friends
- VERB is positive and uses 'can do' messages rather than 'must do' or 'can't do' messages
- VERB encourages trial and praise, for example 'have a go', 'Dad would be so proud of you'
- VERB is solely about physical activity
- VERB is not focused on schools although it can take place in schools. It is activity-focused and fun.

Communication with parents, primarily mothers, is kept separate in order to maintain the VERB brand's 'coolness' amongst tweens. The campaign used extensive national and local media advertising in order to capture the attention and brand loyalty of tweens. Additional motivational tactics, such as participation in community events, competitions and partnerships with corporations, were also undertaken.

Evaluation of the campaign showed a positive impact. Awareness of the campaign was linked to more positive attitudes towards physical activity and more engagement with physical activity.

http://VERBnow.com Web site for tweens

http://www.VERBparents.com Web site for parents including multi-lingual pages

http://www.cdc.gov/VERB Web site for partners and stakeholders

Sources: Wong et al (2004); Huhman et al (2007)

that adopting marketing principles means endorsing these very stereotypes which many health promoters claim are unhealthy. For example, a message about being physically active may be promoted by images of slim young men and women. Such stereotypes reinforce sexism and ageism and damage many people's self-esteem. The alternative for health promoters is to emphasize *moral* values such as responsibility, safety, conformity and social acceptance. It is precisely this difference between the worlds of commerce and health which makes the marketing of health difficult and, in the view of some, inappropriate.

Marketing is predicated on the basis that individuals have the 'freedom' to choose and to buy what they want and that there will be a reward or benefit from the exchange, what is termed a 'voluntary and mutually beneficial exchange'. The consumers get the goods they want at an acceptable price and the manufacturer gets a profit. Yet the process is not straight-forward in health promotion. The product of better public health and quality of life are distant and unlikely returns. The consumer thus sees the marketing of health not as a mutually beneficial exchange but as overt persuasion. Lupton (1995) argues it is this fundamental difference in the 'product', rather than any disparity in available resources between health promotion and commercial companies, which makes for success in commercial marketing and makes health marketing unsuccessful.

 Box 8.11 **Discussion point**

Can health be sold like a washing powder?

Health is a much more complex concept to promote than washing powder. Health is not a physical thing, but a concept with different meanings and values for different people. Finding a message to promote health is difficult, and may require different messages for different groups of people. Washing powder, by contrast, has one use and a similar value for everyone. The target audience for health messages is often the group least interested in it, so it may be difficult to engage with them. For washing powder, the message will attract those most interested in and likely to use the product. The benefits of adopting a health message are often long term, as opposed to the instant gratification obtained from using a product like washing powder. Health messages often involve people giving up something they value (e.g. a favourite pastime, or a familiar way of coping with stress), whereas products only require giving up some money to purchase them. These differences mean that the decision to adopt a health message is much more complex than the relatively simple decision to purchase a product such as washing powder. This in turn means that marketing health is more complex than marketing a product.

It is through attempts to identify the benefits from an exchange that social marketers are led to construct health in ways borrowed from commercial marketing. Health must be seen as both desirable and a product, a tangible thing which it is possible to acquire. Marketers argue they are meeting consumers' needs by identifying what people want from a product or service. Critics argue that marketing is about the artificial creation and stimulation of wants and needs which can be met by commodities. In terms of health promotion, if certain health behaviour is desirable, then people need to be made aware of it and why it is of value and why it would be good for them. Although people value their health as something to have, there is no actual demand for it. In marketing health, health promoters are often trying to get people to give up what they perceive as desirable such as sweet things or cigarettes. The provision of health information is not meeting an unmet demand as a commercial manufacturer would argue about their product.

Box 8.12 **Discussion point**

How could you 'sell' a message about the desirability of active transport to young people?

Communicating with young people about active transport would involve finding out what triggers would motivate them to adopt active transport, and adopting appropriate means of communicating the message. Whilst good health might be a prompt, it is more likely that appeals to financial savings and the effect on body size, fitness and attractiveness would be more relevant to young people. Embedding active transport within young people's culture, perhaps through the use of pop stars and sports champions to adopt the message, might also be an effective strategy. Using communication media that appeal to young people, such as advertising on-line and electronically, is also likely to increase the impact of the message.

It could be argued that the process of surveying needs as a part of social marketing is a participative strategy ensuring better targeting and meeting unmet needs. This is in contrast to the authoritarian paternalism of most health persuasion and health education which Beattie describes as 'employing the authority of public health expertise to re-direct the behaviour of individuals in top-down prescriptive ways' (Beattie 1991, p. 168). On the other hand, critics of a marketing approach to health promotion argue that it is actually a process of constructing needs according to a market model. Health promotion is constructing the individual as a health consumer who wants and needs health (Grace 1991). People are deemed to be consumers with choices about what they use and what they do. They are thus responsible for their own health, preventing ill health by 'purchasing' relevant health information and services when necessary.

Advocates of social marketing in health promotion argue that the consumer is an active participant. People's views are sought to identify needs and then a message is developed *for* them. The lessons from these sophisticated research techniques do not, how-ever, hide the fact that, as Lupton puts it: 'social marketers seek knowledge of consumers better to influence or motivate them, not to ensure that the objectives of social marketing are considered by con-sumers as appropriate' (1995, p. 112).

Empowerment in practice: Dilemmas for the practitioner

Box 8.13 **Discussion point**

When does health education (giving advice and information) and health promotion (trying to get people to adopt healthier behaviour and lifestyles) become disempowering rather than empowering?

For practitioners, there is often a tension between persuading people (perhaps against their will) to adopt a recommended behaviour, or giving them fuller information and enabling them to exercise their free choice. Some practitioners might argue that the long-term benefits of behavioural changes justify the use of coercive measures to bring about such changes. They might also argue that such tac-tics are necessary in order to counter persuasive advertising and marketing of unhealthy products and lifestyles, and to protect bystanders from suffering. The pressure groups that successfully lobbied for smoking bans in public places and stricter controls on alcohol consumption are examples of groups fol-lowing this line of thinking. Others would argue that respecting people's autonomy is paramount, even if the choices that are made are unhealthy. Motivational interviewing, discussed in the previ-ous section, evolved as a method to address con-cerns about forcing people to make changes against their will and thereby disempowering them (even if the changes in question were to adopt healthier lifestyles).

In *Foundations for health promotion* (Naidoo and Wills 2009) we discussed the ethical dilemmas of creating and respecting people's autonomy and the tension between individual choice and the social good. Practitioners have to manage this tension when working with individual clients about healthy choices and lifestyles. Communicating about the probability of risk, the nature of the risk and knowing how people make choices is an important part of a health prac-titioner's skills. Most media, other than print, make the communication of complex information difficult. To convey the contentiousness of much health infor-mation (e.g. the contribution of alcohol as a protec-tive factor in coronary heart disease) demands time (and therefore considerable expense) and a commit-ment to increasing awareness as much as changes in behaviour.

Box 8.14 **Practitioner talking**

We have used financial incentives to reduce smoking and other addictive behaviours. We make the payment when someone first achieves a behaviour change, and there are additional payments when the behaviour change lasts for 6 and 12 months. I believe this incentive has helped to improve our smoking cessation rate, and has also targeted lower income groups in particular, who are particularly at risk of smoking and related illnesses and diseases. It has provided the trigger to implement a behaviour change for many people who want to make the change but find it difficult to achieve.

Commentary

There are pros and cons to this approach. The practitioner has identified the pros, but opponents might argue that such incentives are coercive, paternalistic and, a form of bribery. However, supporters of this approach would argue that many people would prefer to give up their addictive behaviour, but find the attraction of immediate rewards and the habitual nature of their behaviour very difficult to change. Providing financial incentives enables people to act in line with their true preferences, and may be seen as empowering.

Source: Marteau et al 2009

Box 8.15 **Discussion point**

Is empowerment a valued aspect and/or a key target in your work? What contributes to its status?

Empowerment is hard to measure and targets are usually behavioural. There is a growing evidence base to support the use of empowerment strategies to promote health. Chapter 6 argues that community engagement leads to positive health outcomes through participation in decision making. Wallerstein (2006) examines and synthesizes research into the effectiveness of empowerment strategies and concludes that 'empowering initiatives can lead to health outcomes and that empowerment is a viable public health strategy' (p. 2). Empowerment strategies have two major pathways: focusing on the process itself and its positive health effects, and focusing on disadvantaged and socially excluded populations (e.g. women, young people, people at risk for HIV/AIDS, poor people) to reduce health inequalities. Both of these approaches have proved successful. Research into what makes empowerment strategies effective has identified the following characteristics (Wallerstein 2006, p. 4-5):

- Empowering interventions need to be locally nurtured and grown; a standardized 'one size fits all' approach is not effective.
- People need access to information, skills to use information and control over resources.
- Small groups build supportive environments and promote a sense of community.

Health service practitioners often see empowerment as the giving of correct information and communicating with patients. They can, however, play a pivotal role in linking up with other community resources in order to give their clients opportunities to develop skills and self-esteem.

Box 8.16 **Practitioner talking**

I heard about the mother and infant dance therapy group from a health visitor colleague of mine, and went along to find out more. I was really impressed with the group. It started with an open discussion, where everyone had the opportunity to talk about anything that was troubling them. They then moved onto dancing with their babies, finding new ways to relax and bond with them. The facilitator was superb, accepting and supportive. The mothers in the group all stressed how comforting it was to be able to express their feelings truthfully, and own up to the problems they had bonding with their babies without being made to feel deviant or bad. And along the way they learnt how to bond with their babies, and made new friends with each other. It also helped the mums use medical drugs more appropriately. One mum was able to stop her anti-depressives, whilst another realized she really needed to be taking them. It was only one hour a week, but the mothers all agreed it had been life changing for them and their babies. I now regularly refer mums with postnatal depression or with attachment difficulties to the group, and the results are amazing. It must be one of the most cost-effective initiatives going.

Commentary

Empowerment includes being able to be honest about what are seen as obstacles to fulfilment as well as identifying how to address such obstacles. Honest self-reflection, especially when it concerns what is viewed as deviant behaviour, such as not bonding with your baby or alcohol and drug abuse, is often resisted, but may be easier in a group setting with a skilled facilitator as a catalyst. In a group setting, people will be reassured that they are not the only one with a problem. Once the stigma of owning up to such problems is overcome, the way is open to identify and learn how to manage the problem and its ramifications.

Practitioners tend to view empowerment in relation to individual clients or communities, depending on their work remit. However, empowerment, as Labonte and Laverack (2008) state, is a global phenomenon as well. The move towards sustainability and the greening of the environment is a good example of how whole nations, societies and generations can be empowered to take control of global phenomena such as climate warming. The concept of glocalization – think globally, act locally – has evolved to describe initiatives that seek to develop and protect the local environment whilst simultaneously reducing the need for global trading and hence protecting the global environment as well. Community gardens or allotments are an example of glocalization in practice. Such projects seek to be empowering at many different levels, combining the provision of individual activity, access to affordable fruit and vegetables, networking within the local community and reducing food air miles.

 ### Box 8.17 **Discussion point**

Do you see glocalization as part of your work remit?

Adopting an empowering or glocalizing perspective to one's work may appear to be a luxury, embodying as it does a long-term preventive perspective. It may be hard to prioritize such an approach given the daily urgent demands of a case-load. However, such a strategy is likely to be both cost effective and an efficient use of resources, and it is worth taking some time to explore with colleagues how to embed such an approach in your work.

Conclusion

This chapter has discussed the concept of empowerment and how it relates to health. Empowerment is usually defined as individuals or communities taking control over their behavioural choices and lifestyles. However, this chapter argues that empowerment is a much broader concept, encompassing actions to ensure that environments are sustainable and healthy. For most practitioners, the emphasis is on individual empowerment, and this is the focus adopted in this chapter. Empowerment is broken down into four stages – having the correct information, having a sense of self-efficacy, developing skills and being motivated – each of which has been discussed in further detail and illustrated using appropriate interventions. Particular challenges for practitioners adopting this approach have been identified. These challenges include embedding empowerment within professional practice, ensuring ethical values are upheld and building an evidence base for practice. In conclusion, empowerment is central to people's physical and psychological health, and is a legitimate goal for practitioners' practice. Current evidence shows that empowerment works at many different levels – individual, community, society, global – all of which should be considered and supported when possible.

Further discussion

- What tensions are there between being a professional and seeking to empower patients or clients? What strategies can you devise to resolve these tensions?

- Is the use of social marketing empowering and health promoting? Or is it just a more effective means of paternalistic persuasion?

- How could you ensure that your communication with clients and giving of information is empowering (as opposed to authoritarian)?

Recommended reading

- Duman M: *Producing patient information: how to research, develop and produce effective information sources*, London, 2003, King's Fund.
  A guide to patient information and the importance of identifying needs, developing and piloting materials, methods of dissemination, and how to obtain consumer feedback.

- Labonte R, Laverack G: *From local to global empowerment: health promotion in action*, Basingstoke, 2008, Macmillan.

  This book argues that health promoters need to become involved in empowerment at local and global levels. Detailed discussions of empowerment, the political and policy context, and recent economic strategies are presented to support this view.

- Laverack G: *Health promotion practice: power and empowerment*, London, 2004, Sage.

  This text focuses on the social model of health promotion and explores the concept of community empowerment. The book debates the critical role of power and powerlessness in transforming health promotion into a political activity.

- Wallerstein N: *What is the evidence on effectiveness of empowerment to improve health?* Copenhagen, 2006, WHO Regional Office for Europe.

  A synthesis of the evidence supporting empowerment as a health promoting strategy. The report concludes that empowerment is associated with positive health outcomes and is a valid public health strategy.

Useful Web sites:

Re. motivational interviewing:
http://mi.fhi.net
www.motivationalinterview.org
Re. social marketing
www.nsmcentre.org.uk (social marketing in the UK)
www.hc-sc.gc.ca/ahc-asc/activit/marketsoc (Health promotion in Canada)

References

Ajzen I: *Attitudes, personality and behaviour*, Maidenhead, 1988, Open University.

Ajzen I, Fishbein M: *Understanding attitudes and predicting behaviour*, Englewood Cliffs, NJ, 1980, Prentice.

Beattie A: Knowledge and control: a test case for social policy and social theory. In Gabe J, Beattie A, Gott M, Jones L, Sidell M, editors: (1993) *Health and wellbeing: a reader*, Basingstoke, 1991, Macmillan/Open University Press.

Becker MH: The health belief model and personal health behaviour, *Health Educ Monogr* 2:324–473, 1974.

CSDH: *Closing the gap in a generation: health equity through action on the social determinants of health. Final report of the commission on social determinants of health.* Geneva. World Health Organization.

Department of Health (DH): *The Expert Patients Programme*, London, 2007, Department of Health.

Department of Health (DH): *Ambitions for health: a strategic framework for maximising the potential of social marketing and health-related behaviour*, London, 2008, Department of Health.

Dunn C, Derr L, Rivara FP: The use of brief interventions adapted from motivational interviewing across behavioral domains: a systematic review, *Addiction* 96(12):1725–1742, 2001.

Freeman D: *World AIDS Day evaluation report*, London, 1995, Health Education.

Freire P: *Pedagogy of the oppressed*, London, 1970, Continuum Publishing Company.

Grace VM: The marketing of empowerment and the construction of the health consumer: a critique of health promotion, *Int J Health Serv* 21(2):329–343, 1991.

Hastings G, Haywood A: Social marketing and communication in health promotion, *Health Promot Int* 6(2):135–145, 1991.

Huhman ME, Potter LD, Duke JC, Judkins DR, et al: 2007, Evaluation of a national physical activity intervention for children: VERB campaign 2002–2004, *Am J Prev Med* 2007, 32(1):38–43.

Kotler P, Zaltman G: An approach to planned social change, *J Mark* 35:3–12, 1971.

Labonte R, Laverack G: *From local to global empowerment in Action*, Basingstoke, 2008, MacMillan.

Lipstein B, McGuire WJ: *Evaluating advertising: a bibliography of the communication process*, 1978, New York, Advertising Research Foundation.

Lupton D: *The imperative of health*, London, 1995, Sage.

Marteau T, Ashcroft R, Oliver A: Using financial incentives to achieve healthy behaviour, *Br Med J* 338:983–985, 2009.

Martins RK, McNeil DW: Review of motivational interviewing in promoting health behaviours, *Clin Psychol Rev* Feb 23 2009 (Epub ahead of print) www.pubmed.gov accessed 30/04/09, 2009.

Miller WR, Rollnick S: *Motivational interviewing: preparing people for change*, edn 2, 2002, Guilford Press.

Montazeri A: Fear-inducing and positive image strategies in health education campaigns, *Int J Health Promot Educ* 36(3):68–75, 1998.

Naidoo J, Wills J: *Foundations for health promotion*, edn 3, London, 2009, Baillière Tindall.

Nutbeam D: Health promotion glossary, *Health Promot Int* 13(4):349–364, 1998.

Nutbeam D: Health literacy as a public health goal: a challenge for contemporary health education and communication strategies into the 21st century, *Health Promot Int* 15(3):259–267, 2000.

Parker R: Health literacy: a challenge for American patients and their health care providers, *Health Promot Int* 15(4):277–283, 2000.

Pleasant A, Kuruvilla S: A tale of two health literacies: public health and clinical approaches to health literacy, *Health Promot Int* 23(2):152–159, 2008.

Rubak S, Sandbaek A, Lauritzen T, et al: Motivational interviewing: a systematic review and meta-analysis, *Br J Gen Pract* 55(513):305–312, 2005.

Tones K: Health literacy: new wine in old bottles, *Health Educ Res* 17:287–289, 2002.

United Nations Development Programme: Human Development Report, 2007/2008.

Volandes AE, Paasche-Orlow MK: Health literacy, health inequality and a just healthcare system, *Am J Bioeth* 7(11):5–10, 2007.

Von Wagner C, Knight K, Steptoe A, et al: Functional health literacy and health promoting behaviour in a national sample of British adults, *J Epidemiol Community Health* 61:1, 2007.

Wang R: Critical health literacy: a case study from China in schistosomiasis control, *Health Promot Int* 15(3):269–274, 2000.

Wong F, Huhman M, Asbury L, et al: VERB – a social marketing campaign to increase physical activity among youth, *Prev Chronic Dis* 1(3):A10, 2004. Available from http://www.cdc.gov/pcd/issues/2004/jul/04_0043.htm.

World Health Organization (WHO): *Ottawa charter for health promotion*, WHO, 1986, Geneva.

Yeo M: Toward an ethic of empowerment for health promotion, *Health Promot Int* 8(3):225–235, 1993.

Zarcadoolas C, Pleasant A, Greer D: Understanding health literacy: an expanded model, *Health Promot Int* 20:195–203, 2005.

Part Three

Priorities for public health and health promotion

Part 1 of this book explored the key drivers for public health and health promotion and Part 2 discussed core strategies. In Part 3, we take an overview of the current priorities for public health and health promotion. The focus here is on the UK, but many of these priorities are the same for other developed and developing countries. Health is created through the interplay of many factors, including:

* economic status
* the environment
* genetic disposition
* how people behave
* people's ability to satisfy basic needs
* the quality of people's social relations
* access to prevention, treatment and care services.

This gives rise to a broad, and at times bewildering, array of priorities, encompassing and addressing the underlying socio-economic determinants of health, preventing illness through early detection and intervention, improving access to effective treatment and care, reducing the risk factors for ill health and death (smoking, poor nutrition, inadequate physical activity and accidental injury), and meeting the needs of specific population groups who are seen as vulnerable or over-represented in ill health statistics.

The history of public health demonstrates a particular concern with the physical aspects of the environment that may influence health directly, such as water purity and housing quality. Other factors may influence health indirectly and interact with each other – poverty, for example, is associated with poor housing, diet and education. Figure S3.1 illustrates some of the links between socio-economic circumstances and health outcomes, including the ways in which social attitudes and contexts facilitate or hinder individual health behaviours and the resources that promote health.

Public health and health promotion recognizes that a tension exists between agency and structure – whether people are autonomous free agents who choose the behavioural choices that promote or threaten their health, or a deterministic view that sees social and environmental factors as shaping health outcomes. These elements are often seen as discrete and independent variables to be addressed separately. Dahlgren and Whitehead's (1991) diagram, however, shows the health of the population as affected by interlocking factors: broad, societal or

Figure S3.1 ● Socio-economic circumstances and health outcomes, Source: Acheson (1998).

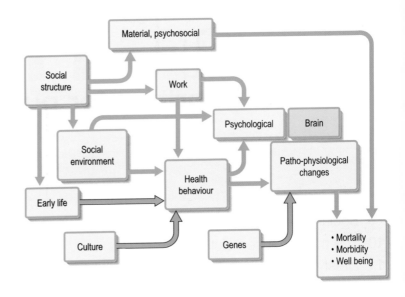

'upstream' forces such as poverty and unemployment, 'midstream' factors that have a direct influence on people's lives and reflect broader social issues such as living and working conditions, and the individual lifestyle or 'downstream' factors that are also affected by the broader conditions in which individuals and families live their lives.

Different theoretical approaches explore the relationship between the social environment and health. Positivist sociologists focus on the impact and constraints of social determinants on individual choices, behaviours and health status. For example, poverty and a polluted environment will disadvantage people, lead to 'poor' health choices, and impact negatively on their health. Postmodernists place greater stress on the cultural meanings and significance of factors affecting health – for example, risk behaviours may be positively valued by some groups, leading to adverse health consequences. Life-course perspectives analyse the ways in which biological risk interacts with economic, social and psychological factors in the development of chronic diseases throughout life. A person's social experience is influenced by genetic endowment, biology and physiology – for example, low birth weight is linked to physical and social disadvantages in later life.

The role of individual lifestyles in determining health status is undisputed, although there are different theories as to what factors affect lifestyles, and how lifestyles impact on health. Whilst the focus is usually on negative effects, the salutogenic approach seeks to explain the factors responsible for creating and maintaining good health. In particular, Antonovsky (1987) focused on how a 'sense of coherence' within individuals can explain the relationship between life stress and health status. The challenge for public health is being able to identify, promote and protect the salutogenic factors that promote health even amongst disadvantaged people.

The medical origins of public health are apparent in the focus on communicable diseases and chronic conditions that impact on quality of life and longevity. This is reflected in policies such as the National Service Frameworks (NSFs) for England and Wales. NSFs set standards for the provision of high quality and evidence-based services relating to major diseases and client groups and also aim to reduce unacceptable variations in care and treatment. NSFs are intended to be inclusive and are developed in partnership with a range of service providers and service users. NSFs currently exist for the following disease conditions: cancer, paediatric intensive care, high blood pressure, coronary heart disease, diabetes, mental health, renal services and long-term conditions. In addition, there are NSFs for older people and children. The control of communicable diseases is another priority in public health, and one that is receiving increased attention as a result of the worldwide increase in HIV and outbreaks such as SARS and swine flu.

Public health refers to the health of the whole population, but within that category, certain groups of people may be prioritized. The rationale for focusing on specific groups is usually that their health potential is not being met. This often emerges from research that demonstrates that a specific population group has a high level of health needs that are often unmet due to problems with service access and availability (e.g. asylum seekers, migrants and travellers). Targeting can, however, stigmatize groups. HIV, for example, is concentrated in social groups that are already marginalized, such as commercial sex workers, injecting drug users and men who have sex with men. It can also lead to oversimplification in categorizing the targeted group. Black, Asian and minority ethnic (BAME) groups, for example, are frequently treated as a homogenous category for interventions.

Interventions to improve health are necessarily complex and inter-linked. A major emphasis is on lifestyles and behaviour change through education and awareness-raising programmes. The focus of many interventions is on defined diseases and is targeted at changing the behaviours of high-risk individuals. In recent years, there has also been a shift towards introducing systemic and structural changes to create environments for better health. Public health and health promotion strategies thus range from the macro structural level via the meso community level to the micro individual level. There are numerous policy initiatives that seek to address the social determinants of health, e.g. housing and transport. The challenge for many public health and health promotion professionals is how to be involved in the political processes and policy making. Adopting the lens of a social model of health through which to tackle priorities is also challenging. At the meso community level, local interventions and projects seek to address priority areas using local knowledge, resources and skills. For many health and welfare workers, individual clients remain the focus. Working with individual clients does not exclude a consideration of how social determinants impact on their health, or how their individual behavioural choices result from community and peer pressures. Whilst it may not be the immediate focus of practitioner-client contacts, recognition of the impact of broad structural factors on individuals can only increase the effectiveness of work with individual clients.

In practice, public health strategies often use a mix of interventions spanning all three levels. For example, food and diet is a public health and health promotion priority area, and poor diet is responsible for a great deal of associated ill health and disease. Food and diet may be construed as an individual lifestyle choice, and many interventions take this approach, focusing on education or weight monitoring to try to effect changes in diet. Many people work with individual clients or patients to raise awareness of health issues and provide information and counselling to change knowledge, attitudes and behaviour. However, research has also pointed out that diet is related to socio-economic determinants of health, and therefore a useful focus may be on communities rather than individuals. Community interventions rely on strategies such as partnership working and building and releasing community capacity and capability. Many of the necessary skills and solutions exist within communities but may require facilitation and networking in order to materialize. For example, interventions such as food cooperatives, food gardens and growing projects and breakfast clubs in schools all rely on the skills and resources that exist within communities. Community interventions seek to model healthier food options and make them accessible and appropriate for local populations. Finally, many of the factors affecting diet are structural, such as the loss of local shops due to supermarkets' aggressive marketing and pricing policies, inadequate food labelling, and poor dietary choices in workplaces and schools. These factors require lobbying and advocacy at local or national levels to tackle relevant structures. An example of successful lobbying and media advocacy is Jamie Oliver's campaign for healthy school meals (http://www.channel4.com/life/micro-sites/J/jamies_school_dinners/, accessed July 2009). Features of successful and effective interventions at each level are identified, and evidence showing that tackling this kind of priority area is effective is collated and presented.

Part 3 therefore explores four public health and health promotion priorities: the social determinants of health, the major causes of ill health and mortality, lifestyles and behaviours, and population groups. Each chapter first explores the rationale for prioritizing this category and then goes on to identify how it has been addressed. Examples are given of work at different levels – macro (structures), meso (communities) and micro (individuals). We hope that Part 3 of this book will prove inspirational in identifying the huge range

of skills, interventions and activities that can impact positively on public health and health promotion. Many of these activities are not primarily concerned with health although they may be pivotal in promoting good health. For example, tackling poverty is a key government policy area because it is seen as crucial to creating a more egalitarian, inclusive and democratic society. However, it is also true that reducing poverty is one of the most effective, if not the most effective, means of promoting the health of the poorer sections of society, and hence of society at large. We therefore hope that everyone, whether or not they work in the health services, will be able to identify in Part 3 relevant issues, skills and interventions which they can use and adapt within their own workplace to improve the health of the people they work with.

References

Acheson D: *Independent inquiry into inequalities in health*, London, 1998, The Stationery Office.

Antonovsky A: The salutogenic perspective: towards a new view of health and illness, *Adv J Mind-Body Health* 4(1):47–55, 1987.

Dahlgren G, Whitehead M: *Policies and strategies to promote social equity in health*, Stockholm, 1991, Institute for Future Studies.

Chapter Nine

Social determinants of health

Key points

Key points

- The influence of social determinants on health
- Approaches to addressing the social determinants of health
  - Legislation and regulation
  - Strengthening disadvantaged communities
  - Supporting individuals
- Tackling social determinants
  - Income and poverty
  - Employment and unemployment
  - Crime and violence
  - Housing
  - Sustainability, regeneration and renewal
  - Transport

OVERVIEW

Health determinants are those factors that influence health. Several models of health have attempted to show the interconnectedness of social, economic, environmental, behavioural and biological factors. Dahlgren and Whitehead's (1991) model, for example (see Figure 9.1 below), defines the determinants of health as individual lifestyle factors, social and community influences, living and working conditions, and general socio-economic and environmental conditions.

This chapter discusses the social determinants of health – those structural factors that impact on health

and are beyond any individual's ability to change. The WHO (http://www.who.int/social_determinants/en/ accessed July 2009) defines social determinants of health as:

the conditions in which people are born, grow, live, work and age, including the health system. These circumstances are shaped by the distribution of money, power and resources at global, national and local levels, which are themselves influenced by policy choices. The social determinants of health are mostly responsible for health inequities – the unfair and avoidable differences in health status seen within and between countries.

Figure 9.1 ● The main determinants of health (from Dahlgren and Whitehead 1991).

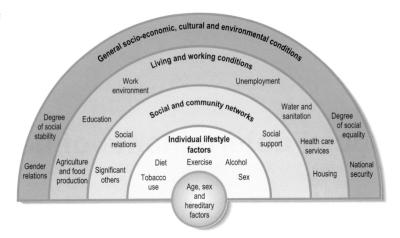

 Box 9.1 **Discussion point**

What factors would you identify as social determinants of health?

Various factors have been identified as social determinants of health by different documents. A UK working group identified social class, stress, early life, social exclusion, work, unemployment, social support, addiction, food and transport as key social determinants (Marmot and Wilkinson 2006). Canadian workers identified aboriginal status, early life, education, employment and working conditions, food security, gender, healthcare services, housing, income, social safety net, social exclusion, unemployment, and employment security as key social determinants of health (Raphael 2008).

These determinants are amenable to change, especially at the collective, community or social policy level. At the macro level the social, economic and physical environment can be changed in significant ways, affording more health-promoting choices and opportunities to people. At the meso level, communities can be supported to address collectively the impact of social determinants on their health. At an individual level, practitioners can work with clients to enable them to overcome the constraints and limitations on their lives and health imposed by social determinants. This chapter first discusses the

concept of health determinants and the evidence showing their impact on health. It then goes on to consider action and interventions at different levels to implement change in health determinants. Evidence demonstrating the effect of interventions tackling socio-economic conditions, environmental conditions, and social and community life on health status and examples of effective interventions are given to illustrate the range of health-promoting activities.

Introduction

Risk conditions are social structures such as poverty or poor quality housing that are associated with poor health. Figure 9.2 shows how the effect of risk conditions (e.g. social marginalization) is directly linked to risk factors (e.g. lack of social support) and is also mediated by risky behaviours (e.g. drug use). Risk conditions and risky behaviours give rise to physiological and psychosocial risk factors that are in turn recognized precursors to many causes of ill health and premature and preventable death. Figure 9.2 also shows how certain groups of people are more likely to experience both risk conditions and risky behaviour, leading to poorer health status. For example, unemployed people are more likely than the general population to be living in poverty and to be socially marginalized. This in turn leads unemployed people to be more likely to participate in risky behaviours such

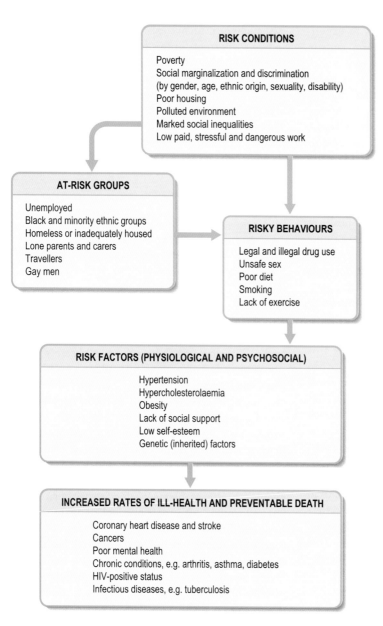

Figure 9.2 ● The relationship between risk and health (adapted from City of Toronto 1991).

as smoking and the use of legal and illegal drugs, and thus to be at increased risk of developing a variety of diseases causing ill health and premature death. Risk conditions, risky behaviours and risk factors tend to cluster together and disproportionately affect certain groups of people.

 Box 9.2 **Discussion point**

Is it possible to target one determinant of health in isolation?

Any one individual or community tends to experience the impact of different health determinants in an integrated way, as 'quality of life' or 'well-being'. Whilst it is possible to isolate the effect of heavy traffic on lifestyles (being unwilling to let children play outside, unwillingness to walk or cycle in busy streets), the sum total of all the effects of traffic become subsumed under concepts such as stress or isolation, which are also affected by many other factors (e.g. housing, income). It is therefore difficult to demonstrate that any one health determinant is the primary cause of ill health. The plus side of this interconnectedness of different determinants of health is that interventions in any one field tend to have ripple effects in other fields. Social and community interventions demonstrate that it is possible to increase health and well-being through building and supporting factors that improve health, such as community safety, social capital and local income.

Addressing the social determinants to enable them to become health promoting is a daunting task that requires many discrete skills. First there is a need to establish the health links, proving that determinants can affect health both positively and negatively. This has already been accomplished by a variety of research studies endorsed by official reports (e.g. Acheson 1998; Wilkinson and Marmot 2003). Most recently, the WHO set up the Commission on the Social Determinants of Health in 2005 to synthesize evidence on how to tackle the social determinants of health in order to achieve health equity, and to prompt different bodies and organizations to strive towards this goal. The Commission published its final report in 2008 (WHO 2008). This report made three recommendations to tackle the social determinants of health:

- Improve daily living conditions – the circumstances in which people are born, grow, live, work and age.
- Tackle the inequitable distribution of power, money and resources – the structural drivers of living conditions – globally, nationally and locally.
- Measure and understand the problem and assess the impact of action – train the workforce to tackle these determinants and raise public awareness about them.

Although the evidence exists, it still needs reinforcing in many different forums because traditionally public sectors have worked in isolation. Establishing that, for example, regeneration and renewal are part and parcel of health development work leads to the next logical step of joint planning, funding and working. This stage still presents many challenges and dilemmas for practitioners, which have been discussed in detail in Chapter 7.

Box 9.3 Activity

Is addressing the social determinants of health recognized as part of your work practice? Do you feel you have the skills and resources to do so effectively?

For those public health practitioners who recognize the social determinants of health, other barriers remain. Acknowledging the scale of the problem can lead to a feeling of helplessness. Healthcare professionals may feel ill-equipped to address such problems, and relevant activities, for example, supporting communal interventions such as food cooperatives, are often seen as falling beyond their remit. Such a situation can lead to low morale and frustration. For many practitioners there is a strong professional ethos of one-to-one intervention that values and respects the individuality of each client. Factors common to people's health problems, such as social isolation or unemployment, tend to be overlooked or are seen as posing additional burdens on health instead of being seen as the fundamental cause of much ill health and premature death. Practitioners may also underestimate the challenges faced by clients in relation to poverty or discrimination due in part to their own distance from such issues. This distance can lead to practitioners imposing advice or information that has little relevance to the lives of their clients.

Structural determinants of health have been recognized by the UK government and included in various health policy and strategy documents. The Acheson Inquiry (Acheson 1998) was a key document that fostered recognition of the need to address health inequalities and their underlying social determinants.

Only 3 out of the 39 recommendations made by the Acheson Inquiry were specifically directed at the health service. This was followed by 'Tackling health inequalities: A programme for action' (DH 2003) and a review of progress (DH 2008). The 2008 review identified five key areas: early years and parenting, work experience, equality of opportunity, mental health services, and coordination of action locally and nationally.

Whilst there is much support for tackling inequalities and health determinants together, certain strategies need to be implemented in order to achieve results (Exworthy et al 2003):

- mainstreaming funding and interventions so that tackling inequalities becomes part of the health or other service's core business
- closer monitoring of the impact of interventions designed to tackle health determinants
- evaluation and research designed to assess the impact and outcomes of strategies.

Legislation and regulation are two of the most effective means to change infrastructure. They demonstrate a common view of what constitutes health risks and what actions should be taken to minimize harm. Legislation often sets minimum standards that have to be met, for example for air quality, wages, safety in the workplace, and housing. This approach requires agreed upon standards based on some form of evidence plus a monitoring and enforcement body to ensure compliance. There also needs to be an adequate infrastructure of trained and resourced inspectors to enforce the standards. Different professions each have a distinctive role to play. For example, environmental health officers (EHOs) are responsible for monitoring and enforcing standards for many health determinants including air pollution, food safety, housing and workplaces, whilst the police force is responsible for public protection and crime detection, and public health specialists are responsible for managing and controlling outbreaks of infectious diseases. Trading standards officers have also been identified as contributing to public health through their role in monitoring faulty goods and workmanship and enforcing the laws regarding the sale of tobacco, alcohol and solvents.

Box 9.4 **Activity**

Is there an enforcement or regulatory aspect to your role? Do you regard it as health-promoting?

There may be tensions in the practitioner-client relationship if the practitioner has an enforcement or regulatory role. Having a regulatory role gives added authority to the practitioner, but this may have a downside. Some practitioners may feel clients will be less open and trusting if they feel they are being checked upon. Conversely, practitioners may feel clients will be more receptive and willing to take advice on board if they know there is an element of enforcement of standards involved.

One of the benefits of legislation is that it is an 'upstream' intervention that directly addresses the social determinants of health. For example, if poor quality housing is upgraded using minimum standards, then eventually no one will be living in substandard housing. This is of course an over-simplification. In practice, standards are constantly being revised, and there is always a shortfall between standards and what happens in real life. Some practitioners feel in addition that tackling determinants of health is a diversion from their primary role and expertise, which is working with individual clients. Many practitioners shy away from activities at a policy level regarding this as political action. As noted in Chapter 4, practitioners are engaged in political activity when they are implementing policy. They also have a clear role in influencing the policy agenda (e.g. the input of learning disabilities nurses into government policy in the White Paper *Valuing People* (DH 2001)) and in monitoring the effects of policy.

Strengthening disadvantaged communities through targeted interventions, regeneration and renewal is another popular approach to addressing the social determinants of health. This aims to strengthen the community fabric, building and releasing social capital and thus enhancing skills and self-esteem. *Foundations for Health Promotion*, edn 3 (Naidoo and Wills 2009) outlines the role and challenges of community development in promoting health including the non-statutory nature of the activity and the ambiguities surrounding professional education and training in a field which aims to break down professional/lay barriers and promote participation and equality.

The third distinct approach is targeted at individuals and aims to provide opportunities for people to tackle or overcome constraining influences on their health. For example, providing opportunities for adult education and training will help people find and retain paid employment, thus enhancing employment and income, two key health determinants. Developing and recognizing skills that people may already have (e.g. child caring) through accreditation may reduce dependency and enhance self-esteem and self-efficacy. Providing services for individuals also has the benefit of providing direct inputs to those most at need. The direct face-to-face interaction implied by such an approach readily conforms to the model of individual client-practitioner relationship underpinning most professional education in the healthcare services. A major limitation of this approach is that it follows a 'downstream' rather than an 'upstream' approach. Supporting people to overcome the constraints of their circumstances will help those individuals, but if nothing is done at source to tackle the causes of their disadvantage, other individuals will take their place, living in poor housing, on low incomes, without secure employment. This cycle will only be disrupted by removing the causes of disadvantage at their source.

In practice, all three approaches are used by practitioners, and the strongest effects are found when the three different approaches build on and complement each other. Most practitioners will feel more at ease with one approach, and this provides another reason for partnership working (see Chapter 7) where different practitioners work together, developing their own area of expertise but working alongside others. So, for example, in any one locality, EHOs may be working to enforce quality standards in housing and minimum exposure to pollutants in the air; youth and community workers may be facilitating and supporting community projects such as walking and exercise programmes or peer education arts projects

to reduce problematic drug use; and health visitors may be providing postnatal support programmes for new mothers to reduce social isolation.

This chapter considers the following socio-economic and environmental health determinants:
- income and poverty
- employment and unemployment
- crime and violence
- housing
- sustainability, regeneration and neighbourhood renewal
- transport.

For each health determinant, the research showing its impact on health is first reviewed, followed by examples of different kinds of strategies and interventions designed to tackle the determinant. In particular, interventions that can be undertaken by health and welfare practitioners are highlighted. Evidence about the effectiveness of different strategies is reviewed and discussed.

Income and poverty

Poverty is acknowledged worldwide as a determinant of ill health. Poor people are unable to afford the basics for good health – for example adequate nutrition, access to clean water, and sanitation. Whilst poverty affects certain regions disproportionately (e.g. sub-Saharan Africa) it also impacts differentially on different demographic groups such as women and children who are typically more vulnerable to poverty and its impact than men.
- 1 billion (out of 2.2 billion) children worldwide live in poverty.
- 25,000 children die each day due to poverty (Leon and Walt 2001).
- 27–28% of all children in developing countries are underweight or stunted.
- In 2003 10.6 million children died before the age of 5 and 1.4 million children die each year due to a lack of safe drinking water and sanitation (http://www.globalissues.org/article/26/poverty-facts-and-stats accessed 1/7/09).

Extreme poverty means that children cannot access a nutritious diet, clean water, adequate sanitation, preventive health services such as vaccination and immunization, or education.

Tackling the problem of global poverty and its impact on health requires sustained and coordinated action by a variety of stakeholders including affected countries, the developed world, financial and banking institutions and the voluntary sector. The Millennium Declaration, endorsed by world leaders in 2000, is an example of coordinated action. The Millenium Declaration set 2015 as the target date for achieving most of its goals (United Nations 2007). At the midway point, progress has been made, although not sufficient to meet the goals.

- The proportion of people living in extreme poverty fell from nearly a third to less than one-fifth between 1990 and 2004.
- Child mortality has declined globally.
- Key interventions to control malaria have been expanded.
- The tuberculosis epidemic appears to be on the verge of decline.

However, many key challenges remain:

- Over half a million women (nearly all in developing countries) still die each year from treatable preventable complications of pregnancy and childbirth.
- There are still many underweight children in Southern Asia and sub-Saharan Africa (almost 30 million).
- AIDS remains a problem, and in 2005, 15 million children had lost one or both parents to AIDS.
- Half the population of the developing world lack basic sanitation.

The current global financial crisis presents a further challenge and will impact negatively on health, with an estimated increase in child mortality of between 200,000 and 400,000, largely driven by malnutrition (http://www.un.org accessed 1/7/09).

Whilst developed countries do not experience the scale of poverty-related health problems seen in developing countries, poverty and income remain key determinants of health status.

In developed countries income is the mediating factor that determines access to a host of variables related to health. The relationship between poverty and ill health is complex and can be seen in:

- reduced access to material resources such as income and good quality housing, neighbourhood and work environments
- constrained behavioural choices such as increased rates of smoking as a coping mechanism or reduced access to healthy food due to price and local availability
- psychosocial factors such as reduced social networks and feelings of low self-worth and self-esteem.

There is now an accepted evidence base that clearly demonstrates that poverty leads to poor health outcomes and excess mortality (Acheson 1998; Benzeval et al 2000; OECD and WHO 2003). There is on-going debate about whether it is low income per se or income inequality that is the key factor determining poorer health and increased ill health (Shibuya et al 2002; Sturm and Gresenz 2002; Wilkinson and Marmot 2003). However, Wilkinson and Pickett (2009) provide robust evidence for asserting that inequality is the key determinant of a range of poor quality of life indicators, including poor physical and mental health.

 Box 9.5 **Activity**

How would you define poverty? Is poverty different to inequality? How?

Income, and hence poverty, is both absolute and relative. Absolute poverty refers to an income that is insufficient to pay for the basics of a healthy life – adequate nutrition, heating and housing (although defining basic minimum needs is not easy and is affected by cultural norms). Relative poverty is 'when (individuals) lack the resources to obtain the types of diet, participate in the activities and have the living conditions and amenities which are customary, or at least widely encouraged or approved, in the societies to which they belong' (Townsend 1979, p. 31). The key issue is whether a poverty line should be set in relation to a basic survival budget, or at a level of income that would enable people to participate in society and meet social and cultural needs. The definition of poverty used by the UK government (DWP 2002) is a household income below 60% of the median income level in that year. Other methods of establishing poverty levels may be the proportion of income needed to cover a basic food basket (used in the USA) or whether people can afford what are perceived to be necessities for life. 'Necessities for life' is a relative concept although there is considerable consensus about basic requirements. For example, a survey conducted by the Joseph Rowntree Foundation (Gordon et al 2001) found beds and bedding for everyone and adequate heating were commonly accepted as necessities for life.

Poverty is both a structural issue, affecting large sections of the population in a patterned and predictable way, and an individual issue, affecting and constraining every aspect of an individual's life. Practitioners need to be aware of the constraints poverty places on people's lives, and take this on board in their interactions with clients living in poverty.

Box 9.6 **Activity**

In what ways do you tackle poverty in your work?

Tackling poverty requires a multi-layered response that addresses the causes and effects of poverty. The government is committed to eliminating childhood poverty by 2020 and there is widespread support for policies to reduce poverty in the UK. Tackling the causes of poverty involves social policies focusing on:

- Providing social protection policies that cover the whole population.
- Interventions to reduce poverty and social exclusion at both the community and the individual level.
- Legislation to reduce vulnerable and minority groups experiencing discrimination and social exclusion.

- Removing barriers to social and health care and affordable housing.
- Reducing social stratification.

Source: Wilkinson and Marmot (2003)

The biggest and most significant anti-poverty policy is the social security system. Each year over £100 billion in social security benefits is distributed to over half the population (Alcock 2002). Universal benefits are paid in the UK on the basis of age or family circumstances, for example pensions and child allowances, but a significant element also constitutes welfare benefits, such as income support or unemployment benefit, which aim to relieve poverty. In addition to social security benefits, policies such as the introduction of a minimum wage, changes to the tax system, for example working tax credit and child tax credit, and changes to the national insurance system, are designed to ensure that being in employment leads to a higher income than being on benefits, and to help working people escape the trap of low income. Practitioners can help to ensure that clients are receiving their full benefit entitlement. Some practitioners may view such work as beyond their remit and area of expertise, but such schemes are practical and effective (see Chapter 5).

Box 9.7 **Example**

Social policy interventions to tackle poverty

Poverty (defined as incomes below 60% of the median) persists within the UK, and is especially prevalent amongst certain groups, for example single parent families and pensioners. In 1999 the government declared its commitment to end child poverty within a generation. Between 1998/1999 and 2003/2004 the number of children living in poverty dropped from 4.1 to 3.5 million (DWP 2005 cited in Asthana and Halliday 2006). In 2002/2003 one-fifth of pensioners were living in poverty and a further 15% were just above this level (Evandrou and

Box 9.7 **Example—cont'd**

Falkingham 2005 cited in Asthana and Halliday 2006) (Table 9.1).

For the working population, greater employment, or 'work for those who can', has made the most significant contribution to reducing poverty, but there is a limit to how much further these measures can contribute. Changes to the tax and benefits system have particularly benefited those with children and low earners but has disadvantaged others, such as those receiving incapacity benefit. Changes in indirect taxation (such as increases in tobacco tax and TV licence) negatively affect those on low income, for whom such taxes represent a significant proportion of total income.

Sources: Sutherland et al (2003), Asthana and Halliday (2006)

At a local level, initiatives such as credit unions or local exchange trading schemes (LETS), which allow local trade by using credits instead of money, are an important means of facilitating and supporting local economies (http://www.letslinkuk.net/). LETS are also intended to maximize employment opportunities by building up skills. Schemes that maximize or increase income, or provide services and stimulate trade via credits, provide the most direct example of tackling the links between poverty and health.

Other strategies to tackle poverty may aim to strengthen individuals. For example, brief behavioural counselling to increase the consumption of fruit and vegetables amongst low income adults was found to be more effective than nutrition education counselling, leading to a 42% increase in the proportion of participants eating five or more portions a day (Steptoe et al 2003). Other interventions may focus on 'living on a budget', such as community kitchens. These schemes can be effective in getting people together to think about common problems and encourage social support networks. The challenge for practitioners is to avoid exacerbating problems by blaming people, explicitly or implicitly, for any unhealthy behaviour.

There is ample evidence of the link between low income and poor health, but historically there has been a separation between health and social care professionals, with income support work being undertaken by social care professionals. However, there are examples of interventions tackling poverty and low income where health practitioners play a key role. With training, support and resources, addressing low income and its effects on health can become a realistic and effective task for health practitioners. At a basic level, awareness and acknowledgement of the effects of low income on clients can enable practitioners' core work, for example health promotion advice and education, to become more sensitive, appropriate and effective.

Table 9.1 The decline in poverty in the UK from 1996/1997 to 2003/2004

		1996/1997	2003/2004
% in relative poverty (income below 60% of contemporary median (%)	All	18	17
	Children	25	21
% in absolute poverty – income below 60% of 1996/1997 median in real terms (%)	All	18	10
	Children	25	11

Source: DWP (2005).

Employment and unemployment

There is a strong link between employment and health. For some people, the work environment can present hazards and health risks. Health and safety legislation covers employers' statutory responsibilities to protect the health of their employees, but occupational ill health remains a significant problem. Social inequalities are reflected in the workplace, with workers from low socio-economic positions, Black, Asian and minority ethnic (BAME) groups and migrant workers disproportionately employed in the most hazardous and unhealthy jobs.

Box 9.8 **The links between work and health**

In the UK conservative estimates of the contribution of work-related conditions to health each year are:

- 2000 premature deaths are caused by occupational disease
- 8000 deaths are caused in part by work conditions
- 80,000 new cases of work-related disease are registered
- 500,000 people continue to suffer from work-related ill health
- ill health accounts for 18 million lost working days
- occupational accidents and ill health are estimated to cost £7 billion.

Worldwide each year:

- 250 million occupational injuries are reported
- 160 million cases of occupational disease are reported.

Source: Watterson (2003)

Box 9.9 **Activity**

Think of your own employment and workplace. What factors there contribute to your health and well-being, and what factors contribute to stress and ill health? What is the workplace response to any case of ill health?

Common mental health problems and musculo-skeletal disorders are the main causes of ill health amongst the working age population. Stress at work plays an important role in contributing to the large differences in health, absence due to sickness, and premature death related to social status (Black 2008). Ill health amongst the working age population is estimated to cost Britain over £100 billion each year – more than the annual budget for the NHS (Black 2008). One way to reduce this burden is to shift practice from the cautionary 'risk avoidance sick note' culture to a more proactive approach focusing on what people can do rather than what they cannot do. A growing evidence base suggests that early interventions directed at people with short-term absence due to sickness is effective in reducing long-term absence due to sickness and the financial costs involved. This approach – the fit for work approach – is recommended in Carol Black's (2008) review of workplace health.

For the majority of people, the association between paid employment and health is overwhelmingly positive. Paid employment provides people with an income, feelings of self-esteem, purpose and self-efficacy, and a social network. Employment provides goods or services that contribute to the national economy. Unemployment is a greater health risk than employment, and is strongly related to ill health and mortality. A good case can be made for targeting unemployed people and supporting them to move into paid employment as a health-promoting strategy.

Getting people into paid employment is a key national policy that is supported by many local initiatives. The approach is many pronged, and includes providing skills and training to enhance employability, helping people apply for jobs, supporting flexible hours through the provision of childcare, and providing transport to enable people to get to work. A pilot project – Pathways to Work – has been shown to be effective in increasing the employment of people on incapacity benefits, with the exception of those whose health condition is a mental illness (Black 2008). Specialist mental health services therefore need to be integrated into all 'back to work' services. Occupational health services need to be reinvigorated and integrated into mainstream healthcare provision.

 Box 9.10 **Example**

Helping people to find employment

The Grimethorpe Jobshop is an example of a local intervention designed to assist people finding paid employment. The Jobshop is based in a community centre and offers help with CVs and applications as well as providing interview skills and further education for clients. Several other projects provide transport for workers and Northolt YWCA offers childcare and work placements to enable mothers to take paid employment.

Source: Social Exclusion Unit (2001)

Another strategy is to provide start-up loans to enable self-employment and the growth of small businesses. This approach was inspired by the example of the Grameen Bank in Bangladesh which has helped millions to set up their own businesses and has a default rate of less than 3%. Community projects offer the benefits of direct accessibility and the provision of services tailored to local needs.

National policy addresses both health and safety in the workplace and unemployment issues. The Health and Safety at Work Act 1974 set out the employer's duty to protect the health, safety and welfare of employees and the wider public with regard to work processes. Dangerous substances used in the workplace are required to be satisfactorily controlled so that they pose no danger to the workforce and members of the public. Employees have a duty to take reasonable care with regard to health and safety issues, and to comply with any safety requirements. This Act also established the Health and Safety Executive and Health and Safety Commission, which are responsible for monitoring the workplace and ensuring that legal minimum requirements are met.

Individually, health workers can try to be more rigorous in considering the impact of employment and unemployment on health when seeing patients who are of working age. Routinely documenting people's employment on their health records can be a first step. Monitoring and audit of records could then attempt to identify any patterns in illnesses related to workplaces. Practitioners can also be proactive about finding out what local back-to-work and fit-for-work initiatives exist, and making appropriate referrals.

Crime and violence

Crime is generally viewed as a social rather than a health issue. However, the known association of crime with inequalities, deprivation, social exclusion and marginalization suggests a health aspect. Violent crime is associated with income inequality (Wilkinson and Marmot 2003). A study of the demographic and spatial factors associated with the rise in the murder rate in Britain between 1981 and 2000 found that the increase was concentrated in the poorest areas (Shaw et al 2004). In the USA, the greater the degree of income inequality, the higher the rates of homicide, robbery and assault. In Scotland, homicides involving knives have been increasing and are of particular concern. Over 20 years, the homicide rate rose 83% whilst homicides involving knives increased by 164% (Leyland 2006). This sharp rise has led commentators to see knife crime as a public health problem (ibid).

Box 9.11 Crime and health

- Police-recorded crime statistics and the British Crime Survey (BCS) both show an overall decline in crime of 9–10% for 2007/2008 compared to the previous year
- Most types of crime have decreased
- The risk of being a victim of crime decreased to 22% in 2008
- 3% of adults had experienced a violent crime in 2008. For young men aged 16–24 this figure was 13%
- 2% households were burgled in 2008
- Illicit drug use is now at its lowest level since statistics were first compiled in 1995, largely due to a decline in the use of cannabis
- Crime levels have fallen by 18% since 2002/2003. This means the Home Office's Public Service Agreement Target 1 to reduce crime by 15% by 2007/2008 has been met
- 53% people think their local police force is doing a good or excellent job
- Around 2 in 3 people believe crime rates have been increasing

Source: Home Office (2008)

Box 9.12 Example

Knife crime in England and Wales

The Tackling Knives Action Programme (TKAP) was launched in 10 pilot areas in England and Wales in June 2008. The aim was to reduce knife carrying and knife crime and related injuries amongst young people, and to reassure the public about the safety of public places. Alongside increased use of stop and search powers and harsher treatment of those found carrying knives, the programme led to significant additional funding for diversionary activities for young people, particularly on weekend nights; £4.5 million was allocated to local community groups to run such activities. Within 2 months of the programme launch more than 55,000 people had been stopped and searched, more than 2500 arrests had been made for knife-related offences, and more than 1600 knives seized. Overall, compared to the previous year, the programme led to fewer knives being found, and those carrying knives were three times more likely than before to go to prison. There was a 27% reduction in related hospital admissions and 17% fewer serious knife crimes against young people.

Source: http://press.homeoffice.gov.uk/documents/ Tackling_Knives_Action_Prog1.pdf?view=Binary accessed 4/7/09

Box 9.13 Discussion point

How do crime and violence impact on individual and community health?

Crime may impact on health by its effects on:
- the physical health of victims
- the psychological health of victims and those who witness criminal acts
- the fear of crime in particular communities that reduces individual well-being and fractures community networks
- its impact on health services.

A public health approach to crime and crime prevention has seen much greater emphasis on community safety rather than policing. Such approaches to crime prevention reflect the importance of the focus on social conditions. Strategies to tackle crime include:

- crime prevention interventions, for example youth work to 'distract' young people from criminal activities; drug and alcohol initiatives such as the arrest referral schemes that refer users from police stations directly to rehabilitation programmes
- crime detection and prosecution strategies, for example closed circuit television (CCTV) and the witness protection scheme
- the identification and support for victims of crime, for example screening for domestic violence in primary care settings, victim support schemes
- treatment and rehabilitation of offenders, for example probation services and community service orders that require offenders to do work in the community, for example gardening or helping in social clubs for the elderly

Such varied activities require partnership working across professionals and agencies, and in particular the active involvement of communities.

Box 9.14 **Example**

Community safety measures

A variety of strategies have been introduced to reduce crime, including Neighbourhood Watch (NW) schemes and closed circuit television (CCTV)

CCTV

Evaluation of the effectiveness of CCTV is mixed. Several local studies report large reductions in crime. For example, the introduction of CCTV into a local authority in Darlington led to a 44% reduction in crime and very positive feedback from residents. However, a systematic review conducted by the Home Office found CCTV led to a non-sigificant reduction in crime of 6%: 'Overall, it might be concluded that CCTV reduces crime to a small degree' (Welsh and Farrington 2002: vii). It has been argued that CCTV involves a number of different context-specific features that will impact on its effectiveness, for example deterrence, displacement of criminal activities elsewhere, greater public safety awareness leading to more defensive behaviour and informal surveillance,

and more effective deployment of resources. Effectiveness measures should therefore include crime detection, conviction of criminals and fear of crime as well as crime reduction.

Sources: Pawson and Tilley (1997), Welsh and Farrington (2002), www.homeoffice.gov.uk accessed 1/07/09

Unlike crime, a neighbour dispute has no legally defined status and may include inconsiderate behaviour such as excessive noise or harassment and intimidation. Noise can undermine quality of life and although it does not necessarily translate into mental health problems it can lead to tension and irritability.

Box 9.15 **Example**

Noisy neighbours

People living next to noisy neighbours may suffer from sleep deprivation, increased aggression and a certain level of mental illness (CIEH 2001; London Health Commission 2003). Noisy neighbours are becoming a more common problem. In the 20 years between 1981 and 2001 the number of complaints about noisy neighbours made to UK local authorities rose more than seven-fold, from 764 per million of the population to 5540 per million of the population. Complaints about neighbours make up approximately 70% of all noise complaints. Approaches to tackling this problem include legal enforcement, education, and community mediation. The Environment Protection Act 1990 (as amended) requires local authorities to investigate complaints about noisy neighbours. Where there is evidence of a nuisance, for example not merely a one-off incident, EHOs may serve a notice requiring noise abatement. Enforcement of the Act can be difficult as an EHO needs to witness the noisy behaviour and this requirement may cause considerable time delays. Other strategies include diversionary activities targeted at young people playing loud music, and education targeted at young people excluded from schools to reduce noisy and anti-social behaviour.

(With thanks to Stephen Young)

Domestic violence is now recognized as a public health priority (WHO 1997). The Home Office defines domestic violence as 'any violence between current and former partners in an intimate relationship … the violence may include physical, sexual, emotional and financial abuse' (http://www.crim-ereduction.homeoffice.gov.uk). Other forms of intra-familial abuse exist, including the abuse of children, parents and the elderly and, rarely, the abuse of men by women. Domestic violence is a common but often hidden problem, with one in four women experiencing domestic abuse at some point in their lives. The health effects of domestic abuse include injury, chronic pain, sexually transmitted infections, mental health problems including depression and post-traumatic stress disorder, addiction and attempted suicide; reproductive disorders and difficulties in pregnancy (Campbell 2002; Plichta 2004). The health services often miss the symptoms of domestic violence, and several programmes have been initiated that focus on training health staff to identify and intervene in cases of domestic violence.

Box 9.16 **Practitioner talking**

Antenatal screening for domestic violence

I'm a midwife and I recently attended a programme on antenatal screening for domestic violence. This involved a taught study day where we practised and developed our skills in asking women about domestic violence and learnt more about interagency working and safety. I learnt about the five stages in antenatal screening for domestic violence:

- *Recognizing abuse as an issue – the wide range of indicators including late booking, repeated attendance in healthcare settings for minor injuries, physical injuries, mental health problems, and emotional or behavioural patterns.*
- *Providing a quiet and private environment for consultation – ensuring privacy and communication, for example using an interpreter for deaf women or women with English as a second language.*
- *Identifying abuse and its effects – questioning women in an open and empathetic manner. Stating in advance that questions about domestic violence routinely included in consultations are helpful, and both direct and indirect questions need to be used appropriately.*
- *Documenting the abuse – ensuring women's consent to any documentation and ensuring that information is confidential and cannot be accessed by the perpetrator, for example using a sealed envelope that is kept separately from women's hand-held records.*

- *Providing information and on-going support to women – advising women of local agencies, liaising with local support services if women want to leave home and drawing up contingency plans if they decide to stay but might need to leave at very short notice.*

The training has made me feel much more confident about asking women about abuse because now I know how to ask, and what to do if women disclose. It is also reassuring to know women feel it is an acceptable topic to broach with them. I know I can get support from other practitioners and agencies and won't be left on my own to deal with any problems that emerge.

(With thanks to Debra Salmon)

Commentary

Practitioners may need to withdraw and seek support if they feel personally threatened. Research has shown that although domestic violence is a very sensitive topic, women do not mind being asked about it as long as the questioning is done by a trained professional in a caring and non-judgemental manner and in a safe and confidential setting (Bacchus et al 2003). Several professional bodies support the introduction of routine antenatal enquiry into domestic violence nationwide (Bewley et al 1997; RCM 1997). Research has also suggested that there is a strong case for advocating routine enquiry into partner abuse, and for providing education and training of practitioners to promote disclosure of abuse and respond appropriately (Taket et al 2003).

The impact of crime and safety issues on health is increasingly being recognized as significant. Partnership working around such issues has the potential to promote the health of communities and individuals. At the individual level, greater awareness of violence and abuse can help practitioners to intervene effectively. Health practitioners working in the area of crime and safety is not unusual, and further networking of good practice examples and provision of appropriate training and support will help establish this topic as part of the health practitioner's remit.

Housing

There is a well-documented association between housing status and health. Owner-occupiers enjoy better health status than people who rent their homes. Owner-occupiers report lower death rates and rates of long-term illness (Flakti and Fox 1995; Gould and Jones 1996). Usually this association is explained in terms of the links between income and housing status, with owner-occupiers enjoying higher income levels and socio-economic status than tenants. There is also a view that the link is due to psychological attributes such as perceived control and deferred gratification. Bonnefoy et al (2004) suggest that housing-related factors that influence health may be divided into four categories:

- Internal housing environment – agents that affect the internal environment, for example indoor pollutants such as asbestos or carbon monoxide.

- Inadequate housing standard – cold or damp housing or poor layout, infestation, noise.
- Social environment – overcrowding, sleep deprivation, poor local infrastructure (e.g. shops and services) and social cohesion.
- Housing and social policy – housing allocation, homelessness, housing investment and urban planning.

The pattern of housing tenure in the UK has shifted dramatically during the last 25 years. The most significant switch is from council tenancy to owner-occupier, fuelled by tenants' right to buy, which was introduced in the 1980s. In 2003/2004 70% dwellings (18 million) were owner-occupied – an increase of 45% since 1981 (Office of National Statistics http://www.statistics.gov.uk/cci/nugget/asp.?id=1105 accessed 28/6/09). By 2003 the number of homes rented in the social sector had declined to just under 5 million (ibid). Figure 9.3 below illustrates possible pathways linking housing tenure and health status.

There is evidence that housing quality impacts both directly and indirectly on health (Ellaway and Macintyre 1998; Macintyre et al 1998). Direct effects include:

- excess winter deaths due to fuel poverty (inability to adequately heat accomodation due to low income and/or poor housing quality) and exposure to disease. This affects elderly people most. In 2007/2008 there were approximately

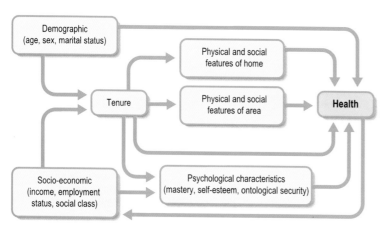

Figure 9.3 ● The relationship between housing tenure and individual health (from Macintyre et al 2000).

25,300 excess winter deaths (Office of National Statistics http://www. statistics.gov.uk/cci/ nugget/asp.?id=1105 accessed 28/6/09)

- home accidents (highest in temporary accommodation for the homeless)
- increases in infectious diseases such as tuberculosis, which are linked to overcrowding
- excess death rates (five times the general population average for people living in houses with multiple occupation and 10 times the average for rough sleepers (Matthews 1999).

Indirect effects are mediated by factors such as crowding, reduced access to amenities, and perception of low social capital in the neighbourhood and include health problems associated with crime, pollution, noise, heavy traffic, and problems for people living in deprived areas accessing health and welfare services. A WHO European Region study (Bonnefoy et al 2003) found numerous links between housing and aspects of health, including mental health, poverty, noise and health, and allergies. The same data have been used to support a link between neighbourhood physical disorder (litter, absence of vegetation, graffiti) and smoking (Miles 2006). Poor housing has been identified as a risk factor for children, increasing the risk of severe ill health and disability by 25% and leading to increased risk of meningitis, asthma and slow growth as well as mental health and behavioural problems (Harker 2006). In the long term, lower educational attainment, unemployment and poverty are all linked to poor housing during childhood.

Unfit housing carries health risks for inhabitants. Unfit housing fails to meet the required standards for a stable structure, adequate heating, lighting and ventilation, satisfactory water supply and waste disposal systems, and adequate bathroom and kitchen facilities. The 2002 English Housing Condition survey estimated that 1.2 million households were unfit (Marmot and Wilkinson 2006). Unfit housing is most common in the private rented sector, and in the owner-occupier sector affects elderly owner-occupiers most. Disrepair is far more common, affecting almost one-third of homes in England. Poor heating and insulation is a significant problem, leading

to 8000 extra deaths for each degree Celsius the temperature falls below average in winter months. Health problems related to unfit housing or housing of poor quality include:

1. Physical health problems, for example
   - respiratory diseases
   - hypothermia
   - ischaemic heart disease
   - gastroenteritis
   - dysentery
   - diarrhoea
   - infections and allergic responses.
2. Mental health problems, for example
   - stress and depression.

There is also a raised risk of accidents, fires and illnesses due to environmental toxins.

Although there is an obvious connection between housing and health, it is difficult to coordinate activity across the housing and health fields. This is due to many reasons, including the difficulty in isolating and quantifying the housing-health link and the historic separation of housing and health functions, professions and agencies, which makes joint working very challenging (Matthews 1999). Nationally what is needed is for housing to become integrated into the public health agenda at all levels. This has started to happen; for example, the 2004 report by the UK Sustainable Development Commission flagged up housing as one of the factors contributing to health (DEFRA 2004 cited in Stafford and McCarthy 2006). However, on the ground, housing and health remain the responsibility of different professions. At present, housing standards are enforced by EHOs who are employed by local authorities and health professionals probably regard the provision of decent housing as outside the remit of the health services.

 Box 9.17 **Activity**

What opportunities are there in your work to address housing issues?

It is health professionals who see the effects of cold, damp housing. Housing and health are obviously linked at the strategic level, but there is also some scope to make links on the ground.

 Box 9.18 **Example**

Links between health and housing in practice

1. Strategic links between health and housing, for example the Director of Public Health's annual report and health commissioning plans, can refer to local housing provision and need, and make explicit the link between housing and health.

2. The housing sector can take the lead in the use of health criteria to prioritize capital work, for example Bexley council, which targeted the council's housing association development programme to provide group homes and wheelchair-accessible housing. Bexley also used empty property to temporarily house high-rise residents experiencing emotional difficulties (Matthews 1999).

3. Practitioners linking health and housing in service delivery to vulnerable people: isolated, old people; those discharged from hospital; and those with mental health problems, for example district nurses who visit older people in their homes should be alerted to the signs of fuel poverty in the home – for example only one room heated or a cold, damp living room (Press 2003).

4. Single assessment, introduced as a central part of the Older People's National Service Framework, replaces multiple assessment of the same client by different health and social welfare agencies. The single assessment is shared between relevant agencies. Single assessment includes consideration of housing and the potential for accidents in the home.

Evaluating housing interventions is extremely difficult, due to the complex relationship between housing and other factors and health, and the practical and ethical problems of using experimental or quasi-experimental methods in this field. A recent systematic review of the health effects of housing improvement interventions concluded that whilst many studies showed health gains, the small study populations and number of confounding factors limit the generalizability of their findings (Thomson et al 2001).

Sustainability, regeneration and neighbourhood renewal

Sustainability means the capacity to endure and the term is used to refer to the responsible use of resources and environments, which does not reduce long-term capacity or threaten future generations. Examples of sustainability include green technology, for example recycling and water purification, and renewable energy, for example solar power or wind turbines. Regeneration or neighbourhood renewal aims to improve disadvantaged urban areas and encompasses a wide range of activities including improved housing and recreation facilities, job creation, community safety interventions, sustainable environments, and the active involvement and participation of local communities in these processes.

Regeneration and renewal is driven by concerns about social and health inequalities and sustainable environments. There is a large gap separating the UK's most deprived neighbourhoods from the rest. In England, four regions (the North West, North East, London, and Yorkshire and Humberside) have particularly high concentrations of deprived neighbourhoods. As the government puts it, 'the goal is to break the vicious circle of deprivation and provide the foundation for sustainable regeneration and wealth creation' (DETR 1997, p. 3). Regeneration of urban areas has a history dating back to more than 30 years. The current programme of regeneration is funded by the Department of the Environment, Transport and the Regions (DETRA) through the Single Regeneration Budget (SRB).

The rationale for regeneration is multi-faceted and includes the following dimensions: economic (to increase local employment); environmental (to develop sustainable local environments); and social (to build a future for local people). The UK Round Table on Sustainable Development identified the following principles to guide regeneration (cited in Fudge 2003):

- Precautionary – if there is a serious environmental threat act immediately to prevent or minimize damage.
- Integration – integrate sustainability into all policy-making areas.
- Polluter pays – those responsible for pollution should pay for its effects.
- Preventative – avoid incurring damage.
- Participative – public partnerships and decision making for sustainable development.

Sustainability therefore needs to be integrated into regeneration and renewal projects in order to protect the environment and build lasting solutions. This is a global issue transcending national or regional boundaries, and concerted action by global partners is required to address the issue. In 2001 the UN adopted eight Millennium Development Goals (MDGs), one of which is 'to ensure environmental sustainability'. Specific targets include:

- Target 9: integrate the principles of sustainable development into countries policies and programs; reverse loss of environmental resources.
- Target 10: reduce by half the proportion of people without sustainable access to safe drinking water.
- Target 11: achieve significant improvement in the lives of at least 100 million slum dwellers by 2020 (UNDP 2008).

Although access to safe water has increased, poor environmental conditions remain the cause of a significant percentage of disease. Worldwide 19% of disease amongst children 0–1 years is caused by contaminated water (mainly via diarrhoea); 10% is due to malaria and 10% due to malnutrition, intestinal infestation and diseases linked to poor environmental conditions (Tulchinsky and Varavikova 2009, p. 334). There are major threats from global warming and climate change including the spread of diseases such as malaria, desertification, disrupted water and food supplies, flooding and bad weather events such as hurricanes.

 Box 9.19 **Discussion point**

How might health professionals be involved in regeneration work?

Tackling the disadvantage that includes lower standards of health involves partnership working with a wide range of organizations and agencies. A key feature of regeneration is the need to involve these partners and adopt an interagency approach. The health services have been identified as a key partner in renewal strategies. For example, health services are a major employer in communities and can thus have an impact on local economies through a commitment to provide training and education to local staff so that their careers can progress. In this way communities become more self-sufficient, local job prospects are improved, and service providers are more in tune with the needs and wishes of service users. There is no definite evidence linking regeneration with health improvement, although the evidence linking poverty and social exclusion with health is extensive.

 Box 9.20 **Discussion point**

Evaluating regeneration programmes

The objective of a regeneration programme is to tackle the broad determinants of health in an area. What would be the indicators of success of the programme for each of the following objectives:
- getting people into jobs
- developing local businesses
- promoting lifelong learning
- developing a high quality living environment
- developing a safer neighbourhood
- promoting health
- empowering communities.

Why might it be difficult to evaluate regeneration initiatives?

A variety of local indicators are already available via local councils, police forces and health organizations. However, there are problems with using these data to evaluate regeneration policies. Harrison (2000) identifies several factors that make such evaluation difficult, including the political nature of urban policy, the complexity of interventions spanning many different policy arenas (such as employment, housing, education and crime reduction), the links between urban decline and national and global processes, the importance of the local context in determining processes and effects, the effect of displacement and migration (so that beneficiaries of regeneration may not be the originally targeted communities), and the need to measure processes as well as outcomes. Despite these confounding factors, there are some studies that show positive outcomes associated with neighbourhood renewal. One example is Blackman et al's (2001) study which showed that mental health can be improved through environmental interventions. Equally it is important to recognize that there are aspects of regeneration that may be damaging to population and individual health:

- the process of decanting residents while housing improvements take place
- the noise, disturbance and stress associated with housing development
- increased housing costs as a result of regeneration programmes
- the effect on populations outside the regeneration area through, for example, the displacement of drug dealing
- increased social divisions.

Regeneration and neighbourhood renewal are important health promoting strategies that directly impact on a variety of socio-economic and environmental determinants of health. Targeting the most deprived neighbourhoods is one means of tackling inequalities in health. Health practitioners have an important role to play as key partners in regeneration and renewal, and the experience of working with communities can also positively influence public involvement strategies used to plan health service provision. A challenge for regeneration is how to balance tackling the short-term and pressing needs of disadvantaged areas with the longer-term planning for sustainability that is required.

Transport

Transport and health are linked in several ways:
- Adequate and appropriate transport increases people's mobility and access to a wide range of services, facilitating choice.
- The dominance of private car transport at the expense of public transport results in high rates of road traffic accidents and air pollution, low levels of physical activity, which in turn leads to increased rates of obesity and the loss of community networks.

Box 9.21 **Transport and health**

- Road traffic accidents account for two-fifths of accidental deaths.
- Heavy traffic reduces physical and social activity, leading to:
  – isolation and the loss of community networks
  – reduced likelihood of people walking or cycling for short journeys
  – sedentary lifestyles and the growth in obesity.
- Pollution from traffic is the major cause of poor air quality in urban areas and contributes to respiratory and cardiac problems.
- In many areas of the UK, transport is the principal source of nitrogen dioxide and particulate matter (PM10) – two major air pollutants.
- It is estimated that air pollution is responsible for the premature death of over 20,000 people each year across Europe (8100 in the UK) and serious ill health affecting many more thousands of people.

Box 9.21 **Transport and health—cont'd**

- Transport produces nearly one quarter of the UK's emission of carbon dioxide, which contributes to environmental damage and global warming.
- Noise pollution and stress from living and working in areas of heavy traffic contributes to mental health problems.

Sources: Kunzil et al (2000), McGrogan (1999), COMEAP cited in HDA (2005)

Between 1986 and 2000 the number of cars registered in the UK increased from 17.4 million to 26.7 million. Today car journeys account for 82% of all journeys by mileage.

Box 9.22 **Activity**

How might you address transport issues within your work practice?

Public health action in the field of transport covers a variety of interventions including promoting physically active means of transport, such as cycling and walking to school and work; promoting the use of public transport to reduce traffic pollution; and measures to enhance the safety of roads, for example pedestrianization, traffic calming and speed cameras. Promoting physically active means of transport is discussed further in the Physical Activity section of Chapter 11.

The most emotive issue, and hence the one likely to legitimize health practitioners' involvement, is probably the reduction of road traffic injuries and fatalities and this priority area is discussed further in Chapter 10. Road traffic accidents are a worldwide problem, affecting both developed and developing countries. In Europe about 127,000 people are killed and 2.4 million injured due to road traffic accidents each year (Racioppi et al 2004). Road traffic accidents are the leading cause of mortality in young people, especially men, and the cost to society is estimated to be approximately 2% of the gross domestic product (ibid). However, there is evidence that traffic fatalities can be reduced through concerted action by a variety of stakeholders including government, businesses and civic institutions. For example, in France the number of traffic fatalities was reduced by 20% from 2002 to 2003 (WHO 2004), and road casualties in Great Britain have also declined (DfT 2009).

Child pedestrian injury arising from road accidents is the leading cause of accidental death in the UK. In 2008, 2807 children were killed or seriously injured on roads (DfT 2009). Social deprivation is strongly associated with child pedestrian injuries, with children from social class 5 being five times more likely to be killed in a road traffic collision than children from social class 1 (Liabo and Curtis 2003). Road accidents are estimated to cost Britain over £16 billion per year. Involvement in such interventions could therefore be justified on the grounds of a concern with children's health, health inequalities and accident prevention.

Box 9.23 **Example**

London Congestion Charge (LCC) Scheme

The LCC was introduced in 2003 to tackle traffic congestion in London. Private cars entering the congestion zone have to pay an additional charge. Camera surveillance is used to monitor car registration plates and check that the charge has been paid. Evaluation of the LCC scheme suggests it has been effective in promoting more active transport methods and reducing traffic congestion. Key outcomes include:

- Increased take-up of public transport instead of private car use (between 35,000 and 40,000 car trips per day switched to public transport).
- Increase in cycling mileage by 28% in 2003 and by a further 4% in 2004.

Box 9.23 Example—cont'd

- Reported improvements in comfort and quality of walking and public transport systems.
- Reinvestment of scheme revenues to finance further improvements in public transport, walking, cycling, and safe routes to school.

Source: NHF (2007)

Transport campaigns tend to be high profile and politicized, which may lead health practitioners to steer clear of them. The private car lobby is very powerful and influential, and has been linked to media campaigns that have tried to discredit road safety campaigns. These tensions are explored in the example of safety cameras below.

Box 9.24 Example

Safety cameras

Excessive and inappropriate speed is the cause of over one-third of the accidents on UK roads. By 2020 road accidents will have moved from ninth to third place in the world ranking of the burden of disease. In Great Britain around 3500 people are killed and 250,000 injured in road accidents each year. Research in Norway, Australia, Canada, New Zealand and the UK has shown that safety cameras affect driving speeds and improve safety. Results from a 2-year pilot scheme in eight areas showed that the number of people killed or seriously injured fell by 35%. Average speed in the pilot areas fell by 10%. There has been a vigorous public media campaign against the introduction of safety cameras, claiming they are being used to raise revenue and are a punitive anti-motorist measure. However, the effectiveness of safety cameras in reducing accidents and injuries is indisputable, and has led to a major expansion of speed cameras. Local safety camera schemes are led by multi-agency Safety Camera Partnerships. A majority of the British public supports safety cameras.

Sources: Dept. of Transport News Release 11 Feb 2003, Pilkington (2003)

Road traffic accidents and fatalities are the most obvious and publicized aspect of the links between transport and health. However, other issues, especially air and noise pollution, are also important, especially in the long term. The reliance in the UK on private cars for transport has led to increases in air and noise pollution. The Environment Act 1995 led to the development of a National Air Quality Strategy that sets targets for the reduction of eight major air pollutants known to affect human health by 2010. The aim is to ensure that everyone can breathe air that poses no significant risk to health or quality of life in public places. Local authorities are required to draw up their own Local Air Quality Management plans to achieve air quality objectives. Local Air Quality Management Areas (AQMAs) and action plans are declared if it is anticipated that targets will not be met. Following the first round of review and assessment, 129 local authorities declared AQMAs; 75% of these AQMAs were purely due to traffic. Local transport plans aim to reduce private car use and encourage other forms of transport such as walking, cycling, and bus or shared car use. Other strategies include regulation to reduce vehicle emissions and improve fuels, tax incentives to use cleaner fuels and vehicles, and the development of an integrated transport strategy that supports sustainable development.

Government agencies are convinced that planning and policy in this area will improve health: 'It is clear that transport and health are inextricably linked. Transport has major health impacts …' (HDA 2005, p. 1). Evaluating transport interventions to promote health suffers from the problems of contamination with other variables and difficulty in isolating relevant factors. However, research into this area does give grounds for optimism. A systematic review of the effectiveness of transport interventions in improving population health (Morrison et al 2003) concluded that the most effective interventions are health promotion campaigns (to prevent child accidents, to increase helmet use and promote the use of children's seats and seatbelt use), traffic calming, and specific legislation to ban drink-driving. A study of the UK national cycling network concluded that environmental modifications (such as the extension of dedicated cycle routes) are often the most effective means of promoting active transport (Lawlor et al 2003). Strategies that have been proven to work in Germany and the Netherlands include better facilities for cyclists and pedestrians, traffic calming, urban design taking into account the needs of non-motorists, restrictions on traffic in urban areas, traffic education and strict enforcement of traffic control legislation to protect cyclists and pedestrians (Pucher and Dijkstra 2003). This suggests that tackling transport does result in significant health benefits, and that a variety of strategies should be used, including environmental modification, legislation, media advocacy, and individual behaviour change.

Conclusion

The social determinants of health have a profound impact on public health. This impact is both direct and indirect, and is often mediated by psychosocial factors such as self-efficacy and social capital. Because social determinants rarely fit the traditional medical disease model of pathogen-host-disease, their effect on health has not always been recognized. In addition, many of the social determinants of health are regulated and addressed by social and environmental services that have historically been separated from health services. However, there is now ample evidence and a general consensus that all the social determinants considered in this chapter – income, employment, housing, crime, regeneration and neighbourhood renewal, and transport – have a significant effect on health.

This chapter has provided a summary overview of some of the evidence linking social determinants to health, followed by examples of interventions designed to address determinants and promote health. Interventions are broad based and include regulation and legislation, environmental modification, community projects and individually based work with clients. Although some of the most important interventions are at a macro policy level, practitioners have discovered a variety of innovative ways of supporting policies locally, enabling clients to address constraints, and supporting communities to overcome limitations. Successful work to tackle the social determinants of health is becoming integrated within health, social and environmental practitioners' workloads. Crucial to the continuing success of this work is effective partnership working and the involvement of communities. The growing evidence base for such work is also important in legitimizing and supporting this approach. There is a huge potential for such an approach to continue to promote and develop public health.

Further discussion

- Consider how you might address a particular social determinant of health within your practice. What resources and skills would you need?

- With reference to your practice, try to assess the impact of one particular determinant of health. What problems do you encounter? Are there ways in which you could collect relevant information routinely, or liaise more with other agencies, making such an assessment less problematic? What would be the advantages of quantifying the impact of this social determinant on health?

- Consider your current networking and partnership work with other services and agencies. Can you identify ways in which this process could become more health promoting for the communities you serve?

Recommended reading

- Marmot M, Wilkinson R, editors: *Social determinants of health*, edn 2, 2006, Oxford University Press.

    This edited book examines different social determinants of health including housing, transport, employment, food, social support and social cohesion, early years, poverty, racial/ethnic inequalities, ageing and sexual behaviour/health. Links with the policy context for each topic are included. This book provides a useful, comprehensive and informative overview of various social determinants of health.

- Russell H, Killoran A: *Public health and regeneration: making the links*, London, 2000, Health Education Agency.

  A short guide that summarizes some of the evidence linking issues such as community safety and housing with health.

- Wilkinson R, Marmot M: *The social determinants of health: the solid facts*, edn 2, 2003, WHO Regional Office for Europe.

  This booklet is the result of a request from the WHO Regional Office for Europe to summarize the evidence around the social determinants of health into 10 key messages for policy makers. The issues that are examined include work, unemployment,

early life, addiction, food, transport, stress, social exclusion, social support and the social gradient.

- World Health Organization Commission on Social Determinants of Health (WHO): *Final Report: Closing the gap in a generation: Health equity through action on the social determinants of health*, 2008.

  This final report presents global evidence of the impact of social determinants of health and their effect on health inequalities. Recommendations to tackle the problem of health inequalities are made, focusing on three areas: improving daily living conditions, tackling the inequitable distribution of power, money and resources worldwide, and research to measure and understand the problem and assess the impact of interventions designed to tackle the issues.

References

Acheson D: *Independent inquiry into inequalities in health*, London, 1998, The Stationery Office.

Alcock P: Anti-poverty strategies. In Adam L, Amos M, Munro J, editors: *Promoting health: politics and practice*, London, 2002, Sage.

Asthana S, Halliday J: *What works in tackling health inequalities? Pathways, policies and practice through the lifecourse*, Bristol, 2006, Policy Press.

Bacchus L, Mezey G, Bewley S: Experiences of seeking help from health professionals in a sample of women who experienced domestic violence, *Health Soc Care Community* 11(1):10–18, 2003.

Benzeval M, Dilnot A, Judge K, et al: Income and health over the lifecourse: evidence and policy implications. In Graham H, editor: *Understanding health inequalities*, Maidenhead, 2000, Open University Press, pp 96–113.

Bewley S, Friend J, Mezey G: *Violence against women*, London, 1997, Royal College of Obstetricians and Gynaecologists Press.

Black C: *Working for a healthier tomorrow: Dame Carol Black's Review of the health of Britain's working age population*, London, 2008, Crown Copyright.

Blackman T, Harvey J, Lawrence M, et al: Neighbourhood renewal and health: evidence from a local case study, *Health Place* 7(2):93–103, 2001.

Bonnefoy XR, SanEng MB, Moissonnier B, et al: Housing and health in Europe: preliminary results of a pan-European study, *Am J Public Health* 93(9): 1559–1563, 2003.

Bonnefoy XE, Annesi-Maesano I, Aznar LM, et al: Review of evidence on housing and health, background document to the Fourth Ministerial Conference on Environment and Health, Budapest, Hungary, 2004, www.euro.who.int/document/HOH/ebackdoc01.pdf

Campbell JC: Health consequences of intimate partner violence, *The Lancet* 359(9314):1331–1336, 2002.

Chartered Institute of Environmental Health (CIEH): *Annual survey into local authority noise enforcement action. England and Wales: noise nuisance*, London, 2001, CIEH.

City of Toronto Community Health Information Section: *Health inequalities in the city of Toronto: summary report*, Toronto, 1991, Department of Public Health.

Dahlgren G, Whitehead M: *Policies and strategies to promote social equity in health*, Stockholm, 1991, Institute of Future Studies.

Department for Work and Pensions (DWP): Opportunity for all: 4th annual report, Cm 5598, London, 2002, The Stationery Office.

Department for Work and Pensions (DWP): *Households below average income – an analysis of the income distirbution 1994/5 to 2003/4*, Leeds, 2005, Corporate Document Services.

Department of the Environment, Transport and Regions (DETR): Regeneration – the way forward, 1997, www.roads.dtlr.gov.uk/roadsafety/strategy/tomorrow

Department of Health (DH): *Valuing people: a new strategy for learning disability for the 21st century,* , London, 2001, The Stationery Office.

Department of Health. *Tackling health inequalities: a programme for action*, London, 2003, DH.

Department of Health (DH): *Health inequalities: progress and next steps*, London, 2008, DH.

Department for Transport. *Road casualties in Great Britain*, London, 2008, DfT.

Ellaway A, Macintyre S: Does housing tenure predict health in the UK because it exposes people to different levels of housing related hazards in the home or its surroundings? *Health Place* 4:141–150, 1998.

Evandrou M, Falkingham J: A secure retirement for all? Older and new labour. In: Hills J, Stewart K, editors: *New labour, poverty, inequality and exclusion*, Bristol, 2005, Policy Press.

Exworthy M, Stuart M, Blane D, et al: *Tackling health inequalities since the Acheson Inquiry*, Bristol, 2003, The Policy Press/Joseph Rowntree Foundation.

Flakti H, Fox J: Differences in mortality by housing tenure and by car access, *Popul Trends* 81:27–30, 1995.

Fudge C: Health and sustainability gains from urban regeneration and development. In Takano T, editor: *Healthy cities and urban policy research*, London/New York, 2003, Spon Press, Ch.4, pp 41–58.

Gordon D, Middleton S, Bradshaw JR: *Millennium survey of poverty and social exclusion 1999*, York, 2001, Joseph Rowntree Foundation.

Gould MI, Jones K: *Housing as health capital: how health trajectories and housing interact*, Cambridge, 1996, Polity Press.

Harker L: *Chance of a lifetime: the impact of bad housing on children's lives*, London, 2006, Shelter.

Harrison T: Urban policy. In Davies TO, Nutley SM, Smith PC, editors: *What works? Evidence-based policy and practice in public services*, Bristol, 2000, The Policy Press.

Health Development Agency: *Making the case: Improving health transport*, London, 2005, HDA.

Home Office: *Crime in England and Wales 2007/8: a summary of the main findings*, London, 2008, Home Office.

Kunzil N, Kaiser R, Medina S, et al: Public health impact of outdoor and traffic-related air pollution: a European assessment, *Lancet* 356:795–801, 2000.

Lawlor DA, Ness AR, Cope AM, et al: The challenges of evaluating environmental interventions to increase population levels of physical activity: the case of the UK national cycle network, *J Epidemiol Community Health* 57:96–101, 2003.

Leon D, Walt G: *Poverty, inequality and health in international perspective: a divided world?* Oxford, 2001, Oxford University Press.

Leyland AH: Homicides involving knives and other sharp objects in Scotland, 1981–2003, *J Public Health* 28(2):145–147, 2006.

Liabo K, Curtis K: Traffic calming schemes to reduce childhood injuries from road accidents and respond to children's own views of what is important, 2003, www.evidencenetwork.org/.

London Health Commission: *Noise and health: making the link*, London, 2003, London Health Commission.

Macintyre S, Ellaway A, Der G, et al: Are housing tenure and car access simply markers of income or self esteem? A Scottish study, *J Epidemiol Community Health* 52:657–664, 1998.

Macintyre S, Hiscock R, Kearns A, et al: Housing tenure and health inequalities: a three-dimensional perspective on people, homes and neighbourhoods. In Graham H, editor: *Understanding health inequalities*, Maidenhead, 2000, Open University Press.

Marmot M, Wilkinson RG, editors: *Social determinants of health*, edn 2, , Oxford, UK, 2006, Oxford University Press.

Matthews G: Why should public health include housing? In Griffiths S, Hunter DJ, editors: *Perspectives in public health*, Abingdon, 1999, Radcliffe Medical Press.

McGrogan G: Transport. In Griffiths S, Hunter DJ, editors: *Perspectives in public health*, Abingdon, 1999, Radcliffe Medical Press.

Miles R: Neighbourhood disorder and smoking: findings of a European urban survey, *Soc Sci Med* 63(9): 2464–2475, 2006.

Morrison DS, Petticrew M, Thomson H: What are the most effective ways of improving population health through transport interventions? Evidence from systematic reviews, *J Epidemiol Community Health* 57(5):327–333, 2003.

Naidoo J, Wills J: *Foundations for health promotion*, edn 3, London, 2009, Baillière Tindall.

NHF: *Building health creating and enhancing places for healthy, active lives: blueprint for action*, London, 2007, National Heart Forum.

OECD WHO: *DAC guidelines and reference series: poverty and health*, Paris, 2003, OECD.

Pawson R, Tilley N: *Realistic evaluation*, London, 1997, Sage.

Pilkington P: Speed cameras under attack in the UK, *Inj Prev* 9:293–294, 2003.

Plichta SB: Intimate partner violence and physical health consequences, *J Interpers Violence* 19(11):1296–1323, 2004.

Press V: *Fuel poverty and health: a guide for primary care organizations and public health and primary care professionals*, London, 2003, National Heart Forum/ Faculty of Public Health.

Pucher J, Dijkstra L: Promoting safe walking and cycling to improve public health: lessons from the Netherlands and Germany, *Am J Public Health* 93(9):1509–1516, 2003.

Racioppi F, Eriksson L, Tingvall C, et al: *Preventing road traffic injury: a public health perspective for Europe*, Copenhagen, 2004, World Health Organization Regional Office for Europe.

Raphael D: Introduction to the social determinants of health. In Raphael D, editor: *Social determinants of health: Canadian perspectives*, edn 2, Toronto, 2008, Canadian Scholars' Press, pp 2–19.

Royal College of Midwives (RCM): *Domestic abuse in pregnancy*, , London, 1997, RCM.

Shaw M, Tunstall H, Dorling D: Increasing inequalities in risk of murder in Britain: trends in the demographic and spatial distribution of murder, 1981–2000, *Health Place* 11(1):45–54, 2004.

Shibuya K, Hashimoto H, Yano E: Individual income, income distribution, and self rated health in Japan: cross sectional analysis of nationally representative sample, *Br Med J* 324:16, 2002.

Social Exclusion Unit: *A new commitment to neighbourhood renewal National Strategy Action Plan Report by the Social Exclusion Unit*, London, 2001, Cabinet Office.

Stafford M, McCarthy M: Neighbourhood housing and health. In: Marmot M, Wilkinson RG, editors: *Social determinants of health: the solid facts*, edn 2, Copenhagen, 2006, WHO.

Steptoe A, Perkins-Porras L, McKay C, et al: Behavioural counselling to increase consumption of fruit and

vegetables in low income adults: randomized trial, *Br Med J* 326:855, 2003.

Sturm R, Gresenz CR: Income inequality and family income and their relationships to chronic medical conditions and mental health disorders, *Br Med J* 324:20, 2002.

Sutherland H, Sefton T, Piachaud D: *Poverty in Britain: the impact of government policy since 1997*, York, 2003, Joseph Rowntree Foundation.

Taket A, Nurse J, Smith D, et al: Routinely asking women about domestic violence in health settings, *Br Med J* 327:673–676, 2003.

Thomson H, Petticrew M, Morrison D: Health effects of housing improvement: systematic review of intervention studies, *Br Med J* 323:187–190, 2001.

Townsend P: *Poverty in the UK*, Harmondsworth, 1979, Penguin.

Tulchinsky TH, Varavikova EA: *The new public health*, edn 2, Boston, 2009, Elsevier and Academic Press.

United Nations Development Programme 2008. *Human Development Report* 2007/2008, UN.

United Nations: *The millenium development goals report*, New York, 2007, UN.

Watterson A: Occupational health. In Watterson A, editor: *Public health in practice*, Basingstoke, 2003, Palgrave/Macmillan.

Welsh BC, Farrington DP: *Crime prevention effects of closed circuit television: a systematic review*, , London, 2002, Home Office Research Development and Statistics Directorate .

Wilkinson R, Marmot M: *The social determinants of health: the solid facts*, edn 2, Copenhagen, 2003, WHO Regional Office for Europe.

Wilkinson R, Pickett K: *True spirit level: why more equal societies almost always do better*, London, 2009, Allen Lane.

World Health Organization (WHO): *Violence against women: a priority health issue*, Geneva, 1997, Women's Health and Development, Family and Reproductive Health, WHO.

World Health Organization (WHO): *World report on road traffic injury prevention*, Geneva, 2004, WHO.

World Health Organization Commission on Social Determinants of Health (WHO): *Final report: closing the gap in a generation: health equity through action on the social determinants of health*, Geneva, 2008, WHO.

10

The major causes of ill health

OVERVIEW

Over the last century, there has been a big shift in the burden of disease – from the infectious diseases of the nineteenth and early twentieth centuries to chronic diseases in the twentieth century and now. Chronic diseases such as coronary heart disease (CHD) and cancer are also strongly related to lifestyle factors such as smoking, poor diet, physical inactivity and alcohol consumption. Changes over time in the burden of disease have shifted the emphasis of public health from health protection measures to tackle infectious diseases towards health promotion policy targeting individual behaviour and lifestyle risk factors, as well as the wider determinants of health, such as poverty and education. Health protection is nevertheless still an important strategy in the context of new, emerging and resurgent infectious diseases (such as HIV, Ebola virus, vCJD, avian and swine flu, and tuberculosis). New diagnostic technologies, including those based on genetics, could also play a role in improving population health. This chapter reviews two key strategies in disease prevention – immunization and screening – and goes on to discuss approaches to some of the major causes of ill health in the twenty-first century – CHD, cancers, accidents, mental illness and HIV.

Introduction

Most international health strategies seek to secure improvements in health by increasing life expectancy and reducing premature death (adding years to life) and increasing the quality of life and minimizing illness (adding life to years). In England, this is achieved by focusing on key health areas that are

- a major cause of premature death or avoidable ill health
- responsive to effective intervention
- amenable to measurement and monitoring.

Saving Lives: Our Healthier Nation (DH 1999a) identified cancers, coronary heart disease (CHD) and stroke, accidents and undetermined injury and mental health as the priority areas. The Public Health Agency of Canada [http://www.phac-aspc. gc.ca] also includes chronic respiratory diseases, diabetes and musculoskeletal diseases. The focus of many strategies is on the prevention of specific diseases rather than the promotion of health in the community as a whole or improvements in the health of specific groups. There are many priority issues, and listing them should not imply that their relationship to behaviours such as smoking is not recognized. Other national strategies focus on risk factors that cause ill health such as smoking, alcohol and diet (e.g. Scottish Office 1998).

The two most common causes of death in the UK are CHD and cancers. Tackling these major causes of ill health is often driven by a medical model which focuses on early diagnosis and treatment of disease or its precursors such as hypertension or diabetes. The National Service Framework for Diabetes (DH 2001a), for example, focuses on the identification of people with diabetes; clinical care; managing diabetic emergencies; the care of people with diabetes in hospital; diabetes and pregnancy; and the detection and management of long-term complications.

However, prevention of diseases requires addressing the risk factors that are common to many diseases:

- reducing smoking prevalence
- improving diet and nutrition
- increasing physical activity
- reducing overweight and obesity.

Chapter 11 discusses how these lifestyle changes are being addressed through health promotion interventions.

The most common way of assessing health improvement is through a reduction in mortality and morbidity. Practitioners may thus find it hard to move outside of this disease-focused framework and think about how they can tackle the major causes of health within a salutogenic approach. For example, the objective for the priority area of mental health is expressed as the promotion of health, but the setting of targets for achievement led to its expression as disease-focused: 'To reduce the death rate from suicide and undetermined injury by at least a fifth by 2010' (DH 1999a).

Disease prevention is only one strand of public health practice. The key purposes of public health identified in the standards for specialist public health practice are

- to improve health and well-being in the population
- to prevent disease and minimize its consequences
- to prolong valued life
- to reduce inequalities in health.

One of the key areas of competence is the surveillance and assessment of the population's health and well-being. This chapter explores two different approaches to disease prevention: screening and immunization.

Approaches to disease prevention

The central question in disease prevention is whether to adopt

- the population approach in which the aim is to lower the average level of risk in the population or
- the high-risk approach in which people at particular risk are identified and offered advice and treatment.

Because most conditions follow a roughly normal distribution in the population as a whole, there are many more people with a risk factor or condition in the main body of the population. The prevention paradox (Rose 1993) suggests that many people need to take protective action in order to prevent illness in a few. There would therefore be more improvement in population health if everyone reduced their risk (e.g. their cholesterol level) than if the few in the high-risk category reduced their cholesterol level to the mean.

Box 10.1 **Discussion point**

What are the implications of the prevention paradox for health improvement?

This supports the whole population approach rather than a targeted approach, which might initially appear the more logical choice. Rose (1993) suggests that many interventions that aim to improve health have relatively small influences on the health of most people and therefore the purported benefits of population programmes are over-stressed to encourage people to take action. This section examines the concept of screening – the process of actively seeking to identify precursors to disease in those who are presumed to be healthy – as a means of preventing disease. Screening has been a recognized and accepted part of general health care but in recent years the cost-effectiveness, efficacy and acceptability of such mass programmes have been questioned.

Infectious diseases account for one-third of all deaths worldwide. Diarrhoea, measles, tuberculosis (TB) and malaria alone account for nearly 10 million and 18% of all deaths in low-income countries (WHO 2008). *Getting Ahead of the Curve*, the UK strategy for combating infectious diseases (and other forms of health protection) (DH 2002a), describes new threats to health:

* the re-emergence of diseases once thought to be conquered (e.g. TB, polio)
* the emergence of new diseases (e.g. most notably HIV, but 2003 saw the emergence of SARS, an outbreak in China that rapidly spread to other countries, and 2009 saw a worldwide swine flu pandemic)
* terrorism.

There are many reasons why infectious diseases have again become a major public health problem, prompting the UK government to set up a Health Protection Agency in 2003 to review new and emerging infectious diseases and strengthen surveillance systems. One factor is the indiscriminate use of antibiotics to treat illnesses and to promote growth in animals which has led to increased microbial resistance. Other factors in the spread of such diseases include population movement, poverty and poor social conditions.

Box 10.2 **Example**

The spread of TB

TB is an example of a disease where worsening social conditions enable the spread of infection. The WHO declared TB a global emergency in 1993, and in 1998 it estimated that one-third of the world's population is infected with mycobacterium tuberculosis. The UK saw a steady decline in TB notifications from 50,000 cases annually in the 1940s to about 5000 cases in the 1980s as a consequence of the introduction of BCG immunization and anti-tubercular therapies.

Yet TB cases have risen by 73% in London since 1987 and the incidence in some London boroughs exceeds 50 per 100,000, the majority of these cases being in people born in countries where the disease is endemic. The spread of HIV infection and the emergence of multi-drug resistance are contributing to the worsening impact of the disease worldwide.

Source: British Thoracic Society (2000)

Immunization has been one of the major strategies to tackle infectious diseases. In Angola, for example, 10 million children were vaccinated against polio in 3 days in 2003. Yet in the same year the UK saw the emergence of serious public concerns over the safety of the measles, mumps and rubella (MMR) vaccination programme (since recognized as unfounded) that saw immunization rates in London drop to 55%. This section examines the dilemmas for practitioners posed by immunization and the challenges of assessing and communicating risk to the public.

Screening

The National Screening Committee defines screening as:

> *a public health service in which members of a defined population, who do not necessarily perceive they are at risk of, or are already affected by a disease or its complications, are asked a question or offered a test, to identify those individuals who are more likely to be helped than harmed by further tests or treatment to reduce the risk of a disease or its complications.*

http://www.nsc.nhs.uk

There are several different types of screening in use:

- mass screening of whole population groups, for example breast and cervical screening of women
- selective screening of high-risk groups, for example the proposed testing of new arrivals for TB and HIV
- anonymous screening used to detect trends in public health, for example diabetic patients in general practice
- opportunistic screening when the opportunity is taken at a general consultation to ask about health-related behaviour
- health screening not linked to a particular disease, but looking at lifestyles in general, for example well woman clinics
- genetic screening investigating inheritable factors in order to assist parenting decisions, for example sickle cell screening
- routine screening in infancy and childhood.

 Box 10.3 **Discussion point**

What screening might take place in a primary care setting? What factors need to be taken into account to determine good practice?

There are particular ethical issues associated with screening and it is not unambiguously a good thing. It may move someone from presuming themselves to be healthy to a state of having an identified disease or condition, with the attendant anxiety and potentially invasive treatment for the patient. Its benefits, therefore, in terms of earlier diagnosis necessitating less radical treatment and reduced morbidity and mortality, must outweigh the disadvantages or costs.

The National Screening Committee has set out a framework for screening that elaborates on the guidelines and principles laid out by the World Health Organization in 1968 (Wilson Jungner 1968):

- The disease should be common and serious.
- The disease should have a recognized latent stage during which early symptoms can be detected.
- There should be a simple, safe, precise and validated screening test.
- The test should be acceptable to the population.
- There should be an effective treatment or intervention for patients identified through early detection, with evidence of early treatment leading to better outcomes than late treatment.
- The screening programme should be effective in reducing mortality or morbidity.
- The benefit from the screening programme should outweigh the physical and psychological harm (caused by the test, diagnostic procedures and treatment).
- The opportunity cost of the screening programme (including testing, diagnosis, treatment, administration, training and quality assurance) should be economically balanced in relation to expenditure on medical care as a whole (i.e. value for money).

Screening programmes may mean that less attention is given to understanding and tackling the causes of the disease. A range of risk factors have been identified as associated with breast cancer including body weight, limited breastfeeding and alcohol consumption.

Screening is a popular service and there is a constant demand for more screening from patients, pressure groups, the media and clinicians. In the UK, there are only three national cancer screening programmes for breast cancer, cervical cancer, and for bowel cancer using faecal occult blood testing. Yet it is only worthwhile when there is an effective intervention or treatment that is more effective if delivered early on in the development of a disease condition. The national screening programmes for

 Box 10.4 **Example**

Screening for prostate cancer

Prostate cancer is the second leading cause of cancer deaths in men in the UK. Each year 34,000 cases are diagnosed and there are over 10,000 deaths. Yet screening for prostate cancer is controversial. By the age of 80, approximately 50% of men will have some form of prostate cancer but more men will die with the disease than of it. Screening for prostate cancer involves the examination of asymptomatic men by blood test for prostate-specific antigen (PSA). Raised levels of PSA are not a very reliable indicator of cancer. This may be followed by a digital rectal examination to detect enlargement or change in the prostate gland. Those who have the disease may be offered prostatectomy or radiotherapy and those with advanced disease may have hormone manipulation therapy to slow or shrink the tumour. These interventions carry risks of increased pain and varying levels of incontinence or impotence. An increased level of testing may lead to a dilemma of whether to treat any cancer aggressively or to adopt a more conservative approach of 'wait and see'. Screening for prostate cancer does not therefore currently satisfy the basic criteria for screening – that testing will improve the prognosis of those with the disease, improve quality of life and that there is an effective treatment available.

Two large international trials into prostate cancer have contradictory conclusions:

The European Randomized Study of Screening for Prostate Cancer (ERSPC) studied 182,000 men aged between 50 and 74 and found that screening could cut deaths by 20% whilst the Prostate, Lung, Colorectal, and Ovarian (PLCO) cancer screening trial reported no benefit.

In 2001, the UK launched an 'informed choice' approach that included new information leaflets and DIPEx (database of individual patient experience). Yet critics argue that the provision of written information to ensure that patients can make informed choices is not sufficient. The information must be understood and framed in such a way that does not suggest there is a right or wrong choice.

Donovan et al (2001) cite several studies that show that decision aids such as videos result in higher levels of knowledge but have varying effects on the decisions themselves. They claim that at least 20 minutes are needed to provide accurate and understandable information. They also raise the problem of communicating risk to the public, arguing that 'strong statements' are needed to explain the uncertainties of the benefits of early detection and treatment of localized prostate cancer.

Sources: http://www.prostatecancercharity.org.uk, http://www.menshealthforum.org.uk, http://www. cancerresearchuk.org, Department of Health (DH) (2000c) The national prostate cancer plan. London, NHS Executive breast and cervical cancer highlight several issues about successful screening programmes in relation to the key principles outlined above. The first of these is whether there is evidence that it reduces mortality. Breast cancer is the largest cause of death in women aged under 65 and accounts for around 12,000 deaths each year (ONS 2009). A number of trials were established to assess the effectiveness of a breast screening programme. The Forrest report in 1986 concluded that there was a case for mammography screening for women aged 50–64 and in 2008 for women aged 47–73. The programme started in 1988, centrally funded and with national quality assurance mechanisms. However, the contribution of screening programmes to any reduction in mortality is constantly questioned. The age-standardized death rate from breast cancer has fallen dramatically from around 42 per 100,000 in 1990 to 27 per 100,000 in 2007. Some studies attribute this to the screening programme but as national coverage was not achieved until 1993 it is likely that the fall is due to improved treatment. An updated Cochrane review (Gøtzsche and Nielsen 2009) concluded there was little evidence from large randomized trials to support mammography programmes.

Screening is not a cost-free activity. There is a delicate balance between detecting all with the disease while protecting those without the disease from false alarms and unnecessary invasive procedures (see Table 10.1).

 Box 10.5 **Discussion point**

What information should be provided about breast cancer screening?

The UK leaflet has the authoritative title 'Breast screening: the facts', which suggests the information can be trusted. An analysis of information given to women in six countries showed that the important harms of screening (over-diagnosis and over-treatment of healthy women) were not mentioned (Gøtzsche et al 2009).

Table 10.1 Benefits and disadvantages of screening

Benefits	Disadvantages
Improved prognosis for some detected individuals	Over-treatment of insignificant or minor abnormalities, for example lumpectomy
Less radical treatment	Expensive
Reassurance for those with negative results	False reassurance for those with false-negative results. Anxiety or unnecessary treatment for those with false-positive results. Problems arising from the screening test itself

Source: Adapted from Chamberlain (1984).

A key principle of screening is that the costs of testing, diagnosis and treatment should be balanced in relation to expenditure on care as a whole. The breast cancer screening programme was estimated to cost £8638 per life saved when it was set up (Clarke and Fraser 1991). Professor Michael Baum, a key figure in the setting up of the breast screening programme, has called for it to be scrapped, arguing that far more attention should be given to more effective treatment for those showing symptoms (Baum 1999).

Particular emphasis is placed on achieving high uptake rates of screening. For example, general practices receive an incentive payment for cervical smears achieved for more than 80% of their eligible female population. Emphasis has been placed in the breast screening programme on systems that reduce the length of time that a woman has to wait for further tests or treatment (all urgent GP referrals should be seen within 14 days).

Another principle of screening is that the test should be socially and ethically acceptable and benefits should outweigh any physical or psychological harm that might arise from testing.

Chlamydia is a common but asymptomatic sexually transmitted infection (STI). Opportunistic screening

Box 10.6 **Discussion point**

What health promotion interventions might improve the wide-scale adoption of cervical screening?

- Targeting those never screened through careful checking of patient records and the Prior Notification List.
- Invitation telephone calls and counselling.
- Improving acceptability of the procedure through better health education information.
- More sensitivity to social and cultural factors.
- Opportunistic screening.
- Patient rewards and incentives.
- Letter from a celebrity.

for those less than 25 years of age is offered in the UK. Studies show (Pavlin et al 2006) the following barriers to uptake:

- ignorance and inaccurate information
- stigma arising from its association as an STI
- fear and anxiety about infertility
- anxiety about partner notification
- discomfort with sample collection.

It is apparent that achieving good coverage of a national screening programme depends on understanding the psychological factors that may influence attendance and ensuring the accessibility and acceptability of the programme itself. Certain groups – working-class women, lesbians and ethnic minorities – are much less likely to attend for either mammography or a smear test.

Immunization

Immunization has been a key strategy in the decline of infectious diseases over the last 100 years and one objective of the Alma Ata declaration (WHO 1978) was to immunize the populations of the world against the majority of infectious diseases. Vaccination works by introducing a small amount of the organism to stimulate the body's immune system to produce antibodies against that disease, resulting in immunity. The aim is to protect the individual against serious disease and to protect the community as a whole (herd immunity) – when members of a community who are not immune to a disease are still protected from it provided sufficient numbers of people in that community are immune. Achieving a high degree of herd immunity (e.g. for measles, 90% of the population needs to be immunized, see http://www.immunisation.nhs.uk) means that unprotected individuals are less likely to encounter the disease, and therefore both immunized and unimmunized individuals are protected.

The success of vaccination programmes against a disease such as smallpox (declared eradicated by WHO) has meant that the introduction of other vaccinations such as influenza or meningitis has been less questioned. However, vaccines have been blamed for adverse health effects. For example, the whooping cough vaccine was linked to brain damage and in the late 1990s a major controversy arose in the UK over the MMR vaccine and a supposed link to autism and Crohn's disease. Public confidence in vaccine safety dropped and MMR uptake fell to 55% in some parts of London (see www.hpa.org.uk).

Box 10.7 **Discussion point**

Should the UK introduce compulsory vaccination?

This concern led to the highlighting of major ethical concerns about immunization programmes. In June 2003 a High Court judge ruled that two girls aged 4 and 10 should be given the MMR vaccination according to their father's wishes and overruling their mother's objections. The judge's decision was not a move to compulsory vaccination but was made in the interest of the children, to which the separated parents could not agree.

Refusing polio vaccination is illegal in Belgium. Vaccination is a condition of school entry in the USA. In this way, individual freedom is curtailed to safeguard population health and all are exposed to the same risks and contribute to the herd immunity.

Of course, the counter-argument is that if there are reasonable grounds for doubt about vaccine safety, individuals should have the right to make their own competent and informed judgement. The challenge for practitioners is how they can enable parents to make informed decisions. The linking of doctors' payments to the number of children immunized may lead to a lack of trust by parents that any advice offered is disinterested.

There are many reasons in addition to current concerns about vaccine safety that explain why individuals may not be vaccinated and these are common to a range of diseases:

- low levels of knowledge about the disease, for example 17% of men who have sex with men do not know that hepatitis means inflammation of the liver and 25% do not know of the existence of a vaccine (Hickson et al 1999)
- low levels of perceived susceptibility
- lack of information about the vaccination process
- lack of understanding how general population risks apply to the individual.

Vaccination against the human papillomavirus (HPV) associated with cervical cancer and genital warts started in the UK in 2008. The vaccine is prophylactic and therefore given in pre-adolescence to girls aged 12 or 13 years. Initial studies of reaction to the programme reveal the main concern of young women to be the vaccination process itself. Those who refused to have their daughters vaccinated were mostly active refusers on the grounds of safety and efficacy (Stretch et al 2008).

Different approaches have been taken to facilitate vaccination uptake including:

- social marketing campaigns promoting vaccination
- health care environments that enable disclosure and full discussion of risk assessment
- use of peer educators.

 Box 10.8 **Discussion point**

How should practitioners communicate risk when discussing immunizations?

Practitioners may find it challenging to negotiate the tension between meeting imposed targets and addressing clients' worries which may have been fuelled by negative media coverage. Arguments about the need to achieve a certain level of herd immunity are unlikely to persuade individual parents.

The prevention of CHD and stroke

 Box 10.9 **The scale of coronary heart disease and stroke**

- CVD is responsible for almost 17 million deaths each year worldwide, and is a major cause of mortality. Nearly 80% of CVD diseases mortality occurs in developing countries.
- Heart and circulatory disease is the UK's biggest killer, causing 39% of deaths in the UK.
- The death rate from CHD continues to fall significantly (for people less than 65 years, they have fallen by 45% in the last decade) but not as fast as in some countries (it fell by 49% in Denmark and 45% in Norway and Austria). Among developed countries only Finland and Ireland have higher death rates from CHD than the UK.
- There are over one million prescriptions of cholesterol-lowering drugs – statins – dispensed in England every month and these now cost the NHS more than any other class of drug with over £440 million spent in 2001 (an increase of £113 million since 2000).
- Around 40% of men and women have raised blood pressure. The Interheart study estimated that 22% of heart attacks in Western Europe were due to a history of high blood pressure.
- Mortality from CHD is around 60% higher in smokers. Exposure to second-hand smoke increases the risk of CHD by around 25%.
- Thirty per cent of CHD and 20% of stroke is estimated to be due to low fruit and vegetable consumption.

Box 10.9 **The scale of coronary heart disease and stroke—cont'd**

- Work stress, lack of social support depression and hostile personality are consistently associated with CHD.
- Sixty-three per cent of heart attacks in Western Europe are estimated to be due to abdominal obesity (a high waist to hip ratio).

Source: World Health Report (2002), British Heart Foundation G30 Coronary Heart Disease Statistics for the UK 2008/09 at http://www.bhf.org.uk
World Health Report (2002)

Cardiovascular diseases, including CHD or ischaemic heart disease and cerebrovascular disease (stroke) and its precursors hypertension (high blood pressure) and angina, are common in the general population. CVD is the second most commonly reported longstanding illness in the UK (after musculoskeletal conditions) (ONS 2008). Registrations from the Quality and Outcomes Framework (QoF) of general practice suggests there are over 1.1 million men living with angina and around 970,000 who have had a heart attack. In 2006, nearly 28% of the UK population reported a cardiovascular condition.

CHD is the most common cause of premature death in the UK. It is often thought of as a disease of affluence – the result of a diet high in fat, excessive alcohol and executive stress. In fact, CHD, like most other diseases, is most common in deprived communities; death rates from CHD among unskilled men are three times higher than among professional men, due partly to higher smoking rates (Acheson 1998).

The National Service Framework (NSF) (DH 2000a) identifies three levels of prevention:
- reducing heart disease in the population as a whole, through reduction in the prevalence of risk factors
- prevention of CHD in high-risk patients in primary care
- secondary prevention to reduce the risk of subsequent cardiac problems in patients admitted to hospital with CHD.

Whilst there is recognition of the broader determinants of CHD, most interventions are underpinned by an individual behaviour change model of health promotion. There is an implicit assumption that it is lifestyle changes that will bring about a reduction in CHD, and the NSF CHD (DH 2000a) focuses specifically on smoking, physical activity and diet as modifiable risk factors.

Box 10.10 **Discussion point**

What are the main difficulties in taking a risk factor approach to the prevention of CHD?

As we have seen earlier, primary prevention can be developed in two ways: by using a whole population approach or through selective targeting of individuals deemed to be at higher risk. Large-scale studies in the mid-1990s looked at the effectiveness of routine screening and lifestyle advice in primary care consultations by practice nurses (British Family Heart Study, Wood et al (1994), and OXCHECK study) and concluded that such preventive checks were of little benefit. The NSF CHD requires that all practices have a systematic approach of identifying those at high risk using an appropriate protocol that would include smoking status, physical activity, body mass index, blood pressure, serum cholesterol and diabetes/plasma glucose. Those with high risk according to such indicators would then be offered tailored advice on how to reduce their risks.

In 2008, the government launched the NHS Health Check, a scheme described as 'predict and prevent', to screen everyone aged between 40 and 74 for vascular risk every 5 years.

Box 10.11 **Discussion point**

The Prime Minister's speech on the 60th anniversary of the NHS (7 January 2008) announced the intention to shift the focus of the NHS towards 'empowering patients and preventing illness'. To what extent is the NHS Health Check programme empowering?

In Chapter 12, we discuss the targeting of population groups for health promotion interventions and how this may mean a focus on lifestyle factors to the exclusion of basic structural factors such as education and income. Chapter 9 discusses how successful health promotion means tackling the broader determinants of health, and Chapter 11 examines approaches to changing lifestyles and behaviour and notes that lifestyle changes depend on more than information provision alone.

Box 10.12 **Example**

Targeting South Asians for CHD prevention

It is a public health conundrum why the death rate from heart disease amongst South Asian men is 38% higher, and amongst women 43% higher, than for the general population. South Asians are a heterogeneous group, yet most studies of CHD treat Bangladeshis, Indians and Pakistanis as a single group. Indians probably have less CHD than Bangladeshis and Pakistanis. The risk factors for CHD are common in South Asians:

- South Asian men smoke more than the general population. Forty-two per cent of Bangladeshi men are smokers (compared to 29% in the general population). One-fifth of Bangladeshi men and a quarter of women chew tobacco.
- Bangladeshi and Pakistani communities eat the least fruit and vegetables of all ethnic groups. Only 15% of Bangladeshi men and 16% of women consume fruit six or more times a week. Only 7% of Pakistani men and 11% of women eat vegetables on 6 or more days a week.
- South Asian men and women are less likely to participate in physical activity than the general population. Only 18% of Bangladeshi men and 7% of Bangladeshi women meet the current recommended physical activity levels (30 min of brisk walking, cycling or swimming at least five times each week).

- The prevalence of diagnosed diabetes is up to five times that of the general population in Pakistani and Bangladeshi men and women (diabetes increases the likelihood of developing CHD by around three times).

Source: British Heart Foundation (http://www.bhf.org.uk/professionals) Bhopal 2007

Whilst individually oriented programmes can help people choose healthier lifestyles, a more effective approach is to introduce community- or society-wide interventions, including health-promoting policies, that change the social determinants of health.

Cancer

Box 10.13 **The scale of cancers in England**

- There are 200,000 new cases of cancer each year.
- Each year 18,000 men and 10,000 women die of lung cancer, approximately 25% of all cancer deaths.
- Each year 11,000 women die of breast cancer, approximately 30% of all cancer deaths in women. Survival rates are lower than in the USA and lower than the average in the European Union.
- Each year 14,000 people die of colorectal cancer, approximately 10% of cancer deaths.
- Death rates from some cancers are improving – the death rate from testicular cancer has fallen by 75% in the last 20 years.
- More than 25% of all deaths from cancer, including 90% of lung cancer deaths are linked to tobacco smoking (Peto et al 2006).

Source: ONS (2006), WMPHO (2002)

The increase in the incidence of cancers worldwide has been thought to be the product of extended lifespans achieved as a result of the decline in infectious diseases. This is only partly true. While the incidence of cancers increases with age, most cases are associated with poverty, disadvantage and deprivation. For example, unskilled workers are twice as likely to die from cancer as professionals are. In part, this reflects a higher incidence of risk factors such as smoking (linked to one quarter of cancer deaths) and low consumption of fruit and vegetables. Survival rates are also lower in deprived areas, in part reflecting difficulties in gaining access to services and poorer service provision in such areas (Comptroller and Auditor General Report 2005).

Cancer, despite being a dreaded disease, is now also seen as a preventable one in many cases. The NHS Cancer Plan (DH 2000b), for example, has a chapter on improving prevention. This focuses on primary prevention (health education and support for behaviour changes particularly in relation to smoking and fruit and vegetable consumption) and secondary prevention (early detection and treatment of pre-cancerous cell changes through the national breast and cervical screening programmes and the possible development of programmes for colorectal, prostate and ovarian cancers). Environmental pollution, exposure to toxic materials such as chemical dyes or asbestos and changes in the quality of food especially linked to the use of pesticides have all been linked to cancer but receive little attention in cancer prevention interventions (Figure 10.1).

Skin cancer is an example of a cancer whose incidence has risen steadily. Intense exposure to sunlight, especially in childhood, is the main cause of deaths. Wealthy lifestyles, with holidays abroad, mean that affluent people are more likely to be at risk, and skin cancer is one of the few cancers that shows rising incidence with rising socio-economic status. However, cheaper holidays overseas, and greater likelihood of outdoor work, mean that lower-income groups, who tend to be less knowledgeable about the risks of skin cancer, are also at risk. Climate change and ozone depletion are likely to play an increasing role in the incidence of skin cancer, due to the time lag of 10–30 years in the development of the condition.

 Box 10.14 **Discussion point**

What elements would you include in a skin cancer prevention programme?

Tackling skin cancer illustrates the main approaches to cancer prevention:
- raising awareness
- environmental measures
- early detection.

In England, the 'Sun Know How' programme, based on the Australian Sunsmart campaign in the State of Victoria, ran from 1994 to 2000. Australia has now recorded a downturn in melanoma mortality rates (see http://www.aihw.gov.au). Raising awareness has been

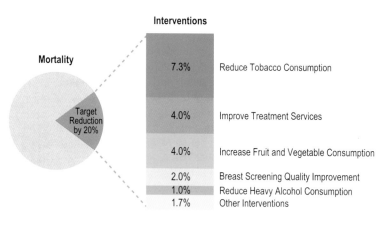

Figure 10.1 ● Improvements in cancer mortality from specific interventions.
Source: Adapted from DH (2001b).

Interventions

Mortality

Target Reduction by 20%

7.3%	Reduce Tobacco Consumption
4.0%	Improve Treatment Services
4.0%	Increase Fruit and Vegetable Consumption
2.0%	Breast Screening Quality Improvement
1.0%	Reduce Heavy Alcohol Consumption
1.7%	Other Interventions

largely achieved through mass media programmes and cues to sun protection such as routinely including UV forecasts in weather reports. Three key actions to halt the increased rates of skin cancer are to

- increase the number of people who are aware of their own skin cancer risk factors
- persuade everyone, and especially people at high risk, to avoid excessive exposure to the sun and artificial sun lamps through the adoption of appropriate sun protection and sun safe behaviour (the 'Slip Slap Slop' campaign slogan referred to slipping on shirts, slapping on hats and slopping on sun protection cream)
- alter people's attitude to a tanned appearance. (see www.who.int/uv/sun_protection/en/)

The challenge for health promoters is that the message to reduce exposure to sunlight is at odds with the lay epidemiology and health beliefs and the behaviour of the public who believe that sunlight is beneficial (e.g. Stanton et al 2004). Whilst the focus of skin cancer prevention is on health education, attention has also been paid to environmental measures and enhancing access to shade is an important aspect of sun-safe policies, especially in schools. Unlike other health issues, such as tobacco and alcohol, where there are strong industries with anti-health interests, the associated vested interests of cosmetic and sunscreen manufacturers are keen to sign up to skin cancer prevention programmes and promote reinforcing messages.

Skin cancer screening illustrates many of the problems common to all screening programmes (see pp. 187–190). Checklists of indicators lack specificity and do not exclude benign lesions or lesions that may not have progressed to invasive cancer if left alone. Screening always attracts those individuals who are more health-conscious and least at risk. Nevertheless, screening programmes for skin cancer typically lead to earlier diagnosis and an increased percentage of skin tumours detected (HDA 2002).

Cancer is a condition that has attracted a great deal of scientific research. Cancer results from the interaction of many different variables, including genetic, behavioural and environmental factors. Yet cancer prevention programmes are skewed towards those that target individuals, and seek to increase knowledge, change behaviour and increase the uptake of screening services. As we have seen in this section, such an approach has limitations, and the potential of broader-based interventions that tackle some of the environmental factors linked to cancer is now being recognized and developed.

Accidents and undetermined injury

Box 10.15 **Discussion point**

The following have been identified as signs of malignant melanoma:

- a mole with three or more shades of brown or black
- an existing mole getting bigger or developing an irregular outline
- a new mole growing quickly
- a mole that becomes inflamed or develops a reddish edge or that starts bleeding, oozing or crusting, or starts to itch or becomes painful.

What problems might be associated with an effective skin cancer awareness campaign?

Box 10.16 **The scale of accidents in England**

- In England, 10,000 deaths each year are due to an accident.
- Unintentional injury is a leading cause of child death and is 13 times higher for children of unemployed parents compared to professional groups.
- Falls are a major cause of disability and the leading cause of injury mortality in people aged over 75.
- Assault is the second leading cause of hospital admissions for young males aged 15–24.

Box 10.16 **The scale of accidents in England—cont'd**

- Each year in England nearly 180 children die and almost 4800 are injured as pedestrians or cyclists. England has one of the worst records in Europe for child pedestrian deaths.
- One-third of all accidents to adults occur in the home. About half of all deaths among children below 5 years happen in the home.

Source: DH (1999a),
http://www.dcsf.gov.uk/everychildmatters/
safeguardingandsocialcare/safeguardingchildren/
stayingsafe/stayingsafe/, Edwards et al (2006)

Risk has become the critical, determining concept in constructing strategies aimed at reducing the major causes of mortality, including accidental injury. Epidemiological research shows that certain factors are associated with an increased risk of accidental injury, so preventive activity addresses itself to removing or controlling those risk factors. At a population level, planned interventions to remove or control risk factors can successfully reduce rates of accidental injury. However, risk factor analysis can never tell us where and when or whom a particular accident will strike, because risk relates to people's perceptions and behaviours as well as to environmental factors. The complex interplay between people's behaviour and the external environment defies accurate prediction. As a unique event, an accident remains unpredictable and, by implication, unavoidable.

Box 10.17 **Discussion point**

The basis of the national strategy on accidents is that they are predictable and therefore preventable. Do you agree?

Over the last 30 years, England has seen an overall downward trend in accidental deaths which can probably be attributed to successful preventive measures and to advances in emergency medical care in hospitals and at the scene of accidents.

Conventionally, accident prevention strategies are categorized as education, engineering or enforcement.

Box 10.18 **Discussion point**

What factors would you address in a campaign to reduce accidents in the home? What strategies would you use?

- *Education* involves raising awareness of hazards and how to avoid them. Examples include Junior Citizen schemes, Traffic Clubs and mass media campaigns, as well as more traditional methods of imparting advice and information, such as leaflets, posters and safety counselling, for example community nurses' safety advice and education.
- *Engineering* refers to technical measures to increase the safety of the environment or product redesign. For example, the provision of cycle paths and pedestrian crossings, child-resistant packaging of medicines, smoke alarms in social housing, the use of fireguards and air bags in cars.
- *Enforcement* is the use of legislation, regulations and standards to reduce accidents or control injury. For example, the compulsory wearing of seat belts or motorcycle helmets, compliance with building regulations, product-testing for conformity with safety standards, for example fire-resistant furniture coverings.

Box 10.19 **Discussion point**

How do you account for the pronounced inverse relationship between the accident mortality rate in childhood and social class? What health promotion interventions might be effective in reducing childhood accidents?

The common theme to emerge from reviews of effective interventions is that engineering and enforcement can be effective, but more evidence is needed about the effectiveness of educational interventions (Towner et al 2001).

Children from lower socio-economic groups are more exposed to hazardous environments than children from higher socio-economic groups. For example, a key determinant of injuries to child pedestrians is the number of roads they cross, and children of families in the lowest quarter of income cross 50% more roads than those of families in the highest quarter. Whilst accident prevention interventions may seek to modify environments, very few directly target social deprivation (Dowswell and Towner 2002).

There is a range of approaches to reduce inequalities and address the social determinants of health (see Chapter 9). In Table 10.2, Dowswell and Towner (2002) show how these may be employed to prevent injuries in house fires. Interventions that focus on environments tend to adopt a universal approach, and may even end up reinforcing inequalities by making safe environments even safer. As Green and Edwards (2008, p. 184) point out, 'strategies to achieve global targets may not be the same as those that will redress inequalities. Indeed efforts to reduce overall levels of risk can exacerbate gradients in inequality'. The other main approach, education and advice, implicitly views accident prevention as a matter of personal responsibility. Thus these types of interventions focus on pedestrian skills training, traffic clubs and cycling proficiency training.

Box 10.20 Activity

As a practitioner, what role do you think you can have in promoting these kinds of interventions?

The World Health Organization's *Targets for Health for All* challenged member states to use legislative, administrative and economic mechanisms to tackle a wide range of health issues, including accidents (WHO 1985). The *Ottawa Charter for Health Promotion* (WHO 1986) further reinforced the idea that health cannot be understood in isolation from social conditions and urged action to ensure safe products, public services and environments. Traffic-calming schemes, remedial highway engineering, child-resistant packaging of drugs, and the compulsory use of seat belts in cars and of helmets on motorcycles have all proved effective in reducing accidental death or injury (Towner et al 2001).

Most practitioners tend to see policy, legislative and enforcement approaches as remote from their everyday practice. There are exceptions – for example, environmental health officers have an enforcement role in relation to many aspects of the environment including food and water safety and

Table 10.2 The prevention of injuries in house fires

Strengthening individuals	Parent education on home hazards (knowledge/behaviour), child education on home hazards (knowledge/behaviour), education on developing escape plans (knowledge/behaviour), parent education on smoking (knowledge/behaviour), parent education on smoke alarms (knowledge/behaviour), installation and maintenance of smoke alarms (environmental change)
Strengthening neighbourhoods	Community-wide smoke alarm giveaway (environmental change), community-wide home inspections (environmental change)
Improving access to services	Developing professional knowledge/skills (knowledge/behaviour), strategies to improve the reach of health promotion activities targeting health promotion at those most at risk
Broad economic and cultural	Safe home design (environment/legislation), safe furniture design (environment/legislation), regulations on smoke alarms in all new/rented/other properties (environment/legislation)

Source: Dowswell and Towner (2002). Reproduced by permission of the authors and Oxford University Press.

occupational health and safety. Chapter 4 discusses in greater detail how practitioners can become involved in the lobbying process, and why an understanding of the policy process is vital to their health-promoting and health improvement work.

 Box 10.21 **Discussion point**

Why might it be important to understand lay explanations for the causes of accidents?

The popular definition of an accident is of an unpredictable chance event. Yet the incidence of accidents is patterned by socio-economic class, exposure to unsafe environments and hazards in the environment, as well as being linked to individual and group behaviours and attitudes. Successful accident prevention campaigns tend to focus on modifying environments, but winning over public opinion through educational campaigns is vital for building a consensus that allows further environmental modification via legislation, regulation or engineering to take place.

Reducing mental illness and promoting mental health

There is increasing recognition of the need to address mental health as an integral part of improving overall health and well-being, and to focus on prevention and promotion in mental health (WHO 2002).

 Box 10.22 **The scale of mental health problems in England**

- 1 in 6 adults have significant mental health problems.
- 2 in 3 children say they are often depressed.
- 1 in 7 older people over 65 has depression which is severe and persistent and affects day-to-day functioning.

- 40% of people who claim incapacity benefit have a mental health problem.
- Each year over 4000 people take their own lives.
- Suicide is the most common cause of death in men under 35.

Sources: UK foresight Project on Mental Capital and Wellbeing http://www.foresight.gov.uk, ONS (2007), http://www.mind.org.uk/information/factsheets/statistics

 Box 10.23 **Practitioner talking**

My role includes mental health promotion but in reality what I mainly do is target those at risk of mental illness such as young people who self-harm, or people with depression. It's frustrating because I am constantly picking up the damaged people instead of preventing the damage in the first place

Commentary

Most strategies to promote mental health have in fact focused on mental illness, being concerned with conditions such as anxiety, depression or schizophrenia. Much less consideration has been given to issues relating to well-being such as isolation, loneliness or low self-esteem. The social environment in which individuals and communities live, and which impacts on people's health behaviours, is an important influence on their mental health (DH 2001a).

 Box 10.24 **Activity**

How would you define mental health?

Mental health is often narrowly defined as the absence of mental illness, but mental health as a positive concept is complex and broad-ranging. Mental health is more than the absence of mental illness or distress. It includes emotional health, mental functioning, self-determination, positive personal relationships and resilience (to manage and cope with the stresses and challenges of life). Given the diversity of concepts of mental health, it is not surprising that definitions of mental health promotion vary widely. Mental health promotion is essentially concerned with:

- how individuals, families, organizations and communities think and feel
- the factors which influence how we think and feel, individually and collectively
- the impact that this has on overall health and well-being (Cattan and Tilford 2006; DH 2001a).

Current national UK strategy includes a target to reduce the death rate from suicide and undetermined injury by at least a fifth by 2010 (DH 1999b). The National Suicide Prevention Strategy (DH 2002b) sets out the ways in which this might be achieved. In addition, the National Service Framework Standard One states that health and social services should

- promote mental health for all, working with individuals and communities, and
- combat discrimination against individuals and groups with mental health problems, and promote their social inclusion (DH 1999b).

Box 10.25 Discussion point

Why might there be criticism of a target to reduce suicide rates as part of a mental health strategy?

Whilst there has been particular concern at the rising trend in suicides amongst young men and in rural communities, the social factors that might explain this trend are largely ignored and suicide is seen as a psychological phenomenon requiring interventions to assist the individual. The *National Suicide Prevention Strategy* for England (DH 2002b) focuses on targeting high-risk groups and reducing the opportunities for suicide. It identifies the following interventions:

- identifying mental illness and depression in primary and social care settings (50% of suicides have visited a doctor within a month of suicide and 25% during the week before death)
- assessment and support for those who have previously attempted suicide (people who have attempted suicide are at particular risk of another attempt in the first year)
- reducing access to methods of suicide, for example sale of paracetamol in blister packs, providing free helplines and environmental modification at suicide 'hot spots' such as bridges, increasing the use of catalytic convertors in cars.

Box 10.26 Discussion point

A target of the National Service Framework for Mental Health (DH 1999b) is to 'promote mental health for all'. What might be the implications of such a target for mental health strategies?

In Scotland, the suicide prevention strategy is called Choose Life and has included a national campaign 'Don't Hide It. Talk About It', which seeks to raise awareness of suicide.

The majority of mental health problems are managed within primary care and a high percentage of problems presented in primary care are psychosocial. Primary care therefore has a crucial role in promoting the mental well-being of people with mild or moderate levels of distress and managing those with severe or enduring mental health problems. A common response is to introduce training to identify early indicators of depression, but as Rogers et al (1996, p. 42) point out, 'despite the common assumption that GPs would be more effective if their psychiatric knowledge were increased and more emotional morbidity identified, from a service users' point of view ordinary relating and practical help may be more important'.

MacDonald and O'Hara's (1996) model (see Figure 10.2) suggests that mental health for all can be promoted by enhancing those factors above the dotted line and by tackling those factors below it. Psychological protective factors for mental well-being include

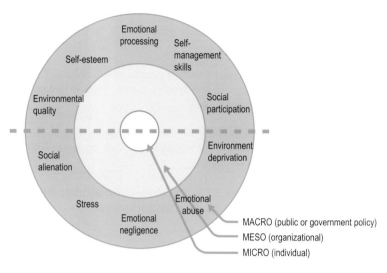

Figure 10.2 ● The elements of mental health promotion. Reprinted from Journal of Counselling and Development 72(2):115–123. ACA. Reprinted with permission. No further reproduction authorized without written permission of the American Counseling Association.

- feeling respected
- feeling valued and supported
- a feeling of hopefulness about the future.

Another important feature is the emphasis on three levels of action beyond the personal level:
1. *Micro* – the individual.

2. *Meso* – groupings such as the family, workplace, peer groups, community groups and small neighbourhoods.

3. *Macro* – wider, larger systems that govern and shape many aspects of our lives such as government (local and national), large and influential companies and organizations like formal religions.

Interventions to strengthen protective factors thus need to take place at all levels and may include:
- *Micro* – strengthening psychosocial, life and coping skills of individuals through, for example, user empowerment, cognitive behaviour therapy, stress, anxiety or anger management, exercise.
- *Meso* – increasing social support as a buffer against adverse life events and reinforcing ways in which people can cooperate together, for example self-help and user-led initiatives, drop-in centres for young people, family and parenting groups.

- *Macro* – increasing access to resources and services which protect mental well-being, for example employment and training opportunities, making mental health services more appropriate and accessible, anti-discrimination strategies.

The comprehensive nature of a programme to reduce the burden of mental illness and unlock the benefits of well-being in terms of physical health, educational attainment, employment and reduced crime is recognised in the 'New Horizons' initiative (DH 2010).

Antonovsky (1987) described people's ability to cope positively with stressful events as a 'Sense of Coherence'. Those with a stronger sense of coherence have what Antonovsky terms 'generalized resistance resources', which include individual skills, social support and good social relationships, cultural stability and money. People with a strong sense of coherence share the following characteristics (Table 10.3):
- better able to understand and explain the origins of their stress (comprehensibility)
- wish to address the stresses and respond proactively (meaningfulness)
- feel that they are able to respond effectively (manageability).

The National Institute for Mental Health (2003) found that the level of mental health problems in children and young people is determined by low household income,

Table 10.3 The sense of coherence

Anna (high SOC)	Barbara (low SOC)
– Discusses with family and friends what is happening in her life and identifies work pressures as stressful	– Is so involved in coping with her stressful job that she hasn't identified its stress-inducing features. Blames herself for feeling tired and irritable all the time
– Is motivated to tackle her stressful job in order to cope with it and avoid 'stress leakage' into other areas of her life	– Believes there is nothing she can do to change her job; that this is the way things are and she is lucky to have a job. All she can do is try to cope and get on with it
– Is confident that she can have an effect on stressful aspects of her work. Recognizes repeating and unhelpful patterns of behaviour. Has in the past made changes to aspects of her life and circumstances (e.g. moved away from her home town)	– Is lacking confidence that anything she can do will affect stress levels but hopes that something will turn up in the future

Reprinted from Antonovsky (1993), Copyright 1993, with permission from Elsevier.

coming from a lone-parent household, being in institutional care and poor school performance. School is therefore a vital setting for promoting the mental health of children. Poor achievement and school performance are risk factors for conduct problems, involvement in crime and substance use (see http://www.nelh.nhs.uk/nsf/mentalhealth/whatworks/knowhow/schools-evidence.htm). The Welsh Mental Health Promotion Network (http://www.publicmentalhealth.org) identifies anti-bullying schemes, the promotion of life skills and self-esteem through mentioning as effective strategies.

In common with strategies tackling other major causes of mortality and morbidity, the focus of mental health promotion has been to target high-risk groups rather than adopting population-based approaches. Young Black, Asian and minority ethnic (BAME) groups men are more at risk of developing mental health problems than their white counterparts. Socio-economic factors such as unemployment, deprivation and racism may contribute to this. There are also cultural differences in the way in which psychological distress is presented, perceived and interpreted and different cultures may develop different responses for coping with psychological distress.

 Box 10.27 **Example**

Evidence of effective mental health promotion interventions among older people

Tackling risk factors:
- home-based support and home visiting
- exercise and music
- reminiscence
- carers' support
- volunteering
- lifelong learning.

Environmental and policy interventions to improve quality of life:
- transport options
- traffic calming to increase pedestrian activity
- housing adaptation
- retirement planning
- planning policy that includes meeting places.

(Cattan and Tilford 2006)

Promoting mental health and reducing mental illness is a complex task, not least because of the multiple meanings of mental health. One response, illustrated by national targets, is to target the most extreme manifestations of mental illness, such as suicide. Well-being is an increasingly widespread concept which includes life satisfaction, realization of potential, resilience and happiness.

Based on Layard's (2006) work on the relationship between the economy and happiness, the New Economics Foundation well-being project (http://www.neweconomics.org) suggests five evidence-based ways to well-being:

1. Connect (social relationships are critical to well-being).

2. Be active (exercise increases mood and protects against cognitive decline).

3. Take notice (awareness of thoughts and feelings can improve well-being).

4. Keep learning (learning encourages social interaction and increases self-esteem).

5. Give (reciprocity and mutual exchange increases social capital and resilient communities).

An alternative, diffuse and longer-term strategy is to promote positive mental health and well-being through programmes aimed at enhancing people's self-esteem and personal relationships. The relationship between the organization of society and the mental health and well-being of the population is interdependent. Strategies to promote mental health and reduce mental illness must therefore take place at all levels: the modification of environments and products, adapting service provision to enhance sensitivity and hence access, community empowerment programmes that build and facilitate social networking and support, and education and skills training for both practitioners and the public. There is also a role for investing in social determinants that promote mental health and well-being, such as employment and good housing.

HIV and AIDS

 Box 10.28 **The scale of HIV and AIDS**

- The increase in HIV/AIDS worldwide has been of epidemic proportions. By the end of 2003 an estimated 34.6–42.3 million people worldwide were living with HIV infection and more than 20 million had died of AIDS.

- Two-thirds of HIV cases occur in Africa, with one-fifth in Asia.

- Since 2000, the global incidence of people living with HIV has stabilized at around 33 million. In sub-Saharan Africa, the rate of HIV has begun to decline, although it is still rising elsewhere.

- Cases of HIV rose sharply between 1999 and 2003 in the UK, although the number of people with AIDS and deaths from AIDS has remained stable and less than the peak in the mid-1990s, largely due to the use of HAART (highly active antiretroviral therapy).

- By the end of 2008, a total of 102,333 diagnoses of HIV in the UK had been reported, with 7370 new cases confirmed in 2008.

- The three main routes of infection are men who have sex with men (44,537 cases); unprotected heterosexual sex, 80% of which are contracted abroad in countries with high rates of HIV (44,617 cases); and injecting drug users (4997 cases).

- In 2001, 0.5% of pregnant women delivering in London were infected with HIV. Eighty-seven per cent of HIV-infected pregnant women were diagnosed before they gave birth.

Sources: Steinbrook (2004), UNAIDS (2008), http://www.avert.org/uk-statistics.htm, http://www.hpa.org.uk

The scale of HIV in the UK is minimal compared to infection rates in Africa or Asia. An estimated 28.5 million people are infected with HIV in sub-Saharan Africa and 11 million children are orphaned by AIDS.

The *Health of the Nation: a strategy for health in England* (DH 1992) identified HIV/AIDS and sexual health as one of five priority areas: a decade later the number of cases had increased. Changes in sexual behaviour over the past 10 years (decrease in the age of first intercourse, increase in lifetime and number of concurrent partners, and decrease in safer sex practices among homosexual men) are likely to further increase infection rates (Second National Study of Sexual Behaviour and Lifestyles, NATSAL II (Erens et al 2001). Other factors including HIV testing, health service utilization and vertical (mother to child) transmission also influence the spread of the disease. The aims of the sexual health and HIV strategy for England (DH 2001c) are to

- reduce transmission of HIV and STIs
- reduce prevalence of undiagnosed HIV and STIs
- reduce unintended pregnancy
- improve health and social care for people living with HIV
- reduce the stigma associated with HIV and STIs.

In common with the other major causes of mortality and morbidity discussed in this chapter, HIV prevention work has targeted risk behaviours and target populations deemed at highest risk:

- *Risk behaviours*
  - increasing the use of condoms
  - recommending a reduction in the number of partners and the number of concurrent partners
  - encouraging intercourse with people of the same HIV sero-status.
- *Risk groups*
  - men who have sex with men (MSM)
  - injecting drug users
  - African communities
  - sex workers
  - prisoners.

Chapter 12 discusses how the categorization of groups into 'high risk' or 'low risk' is often an over-simplification and can lead to a focus on already marginalized groups. Roughly one-third of new HIV infections outside of sub-Saharan Africa arise from needle sharing amongst drug users (UNAIDS 2009); yet this group is the most marginalized, with little recognition or protection from discrimination.

Interventions to reduce the spread of HIV can be categorized into those which seek to

- reduce the risk of infection through information and education about safer sex
- reduce the risk of infection by increasing condom use
- reduce the number of sexual partners and increase safer sex practices through voluntary testing and counselling
- empower people through developing self-esteem and assertiveness skills so that they can negotiate safer sex
- strengthen particular communities (e.g. the gay community) so that safer sex norms, values and behaviours become accepted
- improve treatment for STIs which are thought to increase vulnerability to HIV infection.

Addressing risk behaviours may take place at different levels: individual, group, community or socio-political. Tackling social determinants of sexual health and ill health includes the use of legislation and policy, for example age of consent for gay sex, sex education in schools; and ensuring that there is good access to appropriate information and services, for example provision and labelling of condoms including those for anal sex, provision of accessible services, advice and treatment for STIs. In the USA, for example, programmes that emphasize abstinence till marriage are said to marginalize homosexuality, making unprotected sex more likely. Community-based interventions have been successful in creating peer norms and support favouring safer sex and providing information or skills. In 1992, Rooney and Scott (1992, p. 51) commented that 'The history of the last decade shows that there is a clear correlation between the widespread adoption of safer sex and the existence of a confident and supportive gay affirmative culture providing grassroots community education'. The attachment by gay men to an organized gay community is still one of the most significant factors in maintaining safer sex behaviour.

Box 10.29 **Example**

GMFA, the gay men's health charity

Gay Men Fighting AIDS (GMFA) was founded in 1992 in London to undertake HIV prevention work targeted at gay men. In 2001 GMFA merged with Big Up, the BAME groups gay men's group, and in 2002 extended its remit to include all health issues which particularly impact on gay men. Its mission statement is 'improving gay men's health by increasing the control they have over their own lives', and its guiding principles include empowerment, equity, fairness, and being evidence-based and effective. GMFA is a volunteer-led organization and works in partnership with a range of health and local authority services including genito-urinary medicine (GUM) clinics, community groups and private sector organizations in the gay commercial scene.

Source: http://www.gmfa.org.uk/aboutgmfa/about-us/index accessed 13/7/09

Many interventions which seek to effect behavioural change at the individual level have been shown to increase knowledge but have had little effect on attitudes and behaviour, partly because perceptions of risk are low, especially amongst heterosexuals. Instead, interventions need to address the personal and structural factors that give rise to risk behaviours such as:

- association of condoms with promiscuity or lack of trust
- lack of skills in using condoms or negotiating safer sex
- availability of resources such as condoms or sexual health services
- opinions of peers
- attitudes of society which affect access to services
- poverty, migrant labour and disempowerment of women in poorer countries.

Reducing the rate of HIV/AIDS has been prioritized as a health target, although there are problems with addressing HIV/AIDS separately from sexual health in general. Chapter 11 includes a section looking at sexual behaviour as both a health risk and a health-promoting factor. The narrower focus on HIV/AIDS discussed in this section has been linked to a variety of strategies, including legislative, community development, service development including screening services, and individual education and advice.

Conclusion

This chapter has examined the four priority areas identified in the Our Healthier Nation strategy (DH 1999a) and the additional priority of HIV/AIDS, separately identified in the National Sexual Health and HIV strategy (DH 2001c). These issues represent a large burden of preventable disease and premature death; evidence exists of effective interventions and it is possible to set targets and monitor progress. Despite the recognition (reflected in Part 3 of this book) that a focus on diseases ignores the prerequisites for health such as adequate income, housing and employment and the needs of marginalized or vulnerable population groups, national health strategy has focused on the major causes of mortality and morbidity.

The sections in this chapter illustrate some of the challenges for practitioners in reaching the targets set for disease reduction. Cardiovascular disease, cancers and HIV/AIDS, for example, are diseases that are known to be linked to certain risk factors, some of which are modifiable by individual behaviour change. The key debate for practitioners is the nature of the identified risk factors and the relative emphasis on lifestyle versus structural changes. Accidents constitute a major cause of mortality, but in this case, the notion of risk is debated and contested. Policy interventions have been shown to be most effective in reducing accidental injuries and yet this is an aspect of practice in which practitioners feel least able to effect change (see Chapter 4). By contrast, the key area of mental health poses immediate problems of definition and illustrates the way in which a focus on positive health can be skewed by a disease reduction target.

The sections in this chapter illustrate some of the challenges for practitioners in reaching the targets set for disease reduction. Four main approaches have been discussed:

- whole population health screening and immunization
- individually focused education, advice and counselling to change individual risk factors
- community development approaches to change risk factors relating to norms, beliefs and practices
- environmental modification through legislation and policy.

Health practitioners will probably feel most at ease with the first and second of these approaches, and examples have been given of effective strategies adopting these approaches. Lifestyle approaches are discussed further in Chapter 11. Screening and immunization, discussed earlier in this chapter, remain significant although contested strategies in the drive to reduce major diseases. As health service interventions they are subject to the inverse care law, and tend to be adopted most by those groups at least risk.

Further discussion

- How do the key priority areas in this chapter illustrate the importance of partnership working?

- How appropriate is it to tackle disease reduction in these priority areas through a focus on individual risk factors?

- What can be learned from the examples in this chapter about the strengths and limitations of national screening programmes?

- What are the advantages and disadvantages of medically defined prevention targets?

Recommended reading

- Donaldson LJ, Donaldson RJ: *Essential public health*, edn 3, Oxford, 2009, Radcliffe Press.
- Pencheon D, Melzer D, Muir Gray JA, et al, editors: *Oxford handbook of public health practice*, edn 2, Oxford, 2006, Oxford University Press.
- Detels R, McEwen J, Beaglehole R, et al, editors: *Oxford textbook of public health*, edn 5, Oxford, 2009, Oxford University Press.

These textbooks examine public health issues and how they can be prevented and controlled as well as how to prioritize health issues, how to identify cost-effective strategies and how to mobilize the community through community involvement. The message of all three texts is that a comprehensive rather than an issue/disease-oriented approach is necessary for public health problems.

- Ewles L, editor: *Key topics in public health: essential briefings on prevention and health promotion*, London, 2005, Elsevier.

An accessible text that provides basic information on key issues and how they are tackled at community and individual levels.

References

Acheson D: *Independent inquiry into inequalities in health*, London, 1998, The Stationery Office.

Antonovsky A: *Unravelling the mystery of health*, San Francisco, 1987, Jossey Bass.

Antonovsky A: The structure and properties of the sense of coherence scale, *Soc Sci Med* 36:725–733, 1993.

Baum M: Money may be better spent on asymptomatic women, *Br Med J* 318:398, 1999.

British Thoracic Society: Control and prevention of tuberculosis in the United Kingdom: code of practice 2000, *Thorax* 55:887–890, 2000.

Cattan M, Tilford S, editors: *Mental health promotion; a lifespan approach*, Maidenhead, 2006, McGraw Hill/Open University.

Chamberlain J: Which prescriptive screening programmes are worthwhile? *J Epidemiol Community Health* 38:270–277, 1984.

Clarke PR, Fraser NM: *Economic analysis of screening for breast cancer*, Edinburgh, 1991, Scottish Home and Health.

Comptroller & Auditor General Report: *Tackling cancer in England: saving more lives (HC 2003–04)*, London, 2005, The Stationery Office.

Department of Health (DH): *The health of the nation: a strategy for health in England*, London, 1992, DH.

Department of Health (DH): *Saving lives: our healthier nation*, London, 1999a, The Stationery Office.

Department of Health (DH): *The national service framework: mental health*, London, 1999b, The Stationery Office.

Department of Health (DH): *The national service framework: coronary heart disease*, London, 2000a, The Stationery Office.

Department of Health (DH): *The NHS cancer plan*, London, 2000b, The Stationery Office.

Department of Health (DH): *The national prostate cancer plan*, London, 2000c, NHS Executive.

Department of Health: *Making it happen: a guide to delivering mental health promotion*, London, 2001a, DH.

Department of Health: *National service framework: diabetes*, London, 2001b, The Stationery Office.

Department of Health (DH): *National strategy for sexual health and HIV*, London, 2001c, The Stationery Office.

Department of Health (DH): *Getting ahead of the curve: a strategy for combating infectious diseases*, London, 2002a, The Stationery Office.

Department of Health (DH): *National suicide prevention strategy*, London, 2002b, The Stationery Office.

Department of Health (DH): *New horizons: working together for better mental health*, London, 2010, DH.

Donovan JL, Frankel SJ, Neal DE, et al: Screening for prostate cancer in the UK, *Br Med J* 323:763–764, 2001.

Dowswell T, Towner E: Social deprivation and the prevention of unintentional injury in childhood: a systematic review, *Health Educ Res* 17(2):221–237, 2002.

Edwards P, Green J, Roberts I, et al: Deaths from injury in children and employment status in family: analysis of trends in class specific death rates, *Br Med J* 333:119–121, 2006.

Erens B, McManus S, Field J, et al: *National survey of sexual attitudes and lifestyles II*, London, 2001, National Centre for Social Research.

Gøtzsche PC, Hartling OJ, Nielsen M, et al: UK breast screening: the facts – or may be not? *BMJ* 338.b86, 2009.

Gøtzsche PC, Nielsen H: Screening for breast cancer with mammography, *Cochrane Database Syst Rev* 7(4):CD001877, 2006.

Green J, Edwards P: The limitations of targeting to address inequalities in health: a case study of road traffic injury prevention from the UK, *Crit Public Health* 18(2):175–187, 2008.

Health Development Agency (HDA): *Cancer prevention: a resource to support local action in delivering the NHS cancer plan*, London, 2002, Health Development Agency.

Hickson F, Weatherburn P, Reid D, et al: *Evidence for change – findings from the National Gay Men's Sex Survey 1998*, London, 1998, Sigma Research.

Layard R: *Happiness: Lessons from a new science*, Harmondsworth, 2006, Penguin.

MacDonald G, O'Hara K: *Ten elements of mental health, its promotion and demotion: implications for practice*, Birmingham, 1996, Society for Health Education/Promotion Specialists.

National Institute for Mental Health: *Inside outside: improving mental health services for Black and minority ethnic communities in England*, London, 2003, Department of Health.

Office for National Statistics (ONS): *Mortality statistics: cause. England and Wales 2007*, London, 2009, The Stationery Office.

ONS: *Mortality statistics for England and Wales 2005: cause series DH2, no 32*, London, 2006, ONS.

Pavlin NL, Gunn JM, Pacher R, et al: Implementing chlamydia screening: what do women think? A review of the literature, *BMC Public Health* 6(221):2006.

Peto R, Lopez AD, et al: *Mortality from smoking in developed countries 1950–2000*, edn 2, 2006 http:\\www.deathsfromsmoking.net.

Rogers A, Pilgrim D, Latham M: *Understanding and promoting mental health*, London, 1996, Health Education Authority.

Rooney M, Scott P: Working where the risks are: health promotion interventions for men who have sex with men. In Evans B, Sandberg S, Watson S, editors: *Working where the risks are: issues in HIV prevention*, London, 1992, Health Education Authority.

Rose G: *The strategy of preventive medicine*, Oxford, 1993, Oxford University Press.

Scottish Office: *Working together for a healthier Scotland*, London, 1998, The Stationery Office.

Stanton WR, Janda M, Baade PD, et al: Primary prevention of skin cancer; a review of sun protection in Australia & internationally, *Health Promot Int* 19(3):369–378, 2004.

Steinbrook R: The AIDS epidemic in 2004, *N Engl J Med* 351:115–117, 2004.

Stretch R, Roberts SA, McCann R, et al: Parental attitudes and information needs in an adolescent HPV Vaccination Programme, *Br J Cancer* 99:1908–1911, 2008.

Towner E, Dowswell T, Mackreth C, et al: *What works in preventing unintentional injuries in children and young adolescents? An updated systematic review*, London, 2001, Health Development Agency.

West Midlands Public Health Observatory: *West Midlands health issues: cancers*, Birmingham, 2002, WMPHO. (http://www.wmpho.org.uk).

Wilson JMG, Jungner G: *Principles and practice of screening for disease*, Geneva, 1968, WHO.

Wood DA, Kinmouth A, Pyke SDM, et al: Randomized controlled trial evaluating cardiovascular screening and intervention in general practice: principal results of British family heart study, *Br Med J* 308:313–320, 1994.

World Health Organization (WHO): Report on the international conference on primary health care, Alma Ata, 6–12 September, Geneva, 1978, WHO.

World Health Organization (WHO): *Targets for health for all*, Copenhagen, 1985, WHO.

World Health Organization (WHO): *Ottawa charter for health promotion*, Copenhagen, 1986, WHO.

World Health Organization (WHO): *Prevention and promotion of mental health. Department of Mental Health and Substance Dependence*, Geneva, 2002, WHO.

World Health Organization (WHO): *World health report–reducing risks, promoting healthy life*, Geneva, 2002, WHO.

World Health Organization (WHO): *Global burden of disease 2004 Update*, Geneva, 2008, WHO.

UNAIDS: *AIDS epidemic update*, Geneva, UNAIDS/WHO, http://data.unaids.org/pub/Report/2009/Jci700_Epi_Update_2009_en.pdf.

Chapter Eleven

Lifestyles and behaviours

- Social construction of risky behaviours and risk perception
- Tackling lifestyles and behaviours
    - Smoking
    - Diet
    - Exercise and physical activity
    - Alcohol and drug use
    - Sexual health

OVERVIEW

The shift in disease patterns in developed countries, from communicable diseases to chronic diseases, has highlighted the importance of lifestyles and behaviours as potential contributors to disease or health. Many practitioners see their role as giving information and advice about healthy lifestyles to their clients. Behavioural lifestyle choices, such as diet, exercise and the use of recreational drugs are major factors in determining health status. A single lifestyle behaviour, such as diet, can affect the likelihood of developing a range of conditions, including life-threatening illnesses such as cancers of the digestive system, severe chronic conditions such as diabetes and many more minor conditions such as irritable bowel syndrome and dental decay. It has therefore become a common strategy in public health and health promotion to target behaviours.

This approach aims to persuade people to change unhealthy behaviours and adopt health-promoting behaviours. Chapter 4 showed how neoliberal policies in many developed countries privilege individualist approaches and have favoured public health programmes that target healthy lifestyles rather than social determinants of healthy. This chapter explores approaches to behaviour change and their popularity and then goes on to examine in more depth five key areas where behaviours impact significantly on people's health – smoking, diet, exercise, drugs and alcohol use, and sexual behaviour.

Introduction

Certain behaviours have become labelled as 'risky behaviours' associated with negative health outcomes. Such behaviours include smoking, excessive use of alcohol and other recreational drugs, unsafe sex, poor diet (high fat and high sugar diet) and sedentary lifestyles. These have all been the subject of the UK national health strategies. Risky behaviours are often linked to a range of illnesses and conditions. For example, smoking is linked to lung cancer, coronary heart disease, chronic obstructive lung disease and asthma. Lifestyle risk behaviours have been associated with most of the common chronic diseases in developed countries. These conditions (e.g. diabetes, coronary heart disease and cancers) represent a significant disease burden and are very costly to manage and treat. The Coronary Heart Disease National Service Framework (NSF) (DH 2000a) highlighted the importance of tackling lifestyle behaviours as a means towards reducing the incidence of coronary heart disease. Funding for smoking cessation groups, local exercise action pilots (LEAPS) in deprived areas, a ban on advertising tobacco, and free fruit for primary school children were all introduced to support the coronary heart disease NSF.

As discussed in Chapter 10, most research into the prevention of risk factors for disease has focused on 'downstream' interventions that aim to affect the lifestyle and behaviour of individuals, rather than 'upstream' interventions such as policies that seek to influence the broader determinants of health. This has led to greater evidence for individually focused interventions than for social policy interventions. Targeting lifestyles has therefore been viewed as both an effective and an efficient strategy to promote health.

Targeting lifestyles has a long history: 'The way in which people live and the lifestyles they adopt can have profound effects on subsequent health. Health education initiatives should continue to ensure that individuals are able to exercise informed choice when selecting the lifestyles which they adopt' (DH 1992, p. 11). The lifestyles approach is popular because it is focused on individuals and can therefore be integrated into one-to-one contacts between practitioners and their clients. It also reinforces the popular concept of individual freedom and autonomy in lifestyle choices. However, it has also been criticized for taking behaviours out of their social context and ignoring the effect of structural constraints (such as income) and the regulatory context (e.g. banning smoking in public places) on behavioural choices.

The lifestyles approach also assumes that people make rational choices based on weighing up the pros and cons of adopting a specific behaviour, and this too has been criticized for failing to take into account custom, habit, identity and the meaning of behaviours within people's lives. Behavioural change models, such as the Stages of Change model, that assume individual autonomy and choice have been seen as unrealistic. These critiques of the behavioural change approach are discussed in greater detail in Chapter 11 of *Foundations for health promotion*, edn 3 (Naidoo and Wills 2009). Empowerment strategies that educate and enable people to take control over their health are discussed in Chapter 8 of this book.

The construction of certain behaviours as risky is, however, problematic. In particular, there is a gap between epidemiological and lay perceptions of risk. Epidemiological risks are scientifically calculated and presented as statistical probabilities. However, people interpret epidemiological risks within their own behavioural landscape, according to their own circumstances and priorities (Lupton 1999). For example, someone may have unsafe sex and underestimate the risks of so doing, because they want sex to be spontaneous and not negotiated, and because it is the norm amongst their peers.

Lupton (1995, p. 9) argues that risk has replaced the notion of sin. Taking risks is attributed to lack of will power and moral weakness and as a result people do not seek advice because they fear they will be 'told off'. Research suggests that health risk behaviours should not be perceived as 'wrong' lifestyle choices, but as rational coping strategies adopted in the context of the demands of caring and the constraints of poverty (Graham 2003). People have very different constructions of risk, and people's personal 'landscapes of risk' vary according to their social situation and status. For example, smoking is a high-risk behaviour but its risk may be downplayed and offset against its positive role, for example as a stress management and coping tool, within people's lives. In this way, epidemiological risk factors such as smoking or poor diet may be overridden by more immediate risks and more urgent problems. The link between unhealthy lifestyles and poverty has been recognized in official government documents:

The key lifestyle risk factors, shared by coronary heart disease and stroke, are smoking, poor nutrition, obesity, physical inactivity and high blood pressure. Excess alcohol intake is an important additional risk factor for stroke. Many of these risk factors are unevenly spread across society, with poorer people often exposed to the highest risks.
DH (1999, p. 74)

 Box 11.1 **Activity**

Do you engage in any behaviour that might be deemed to carry a risk? (If yes) How do you justify continuing with these behaviours?

Risk perception is also influenced by role models. 'Candidates' for premature death who in fact lived to a ripe old age (e.g. 'granddad smoked 40 a day and lived to 93') and 'victims' who lived healthily but died prematurely (e.g. 'my aunt never smoked, ate healthily all her life, and then died of breast cancer aged 48') are referred to as reasons for treating epidemiological risk assessments sceptically (Davison et al 1992). In our companion book, *Foundations for health promotion*, the sociopsychological models of behaviour that explain health-related decision making are discussed in depth (Naidoo and Wills 2009). Lay perceptions of risk are also affected by social and cultural norms. If, for example, one's peer group values a risky behaviour, for example binge drinking among young women, its risk is likely to be underestimated or offset against other immediate benefits, such as belonging and peer approval. Illegal behaviours are also likely to be assessed as much more risky than legal behaviours, regardless of the evidence. For example, the use of the illegal drug ecstasy is generally viewed as more risky than the use of alcohol, although alcohol represents a much more significant health risk.

Recent guidance from the National Institute for Health and Clinical Excellence (NICE) states that interventions to change behaviour can be divided into four main categories:

* policy – such as legislation, workplace policies or voluntary agreements with industry

* education or communication – such as one-to-one advice, group teaching or media campaigns
* technologies – such as the use of seat belts, breathalysers or childproof containers for toxic products
* resources – such as leisure centre free entry, free condoms or free nicotine replacement therapy (NRT).

 Box 11.2 **Discussion point**

Many practitioners will suggest education as a strategy to improve health. Why are educational interventions so popular?

Educational interventions are valued and popular with practitioners because they:

* empower people, enabling them to make desired changes and increase their control over their health
* involve working directly with people, enabling communication and feedback, which in turn can be used to fine-tune the intervention, enhancing its effectiveness.

Educational and behaviour change approaches have been criticized for

* failing to take sufficient account of the social and environmental context in which behavioural choices are made
* reinforcing health inequalities because educational and motivational messages are more likely to be acted upon by those with the most resources, who already enjoy better health due to their more advantaged circumstances
* being 'victim-blaming' – holding people responsible for their lifestyles when change is very difficult or even impossible to achieve has been viewed as unethical because it blames people for circumstances beyond their control
* assuming a direct link between knowledge, attitudes and behaviour
* encouraging state intervention and interference in people's private lives.

The educational approach is discussed in more detail in Chapter 8.

Practitioners will often need to discuss behavioural lifestyle changes with their patients or clients. This may be in the form of information, advice or a more structured and client-led examination of opportunities for change. People may reject education or advice because it runs counter to their intuitive understanding, their life experience, or the example of significant others. However, even when a message is understood and accepted, it may still not be acted upon. Being exposed to behavioural change messages that are accepted but impossible to achieve is likely to lead to loss of self-esteem and feelings of inadequacy. The alternative is to reject or deny such messages.

Box 11.3 **Activity**

Think of a patient or client you regarded as 'difficult' because they resisted or didn't follow your advice. Can you identify why they may have been like this?

Another criticism of the lifestyles approach is that it interferes with people's private lives. This argument holds that people freely choose their lifestyles and behaviours, and that unless this impacts negatively on the quality of others' lives, it concerns no one but themselves. This is an example of individualism, a highly valued concept in modern developed countries, which stresses the autonomy and freedom of individual people. The degree to which individual

Box 11.4 **Discussion point**

Should practitioners encourage clients to change their lifestyles?

lifestyles impact on others is hard to determine. It is arguable whether lifestyles are a matter of choice. In addition to the constraints on choice imposed by the socio-economic context, some behaviours, for

example smoking and excessive alcohol use, are addictive. People may not have all the relevant facts at hand when making behavioural choices, and access to more information may change their choices. The behaviour of significant others has an impact on lifestyles, and advertising and marketing are also significant factors determining individual behavioural choices. Recognition of the persuasive effect of mass media techniques has led health promoters and public health practitioners to adopt techniques such as social marketing to try to achieve healthy lifestyle changes (see Chapter 8 for further discussion of this topic).

Individually focused educational and persuasive approaches have been used to try to change many behaviours. In addition, many other approaches have been used, including legislation and regulation, policy formation and implementation (discussed in more detail in Chapter 4), and community development. The following sections examine a range of strategies addressing smoking, diet, exercise, alcohol and drug use, and sexual health. Within each section, the contribution of this behaviour to ill health is first outlined, followed by a discussion of approaches used in practice and evidence as to their effectiveness.

Smoking

Although the detrimental effects of smoking on health have been known for half a century, smoking remains a common habit that significantly affects the health of the population, both in the UK and worldwide.

Box 11.5 **The prevalence of smoking**

In 2006, 22% of adults aged 16 and above in the UK (23% of men and 21% of women) were current cigarette smokers (http://www.ic.nhs.uk/pubs/smoking08).
- Cigarette smoking continues to be most common among younger age groups (32% of 20–24-year-olds and 31% of those aged 25–34 were current smokers) and least likely amongst those aged 60 and above (14% were current cigarette smokers).

Box 11.5 **The prevalence of smoking—cont'd**

- Although smoking rates are declining, the strong social class gradient in smoking persists. In England in 2008, 27% of those in manual groups were smokers, compared to 16% of those in the non-manual groups (Robinson and Bugles, 2010).

Smoking has been identified as one of the greatest causes of the health divide between the rich and the poor. Due to its expense, smoking also has a significant financial impact on low-income households, and money spent on cigarettes may lead to shortages in essential items such as food, heating and clothing.

The evidence relating to the harmful health effects of tobacco has been well documented for over half a century dating back to Doll and Hill's (1950) original work, published in the *British Medical Journal* in 1950, which demonstrated the link between smoking and lung cancer. The 1963 Report by the Royal College of Physicians, which led to the setting up of the pressure group ASH (Action on Smoking and Health) and the Froggatt Report on passive smoking published in 1988, summarized the available evidence and made the case for stronger controls on smoking in public places and the advertising and promotion of tobacco. The government finally acted on this evidence base and in 1998 published the White Paper *Smoking Kills* (DH 1998).

Box 11.6 **Smoking and health**

- Smoking tobacco is the single most important preventable cause of ill health and premature death.
- Around 82,800 people in England die from smoking each year, accounting for around one-fifth of all deaths.
- Almost one-third (29%) of all cancer deaths are caused by smoking.
- Eighty-eight per cent deaths from lung cancer, 17% deaths from heart disease and 30% deaths from respiratory disease are caused by smoking.
- One in two long-term smokers will die prematurely due to their smoking habit.
- It is estimated that between 1950 and 2000, 6 million Britons and 60 million people worldwide died from tobacco-related diseases.
- Smoking causes ill health and reduces the quality of life. For every death caused by smoking, approximately 20 smokers suffer from a smoking-related disease.
- In 2006/2007, it is estimated that 445,100 adults over the age of 35 were admitted to NHS hospitals in England as a result of smoking.
- Passive smoking, or exposure to the tobacco smoke of others, affects the health of non-smokers including children.
- Children who are passive smokers due to parental or carers' smoking are at increased risk of respiratory disease, asthma, glue ear, sudden infant death syndrome and school absences.
- Second-hand smoke causes lung cancer and heart disease in adult non-smokers.
- Smoking is estimated to cost the NHS approximately £2.7 billion each year.

Source: http://www.ash.org.uk

Smoking is a global health issue affecting all countries. The WHO global burden of disease study (Ezzati et al 2002) found that in developed countries tobacco is the leading cause of disability adjusted life years (DALYs), and tobacco remains a significant cause of disability and a major health risk factor in developing countries. The WHO recognized the global impact of tobacco and negotiated the Framework Convention on Tobacco Control (WHO 2003), its first global health treaty. The Framework Convention is a legal instrument based on evidence that is intended to be incorporated in law and implemented in different countries.

Box 11.7 **WHO framework convention on tobacco control (2003)**

1. Measures relating to reducing demand for tobacco:
   - price and tax measures
   - protection from exposure to environmental tobacco smoke
   - regulation and disclosure of the contents of tobacco products
   - packaging and labelling
   - education, communication, training and public awareness
   - comprehensive ban and restriction on tobacco advertising, promotion and sponsorship
   - tobacco dependence and cessation measures.
2. Measures relating to reducing the supply of tobacco:
   - elimination of the illicit trade of tobacco products
   - restriction of sales to and by minors
   - support for economically viable alternatives for growers.

Recent years have seen a raft of smoke-free legislation in the UK:
- 2003 Advertising of tobacco banned except limited advertising at the point of sale
- 2003 Tobacco sponsorship of domestic sporting events banned
- 2005 Tobacco sponsorship of international sporting events banned
- 2007 Sale of tobacco products to under 18-year-olds banned
- 2007 Smoking in virtually all enclosed public places and workplaces banned
- 2008 Mandatory written and pictorial health warnings on all tobacco products.

The European Union banned all tobacco advertising and sponsorship in 2008. Smoke-free legislation has been supported by an increasing percentage of the population – 81% in 2008 compared to 51% in 2004 (http://ash.org.uk/files/documents/ASH_119.pdf).

Box 11.8 **Discussion point**

Which of the measures in Box 11.7 do you think has most impacted on smoking rates?

WHO reports that the most cost-effective option in all countries is taxation on tobacco products, followed by comprehensive bans on advertising tobacco. Together, it is calculated that these two measures could reduce the global burden of tobacco by 60%. In countries such as the UK, where these two measures are already in place, additional measures such as education and smoking cessation interventions become cost-effective.

Box 11.9 **Example**

Evidence of effective smoking cessation

Effective methods of smoking cessation include advice from doctors, structured interventions including brief interventions (see Box 11.12) by nurses, individual and group counselling either face-to-face or by telephone, standard and personalized self-help materials, and pharmacotherapies (NRT). Recent guidance from NICE (2008) provides a review of the evidence relating to each of these interventions and considerations involved in their provision. NRT increases the rate of quitting by 50–70%, regardless of the setting (Stead et al 2008). The effectiveness of NRT appears to be largely independent of additional support, although NRT combined with cessation support is effective in increasing quit rates amongst those who feel unable or unwilling to quit abruptly (Wang et al 2008).

Tobacco use is unique in that its effects are unequivocally negative, both for the immediate user and for others exposed to tobacco smoke. Strategies to reduce tobacco use are correspondingly well advanced and multi-pronged, including legislation to ban tobacco advertising and promoting access to nicotine replacement drugs on prescription. The American social marketing youth campaign 'Truth', with its message that 'tobacco will control you', recognizes the pervasive influence of the tobacco industry and the addictive nature of tobacco. The WHO Framework Convention demonstrates the potential for global strategies to change unhealthy behaviours. A range of strategies is necessary because the addictive nature of tobacco means that education and advice alone are insufficient. However, the use of complementary strategies at different levels (individual, community, national, global) has been shown to be effective in reducing tobacco use.

Diet

Diet is a crucial factor contributing to health. Malnutrition and underweight is a problem for the developing world, and the Millennium Development Goal 1 is to reduce by 50% the number of people who suffer from hunger. Nine hundred and forty-seven million people in the developing world are undernourished, leading to a failure to grow and thrive and an increased likelihood of becoming ill and dying prematurely (Bread for the World 2009). In 2006, about 9.7 million children died before the age of 5 years. Four-fifths of deaths occurred in sub-Saharan Africa and South Asia, the two regions where people suffer most from hunger and malnutrition (UNICEF 2008).

Box 11.10 Obesity in the UK

- Obesity has nearly trebled in the UK since 1980 and is still increasing.
- In 2006, 24% of adults aged 16 or above and 16% of children aged 2–15 years in England were classified as obese.
- Obesity is linked to social disadvantage and poverty, with higher rates for overweight and obesity amongst Asian groups, lower social classes, and people living in Wales and Scotland.
- Obesity is responsible for 2–8% of health costs and 10–13% of deaths in Europe.
- In 2004, over £30 million was spent on drugs to treat obesity. It is estimated that treating obesity-related conditions (ischaemic heart disease, stroke, diabetes mellitus and some cancers) costs England over £3 billion each year.

Sources: http://www.euro.who.int/obesity British Heart Foundations Statistics Website The Information Centre 2008 http://www.heartstats.org accessed 13/7/09

In many countries, there has conversely been an epidemic rise in the incidence of obesity. Diets in Western developed countries have changed rapidly, alongside changes in farming, cooking habits, processing, and the availability of prepared and packaged food. Unhealthy diets, characterized as high fat, high sugar and high calorie diets, are linked to the rise in obesity, which itself is implicated in a host of diseases and illnesses including diabetes, coronary heart disease and some cancers.

Although obesity is a problem in developed rather than developing countries, it is the poorest members of society who are most likely to be obese and suffer related ill health and premature death. Substantial evidence shows how poverty affects food choice:

- Many low-income neighbourhoods in the USA and Canada have become 'food deserts', with the loss of local retailers resulting in less availability of healthy affordable food (Cummins and Macintyre 2006).
- In 2006, only 28% of men and 32% of women, and 19% of boys and 22% of girls aged 5–15 years consumed five or more portions of fruit and vegetables daily, with the proportion doing so increasing with age and income (NHS Information Centre 2008).
- People living in the most deprived neighbourhoods are unlikely to have access to a car, and local shops charge more than supermarkets for basic foods including fruit and vegetables (Lang 2005).

Box 11.11 **Discussion point**

Is the '5-a-day' message to eat five portions of fruit and vegetables a day relevant and realistic for families on a low income?

For low-income families whose budgets only just cover basic food requirements, experimenting with unfamiliar fruits and vegetables in the family diet may not be a feasible option. To make '5-a-day' a viable option for all families, attention needs to be paid to the availability, accessibility and price of fruit and vegetables. Reducing the price of fruit, or ensuring it is available daily in school meals, may be more effective than educational advice on the nutritional benefits of fruit, although brief counselling interventions have also been shown to be effective.

 Box 11.12 **Example**

Fruit and vegetable project for adults on low incomes

The most common techniques of health promotion (providing information and facilitating goal-setting) may be helpful for low-income groups. Personalized information, combined with professional consultation or advice, can improve knowledge and recall. Disadvantaged populations benefit from this approach more than other groups, possibly because their knowledge base is less, and so they have more to gain from health information (King's Fund 2008). For example, brief counselling interventions by primary care nurses have been shown to be effective in increasing the consumption of fruit and vegetables among adults with low incomes. The intervention consisted of nutrition or behavioural counselling involving two 15 min consultations a fortnight apart supplemented by written information. A randomized trial has shown that the most effective intervention is behavioural counselling based on social learning theory and the Stages of Change model, although nutritional counselling is also effective.

Source: Steptoe et al 2003 cited in Press and Mwatsama (2004)

Figure 11.1 shows how diet is determined by a number of different interweaving factors. Simply improving knowledge about healthy foods does not necessarily lead to changes in consumption. Such foods need to be accessible and available and people need the skills and confidence to prepare these foods. The UK government has recognized the negative impact of fast food outlets on the nation's diet, and in a recent strategy document stipulates that local authorities can and should use existing planning powers to control the number and location of fast food outlets in their local areas, especially in relation to parks and schools (HM Government 2008).

The environments in which people work or live can promote or inhibit healthy behaviours. (For a more detailed discussion of the policy context see Chapter 4 and the section on settings in our companion volume, *Foundations for health promotion* [Naidoo and Wills 2009].) The 5-a-day programme has taken these factors into consideration. Included in the programme is a national school fruit and vegetable scheme, which, following a positive evaluation of several pilot schemes, has now been rolled out throughout England. The school fruit and vegetable scheme offers a free piece of fruit or vegetable to all 4–6-year-olds at nursery and school. Nearly 2 million children in more than 16,000 schools are now involved in the scheme (http://www.dh.gov.uk). The reintroduction in 2006 of nutritional standards for school meals states that fresh fruit and vegetables should be available each day as part of the school meal. Catering outlets also need to be targeted, as 10% of people's total food intake is now eaten outside the home (Office for National Statistics 2000).

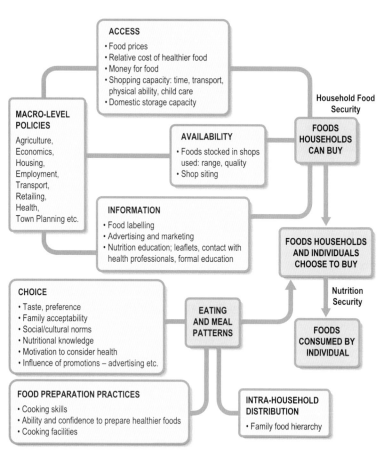

Figure 11.1 ● Determinants of food and nutrition consumption. Source: DH (1996, p. 4).

 Box 11.13 **Example**

Social marketing to address obesity

Romp and Chomp is an initiative of the Sentinel Site for Obesity Prevention, a WHO collaborating centre within Deakin University. The Romp and Chomp project, based in Geelong, Australia, is a community-based intervention addressing obesity. About 20% of Australian children are obese, and lack of physical activity and poor eating habits amongst the under fives sets a pattern for later life that is difficult to remedy. Staff taking care of early childhood needs lack the knowledge, confidence and skills to initiate physical activity programmes. Romp and Chomp uses social marketing techniques to promote healthy active lifestyles to families with children aged up to 5 years. The Romp and Chomp family provides a role model to encourage daily physical activity and healthy eating. Once families identify with the Romp and Chomp family, support messages (e.g. how to increase active play opportunities for children under 5) can be delivered. Romp and Chomp works with a variety of partners including day care facilities, families and physical activity providers.

Sources: Riethmuller et al 2009; http://www.deakin.edu.au/hmnbs/who-obesity/about-us/publications/flyers/romp-chomp-brochure-dec-2005.pdf

The rise of fast food, takeout meals and the loss of practical food preparation skills in schools' curricula has led to a focus on providing cooking skills. Cooking skills programmes seek to encourage people to practise food preparation in a safe environment and stimulate home cooking using fresh foods.

Box 11.14 **Example**

Cookery classes for homeless people

Centrepoint, a registered charity and housing association for young homeless people in Greater London, has launched a comprehensive project to improve the diet of the young people with whom it works. The project was initiated following research in 2002 that flagged up the problem of food poverty and poor diets amongst its clients. In addition to improving the nutritional quality and variety of the food it provides and ensuring that its kitchen and dining facilities are of a high standard, Centrepoint has initiated a free programme that includes cooking workshops run by a chef who focuses on how to cook nutritious meals using cheap available ingredients. The workshops are run every week and young people can attend as often as they like. Workshops on 'budgeting for food', which support young people to use their limited money most effectively when shopping for food, and food hygiene sessions have also been instigated. Attendance at the cooking and shopping workshops has been high and feedback from young people has been very positive.

Source: http://www.foodvision.gov.uk/pages/cookery-courses-for-the-homeless accessed 8/7/09

Integrated programmes that adopt a variety of strategies including individually based education and persuasion and community-based structural programmes focusing on access and availability are most effective. Interventions may also target providers further up the food chain, for example the sourcing of locally grown produce sold in farmers' markets, or food labelling to ensure that consumers can easily compare fat and sugar contents of processed foods. Practitioners can play an important role in supporting and reinforcing such programmes through the provision of dietary education and advice. In addition, practitioners can take a lead in implementing appropriate interventions within the healthcare service setting and referring clients to local programmes.

Physical activity

Physical activity is associated with positive health benefits as well as reducing the risk of coronary heart disease:

> *The public health importance of physical activity is clear, as adults who are physically active have 20–30% reduced risk of premature death, and up to 50% reduced risk of developing the major chronic diseases such as coronary heart disease, stroke, diabetes and cancers.*
>
> CMO (2004, p. 1)

The British Heart Foundation (2003) estimates that 37% of deaths from coronary heart disease could be attributed to inactivity. The degree of risk of inactivity is comparable to the relative risk associated with the three main risk factors for coronary heart disease, i.e. smoking, high blood pressure and high cholesterol. Inactivity is the biggest risk factor for the population as a whole and has one of the largest potentials for improvement. In common with debates over dietary recommendations regarding the desired quantity of daily fruit and vegetables, recommendations relating to levels of physical activity have varied. Current advice is a recommended minimum of 30 minutes of moderate exercise five times a week, but there is flexibility in how this is achieved. For example, incorporating exercise into everyday life in 10 min blocks can be equally effective. Children and young people should undertake a range of moderate to vigorous activities for at least 60 min every day. At least twice a week this should include weight-bearing activities that produce high physical stress to improve bone health, muscle strength and flexibility (NICE 2009). Recent research shows that the majority of the population is not taking adequate exercise.

Box 11.15 **Example**

Levels of physical activity in England in 2006

The Active People Survey is conducted by Sport England, with the first survey taking place in 2005/2006.

- 21% of adults take part in at least three moderate intensity 30 min sessions of sport and physical activity every week
- Walking was the most popular recreational activity for people in England. Over 8 million adults aged 16 and above (20%) had walked for at least 30 min during the previous 4 weeks
- 5.6 million people (13.8%) swim at least once a month

- 4.2 million people (10.5%) go to the gym
- More men (23.7%) regularly take part in sports than women (18.5%)
- Over 2.7 million people put some voluntary time into sport – with an estimated 1.8 million hours unpaid support every week of the year. This equates to over 54,000 full-time equivalent jobs
- 4.7% of the adult population (1.9 million) contributes at least 1 hour a week volunteering to sport

Source: http://www.sportengland.org/research/active_people_survey/

Box 11.16 **Example**

Approaches towards promoting physical activity amongst adults

The promotion of physical activity amongst adults through primary care has included subsidized access to leisure facilities, the use of pedometers and walking or cycling schemes, and on-going support and advice to inactive people from practitioners.

'Exercise on prescription' or exercise referral schemes have been widely established. However,

no evidence has been found in the review from NICE (2007a) to suggest that exercise referral schemes are effective in increasing physical activity levels in the longer term (over more than 12 weeks) or over a very long time frame (over more than 1 year). Their guidance suggests that new exercise referral schemes should not be established other than as part of such an evaluation programme or other relevant evaluative study.

However, brief interventions from primary care practitioners have been shown to be effective (NICE 2007a). Lawton et al (2008) found that a brief intervention by the practice nurse with a 6-month follow-up visit and monthly telephone support over 9 months was effective in increasing physical activity and quality of life for women aged 40–74 over a 2-year period (although there were also more falls and injuries). A cluster randomized trial of a primary care intervention that involved physicians providing advice and prescribing physical activity during an additional appointment found this intervention to be effective (Grandes et al 2009). Although the overall clinical effect was small it would have a significant impact if rolled out across the population.

Although both the Health Survey for England (NHS Information Centre 2008) and the Active People Survey (http://www.sportengland.org) have found that the proportion of men and women achieving recommended exercise levels has been increasing steadily, only 6% of men and 9% of women knew what the recommended level is, with around one quarter thinking it was greater than it is and most people either unaware of the recommendation, or thinking it was less than it is. The most commonly cited barriers to doing more physical activity were work commitments (cited by 45% men), lack of leisure time (cited by 37% women), and caring for children or older people (cited by 25% women). Around 15% of people cited lack of money, and around 12% cited poor health, as barriers.

Children are a particular target group for increased physical activity. The rise in passive hobbies and leisure pursuits, such as using the computer or watching TV, together with fears about road safety and the loss of sports activities in school (driven out partly by the demands of the national curriculum) have all combined to reduce the physical activity patterns of a whole generation. Behavioural patterns established in childhood exert an influence on later adult behav-

iour and cardiovascular risk factors have their origins in childhood. Positive changes within a school setting are associated with the following characteristics (HDA 2001; Canadian Cancer Society 2008; NICE 2009):

- appropriately designed, delivered and supported physical activity curriculum
- access to suitable and accessible facilities and opportunities for physical activity
- involvement of young people in planning programmes
- self-management programmes
- complementary classroom curricula focusing on physical activity
- family involvement programmes.

Box 11.17 **Example**

Walk to school

Walking to school provides not only valuable exercise but also the opportunity for social contact and bonding between children and their parents and peer groups. More active transport methods are also good for the environment. During national walk-to-school weeks the number of pupils walking to school increases by about a third. Over 6,380 schools, involving 1,719,558 pupils, currently take part in walk-to-school schemes, which are promoted by 2 out of 3 local authorities.

Walk to school on one day a week (WoW), first launched in Gloucestershire in 1999 and later adopted by six London boroughs in 2004, aims to achieve a permanent shift in commuting patterns. WoW is supported by a variety of partners including

the Department for Transport, Transport for London, Living Streets, and various local partners.

http://www.livingstreets.org.uk/

There is evidence that walking buses (volunteer-led walking groups supported by parents and teachers plus the involvement of the local highways or transport authority) led to increases in self-reported walking among 5–11 year olds, and reduced car use for children's journeys to and from school. However, the provision of a walking bus may in itself not be sufficient to stem a more general decline in walking to and from school. Retaining volunteers to act as coordinators for these schemes appears to be a key factor in the sustainability of walking buses (NICE 2009).

Health promotion and public health interventions have focused on targeted interventions that reduce barriers to exercise rather than promoting physical activity. However, more integrated approaches that are multi-level and include local travel plans and the

use of open spaces are being proposed. More often a settings approach is used, as in the school setting in the example above, and increasingly a targeted focus on a particular group (e.g. young women) in a particular setting is adopted.

Alcohol and drugs

Alcohol and drug use is associated with many health and social problems including violence, burglary, hazardous driving and public disorder in addition to physical and mental health problems. The links with criminal justice tend to receive a higher profile than the health issues. This is illustrated by the public focus on drugs, especially illegal drugs, rather than alcohol, although alcohol poses a more serious risk to the public health.

Box 11.18

Alcohol consumption in the UK

- Current recommendations are that men should not regularly drink more than 3–4 units per day and women should not regularly drink more than 2–3 units per day. A unit of alcohol is equivalent to half a pint of beer, a glass of wine or a measure of spirits.
- The General Household Survey shows that in 2007, 37% exceeded the recommended level and 20% of adults consumed more than double the benchmark at least once during the preceding week.
- Men drink more than women (41% of men exceeded the daily limit at least once during the previous week compared to 34% of women).
- People in 'managerial and professional' households are more likely than those in 'routine and manual' households to have exceeded the daily limit at least once during the preceding week (43% and 31%, respectively).
- People are most likely to be drinking at home on the days they drink the most.
- Over four-fifths of people (86%) had heard of alcohol units but only about two-fifths of people knew the correct recommended daily maximum for men and women (38% men and 44% women).

Source: http://www.statistics.gov.uk/StatBase/Product.asp?vink=5756

Box 11.19 Discussion point

In 2009, the Chief Medical Officer called for a minimum pricing policy for alcohol of 50 pence per unit of alcohol. What might be the objections to such a policy?

There is considerable ambivalence in the UK about tackling alcohol. On the one hand, there is evidence of alcohol abuse and a recognition that reducing consumption is a legitimate policy aim. On the other hand, the UK alcohol industry employs more than one million people and is the fourth largest producer of spirits and the sixth largest producer of beer in the world. Alcohol constitutes over 3% of total tax revenue.

Health messages relating to alcohol may be ambiguous and confusing because a limited intake of alcohol is associated with reduced risk of coronary heart disease. However, excessive use of alcohol is linked to a variety of health and social problems. The rise in alcohol-related health and social problems has been fuelled by increases in alcohol consumption, especially amongst young people and women.

Box 11.20 Discussion point

What are the benefits and disbenefits of alcohol consumption to:
- **a.** society at large
- **b.** communities
- **c.** trade and industry
- **d.** health and social care services
- **e.** individuals and families.

Box 11.21 Alcohol and health

In 2006, in England there were over 6500 deaths directly linked to alcohol, of which two-thirds were men.

In 2006/2007, there were 207,788 hospital admissions with a primary or secondary diagnosis

Box 11.21 Alcohol and health—cont'd

related to alcohol, with 9% of these involving patients under 18 years.

Excessive use of alcohol is linked to many health problems including raised blood pressure, certain types of cancers, strokes, fertility problems, gastritis, pancreatitis, liver disease, mental health problems, accidents and suicides.

Excessive use of alcohol is also linked to social problems such as violence and crime.

In 2006/2007, just over a half of violent attackers were believed to be under the influence of alcohol at the time of the attack.

In 2004, alcohol misuse was estimated to cost the health service between £1.4 and £1.7 billion per year.

Recent estimates put the total cost of alcohol-related harm at around £20 billion per year.

NHS Information Centre for Health and Social Care 2008.
Cabinet Office 2004.

Box 11.22 Practitioner talking

It is so depressing being on the weekend night shift at hospital and each week seeing the same avoidable injuries, accidents and deaths, all caused by alcohol. Last week was freshers' week at the university and was even worse than usual. We were stretched to the limit, and then on top of it all you have drunken young people causing disruption in hospital and being offensive to the people trying to help them. If they're bright enough to go to university, surely they're bright enough to know about sensible drinking limits? Although a lot of it is down to irresponsible marketing and promotion by the drinks industry. All around town and the university, there are notices offering cheap drinks and happy hours, and these students think it's great.

Commentary

Current research and policy supports a multi-partner and multi-factorial approach to alcohol misuse and related harm. The current approach seeks to preserve individual freedom and choice whilst promoting self-regulation. Many countries focus on limiting intoxicated behaviour and the criminalization of some drinkers (e.g. those in public places). Demand reduction is anticipated following a health education programme of recommended sensible drinking levels. Yet there is a persistent credibility gap between messages such as 'safe, sensible and social' and contemporary alcohol-related attitudes and behaviours. In relation to supply, government seeks a more responsible approach to marketing and promotion by the drinks industry, notwithstanding the liberalization of licensing laws. Alcohol impacts on local communities, crime and disorder, and health and social care, so tackling alcohol misuse and its effects requires close partnership working across a variety of agencies and services to promote a safe night-time economy through the promotion and enforcement of responsible retailing and enhanced public protection measures. There is a role for many different strategies including legislation, mass media campaigns, community action and individually tailored education and advice. This is illustrated in the following example of England's alcohol harm reduction strategy.

A national alcohol harm reduction strategy for England, announced in 2004, identified the following approaches (ibid):

- Better education and communication, for example the 'Know Your Limits' binge-drinking campaign and the 'THINK' drink-driving campaign.
- Improving health and treatment services.
- Combating alcohol-related crime and disorder through the use of new enforcement powers in the Licensing Act 2003 and the Violent Crime Reduction Act 2006.

- Working with the alcohol industry to promote sensible drinking and curb irresponsible advertising and marketing of alcohol.

In 2007, this strategy was reviewed by several government departments (DH, Home Office, DES and DCMS 2007), who announced the next steps in the national alcohol strategy:

- Sharpened criminal justice for drunken behaviour.
- A review of NHS alcohol spending.
- More help for people who want to drink less.
- Tougher enforcement of underage sales.
- Trusted guidance for parents and young people.
- Public information campaigns to promote a new 'sensible drinking' culture.
- Public consultation on alcohol pricing and promotion.
- Local alcohol strategies.

 Box 11.23 **Discussion point**

Do you think that the current policy employs an effective mix of legislation, media advocacy and education?

The BMA (2008) concluded that education and health promotion had only a limited effect on drinking behaviour, and advocated instead more emphasis on the early intervention and treatment of alcohol misuse within primary care and hospital settings. At present, there is no routine screening for alcohol misuse, although alcohol misuse questionnaires are an efficient and cost-effective means of detecting alcohol misuse. Brief interventions delivered in healthcare settings are effective for people who are not dependent on alcohol. For alcohol-dependent people, specialized alcohol treatment services are vital and need to be provided and adequately funded throughout the UK (BMA 2008).

NICE (2007b) guidance on school-based interventions on alcohol concluded that a whole school approach involving a range of local partners should be adopted. Interventions should include addressing alcohol education in the curriculum, policy development and the school environment, and staff training. Children and young people thought to be at risk of alcohol misuse should be offered one-to-one advice or be referred to an appropriate external service. Legislation continues to be one of the most effective strategies in combating alcohol misuse. A combination of alcohol taxes, restrictions in availability, and drink-driving countermeasures is effective in reducing alcohol misuse and its effects (Room et al 2005).

Drugs

The numbers of problematic drug users is hard to estimate but is in the region of 200,000 in England and Wales. Problematic drug use is therefore a low prevalence risk behaviour but it is associated with many health and social problems and high levels of mortality. For example, the standardized mortality ratio for Scottish drug users is 12 times as high as for the general population and the higher prevalence of problematic drug use in Scotland compared to England accounts for a third of Scotland's excess mortality over England (Bloor et al 2008). The new National Drug Strategy (COI 2008) focuses on six key areas:

1. target drug-misusing offenders who are the source of crime in communities and take away their proceeds

2. focus on people at the top of the drug supply networks

3. ensure that the police listen and respond to community concerns

4. offer more support to families, especially where there are parents misusing drugs

5. provide better information to parents and young people, with compulsory drug education in schools and local information campaigns

6. provide better drug treatment services that help drug users stay drug-free and reintegrate into society.

Box 11.24 **Example**

The FRANK campaign

Caught between media hysteria, adult denial, and anecdotal stories from peers, young people can find it hard to be informed about drugs. In 2008/2009, £6.6 million was allocated to the FRANK campaign, using TV, radio and online advertising to reach young people. The social marketing campaign was developed from young people's concepts of risk to develop clear information. The website offers free and impartial information and advice about drugs, and individual queries can be e-mailed. A number of sources of help are signposted from this website. The FRANK campaign is jointly funded by the Home Office and the Department of Health, working closely with the Department for Education and Skills. The recent FRANK campaigns on cannabis and cocaine have been hailed as a success, with the cocaine campaign featuring Pablo, a dog used to traffic the drug, being viewed more than 700,000 times on the YouTube website. Research shows that 89% of young people recognized the campaign and over half the young people interviewed (53%) would turn to FRANK for information about drugs.

Source: http://www.talktofrank.com HM Government (2009)

Local communities bear the brunt of drug-related disorder and crime. Coordinated action between local people and agencies and local police can have a dramatic effect on the local availability of drugs and associated problems. Drug arrest referral schemes, in which users are offered early interventions and support through local police stations, self-referral, and the courts, have been widely adopted. Following consultation with local people living in the London Road area of the city, Sussex Police and Brighton and Hove City Council launched Operation Reduction in 2005. Operation Reduction targeted drug dealing and aimed to cut demand by getting drug users into treatment. The campaign has been a success, with nearly

500 arrests and almost 300 people being referred to drug treatment services. The area has become safer and a more pleasant environment (HM Government 2009, p. 8).

Box 11.25 **Activity**

How easy and ethical is it for practitioners to adopt a harm reduction approach?

Treatment is a crucial part of the overall strategy. Treatment is both effective and cost-effective – for every £1 spent, an estimated £3 is saved in criminal justice costs alone (Home Office 2002). The National Treatment Agency oversees treatment services that are locally coordinated and provided by Drug Action Teams. Services range from in-patient detoxification and prescribing to structured counselling and residential rehabilitation. The aim is to provide a positive route out of addiction and crime for drug users.

Harm reduction is another important aspect of strategy. There are many definitions and approaches to harm reduction but essentially it is a package of measures and approaches that enable people to reduce their risks. Some practitioners may find such an approach difficult because it acknowledges people's right to make unhealthy or illegal decisions. It also does not presume a goal of abstinence. For some, this may be an unethical stance and one they cannot endorse. For others, using such an approach can provide a useful way to contribute effectively to reducing risks without having to adopt an unrealistic 'all or nothing' approach.

Box 11.26 **Discussion point**

Why do you think there are separate national strategies for alcohol, tobacco and drugs?

Alcohol and drug use presents law and order challenges as well as health problems. The most effective approaches combine the use of different strategies targeting different aspects of the problem. The use of legislation, regulation and the criminal justice system is an important adjunct to the individual health screening, education, advice and medication provided by practitioners. The evidence demonstrates that specific targeted interventions by health practitioners are effective and contribute to the reduction of the disease burden caused by alcohol and drug use.

Sexual health

The term sexual health has many contrasting definitions that are influenced by beliefs about concepts such as health and sex. Definitions may range from a focus on the clinical causes of ill health, such as infections, to a celebration of pleasure.

 Box 11.27 **Activity**

How would you define sexual health? Does your definition impact equally on men and women? On heterosexual and homosexual people?

Sexual health has been defined in various ways. Whilst there is often a focus in service provision on sexual ill health and disease, most definitions refer to a holistic positive concept of sexual health. For example, the World Health Organization refers to 'the integration of the physical, emotional, intellectual and social aspects of sexual being, in ways that are enriching and that enhance personality, communication and love. Fundamental to this concept are the right to sexual information and the right to pleasure' (WHO 1975). The Department of Health reinforces the holistic concept of sexual health whilst acknowledging the need to avoid unintended consequences of sexual activity including disease.

Sexual health is an important part of physical and mental health. It is a key part of our identity as human beings together with the fundamental human rights to privacy, a family life and living free from discrimination. Essential elements of good sexual health are equitable relationships and sexual fulfilment with access to information and services to avoid the risk of unintended pregnancy, illness or disease.

DH (2001b, p. 7)

Gender is an important factor affecting sexual health. 'The differential power of men and women is evident in most sexual intercourse as it is in the wider context of male–female relations' (Doyal, 1995, p. 62). Women's capacity to enjoy and express their sexuality is limited by the fundamentally unequal relationship between men and women. Women may have to negotiate their concerns about fertility and safer sex and may be threatened with violence, harassment or abuse from their partners. A survey of young women's sexual attitudes concludes that for 'a young woman to insist on the use of a condom for her own safety requires resisting the constraints and opposing the construction of intercourse as a man's natural pleasure and a woman's natural duty' (Thomson and Holland 1994, p. 24). Homosexuality remains a less socially valued and more discriminated against sexual identity compared to heterosexuality. Activities that heterosexuals take for granted, such as public recognition and acceptance of their sexual partners, can be problematic for homosexuals. The rights of homosexuals are prescribed by law, for example the age of consent for homosexuals is 18 compared to 16 for heterosexuals.

The element of sexual health that is defined as being free from sexually transmitted infections (STIs) has declined in recent years. All STIs have increased in the past decade (1998–2007), especially gonorrhoea (42% increase), chlamydia (150% increase) and syphilis (increased by a factor of 19) (http://www.avert.org/stdstatisticuk.htm). The incidence of STIs is linked to ethnicity (in 2005 Black Caribbeans accounted for 18% gonorrhoea diagnoses) and homosexuality (in 2007 55% syphilis cases were acquired through sex between men) (ibid). The incidence of HIV/AIDS has also increased significantly; for further details see Chapter 10.

The UK has the highest rate of teenage pregnancies in Western Europe. Teenage pregnancy is linked to poverty and disadvantage, and is more common in lower socio-economic families living in deprived areas. It is also more common amongst some ethnic groups (e.g. Caribbean, Pakistani and Bangladeshi young women), young people with below average educational achievement, young people who have been in care, socially excluded from school, or involved in crime, and children of teenage mothers. Teenage pregnancy is linked to a number of negative outcomes (health problems for babies, lower educational attainment and employment rates of mothers, lone parenthood and social isolation), and is one of the mechanisms which perpetuates cycles of deprivation throughout generations (Swann et al 2003).

England launched a Teenage Pregnancy Strategy in 1999 with an ambitious target to halve teenage pregnancies by 2010. Since 1998 there has been a 13.3% reduction in conceptions amongst under 18 year olds, with reductions in more than 120 local authorities. More than 20% of local authorities have had decreases of at least 25% in teenage pregnancy rates. A new strategy "Teenage Pregnancy Strategy: Beyond 2010" has been launched. (http:www.dcsf. gov.uk/everychildmatters/healthandwellbeing/ teenagepregnancy) A review of evidence found the following interventions to be effective (Swann et al 2003):

- sex education in schools, particularly when linked to contraceptive services
- community-based education, development and contraceptive services
- youth development programmes focusing on personal and vocational development and education
- family outreach involving parents of young people.

Responsive local services that are accessible and staffed by trained and committed staff are also vital. Peer education, ensuring age-appropriate interventions tailored to young people with clear messages and partnership working are all factors flagged up as contributing to effective interventions. Abstinence-based interventions (which advocate no sexual activity before marriage) have been widely supported in the USA but are shown to be ineffective, and have

also been criticized for adopting a moralistic stance and treating young people as immature and lacking in autonomy. Sex education programmes in the UK are supporting young people to delay sexual activity.

A review of the government's 10-year sexual health strategy, launched in 2001, pinpointed five key strategic areas where priority action was needed (MedFASH 2008):

- Prioritizing sexual health as a key public health issue and sustaining high-level leadership at local, regional and national levels.
- Building strategic partnerships with health services, local authorities and the third sector (voluntary sector).
- Commissioning for improved sexual health.
- Investing more in prevention through commissioning and resourcing sexual health promotion, making personal social and health education in schools statutory, and improving dissemination of effective interventions.
- Delivering modern sexual health services.

 Box 11.28 Activity

Why do sexual health services remain the Cinderella of the NHS – underfunded, understaffed and relatively invisible?

Health promotion and public health interventions aimed at changing sexual behaviour face particular challenges due to the sensitive nature of the subject and the power of gender and sexual orientation in shaping people's perceptions and attitudes. Sexual health is also a complex area and includes both fertility and STIs. The focus of the national strategy is on increasing access, availability and acceptability of NHS sexual health services. This may involve practitioners developing more client-centred, flexible approaches to service delivery. The priorities remain, however, more focused on sexual ill health – to reduce STIs and HIV, and also to reduce the teenage pregnancy rate.

Conclusion

Lifestyles and individual behavioural choices have a long history of being targeted for change by health promoters. The significance of behaviours such as diet, exercise, smoking, alcohol and drug use, and sexual activity in affecting or even determining health outcomes is widely accepted. What is disputed is the effectiveness of different kinds of approaches to changing lifestyles and whether they are ethically defensible. Lifestyles are generally viewed as an individual choice that should be respected unless they directly infringe on someone else's freedom to choose. The impact on others is generally easier to appreciate when it involves aspects such as safety and crime (linked to alcohol and drug use) rather than aspects such as health (linked to smoking). However, the counter case may be made – that the government has a duty to protect people from known health risks, especially when these are socially patterned and linked to socio-economic inequalities. When behaviours directly impact on others, it is much easier to get support for legislation and regulation to control such behaviours. When the effects are more diffuse, the case for legislation is correspondingly more difficult. This can be demonstrated by comparing the existence of laws regulating drunkenness in public places and whilst in charge of vehicles with the long battle to ban the advertising and promotion of tobacco products. Whilst smoking causes ill health and distress to passive smokers as well as to smokers, it is not associated with visible anti-social behaviour. The campaign to ban tobacco advertising therefore took a long time to build the evidence and win support, and a ban on smoking in virtually all public places and workplaces was only introduced in 2007.

Whilst legislation and regulation may be the most effective means of changing lifestyles, in many cases they are seen as inappropriate because of the right to individual freedom and liberty. In these cases, education and persuasion through the use of mass media campaigns may be the appropriate strategy. Health practitioners have an important role to play in using educational and motivational strategies with individual clients, and also with groups and local communities if the opportunity arises. These techniques seek to change people's behaviour voluntarily as a result of education, information, support and advice. An evidence base of effective techniques to use in educational and motivational interventions is growing. A combination of different strategies that includes legislation and regulation is the most effective means of achieving behavioural changes.

Further discussion

- Identify the opportunities and barriers to working with individual clients to change one of the behaviours discussed in this chapter.

- What criteria would you use to determine whether or not individual behaviours (such as smoking and alcohol and drug use) should be the subject of legislation and regulation?

- Discuss the relative contribution of individual education and advice, mass media campaigns and legislation in achieving behavioural change.

Recommended reading

- Ewles L, Simnett I: *Promoting health: a practical guide*, edn 5, Edinburgh, 2003, Baillière Tindall.
  This popular book includes sections on how practitioners can assess needs and help their clients change their behaviour and lifestyles.

- NICE: Behaviour change at population, individual and community levels, 2007, at http://www.nice.org.uk/Guidance/PH6.
  This guidance identifies how to plan and run relevant initiatives based on evidence from different theoretical perspectives and research.
  Summaries of evidence of effective interventions to tackle a range of public health issues are available on the NICE website http://www.nice.org.uk and currently include:

- School-based interventions on alcohol (PH7)
- Brief interventions and referral for smoking cessation (PH1), smoking cessation services (PH10) and smoking cessation in the workplace (PH5)
- Maternal and child nutrition (PH11)
- Four commonly used methods to increase physical activity (PH2), physical activity in the workplace (PH13), physical activity and the environment (PH8), promoting physical activity for children and young people (PH17)
- Prevention of sexually transmitted infections and under 18 conceptions (PH3).

- Press V, Mwatsama M: *Nutrition and food poverty toolkit*, National Heart Forum, 2004.

This toolkit is aimed at a wide range of professionals presenting the evidence for food poverty and the role of poor nutrition in a wide variety of health problems. Examples of good practice and other sources of guidance are flagged up to help with the development of local strategies.

- Rollnick S, Mason P, Butler C: *Health behaviour change: a guide for practitioners*, London, 1999, Churchill Livingstone.

  A practical guide to support practitioners working with clients to change behaviours.

References

Bloor M, Gannon M, Hay G, et al: Contribution of problem drug users' deaths to excess mortality in Scotland: secondary analysis of cohort study, *Br Med J* 337:a478, 2008 Published online 2008 July 31. doi:10.1136/bmj.a478.

Bread for the World: *Global development: charting a new course*, Hunger Report 2009, 2009. http://www.bread.org/learn/hunger-basics/hunger-facts-international.html accessed 7/7/09.

British Heart Foundation: *Coronary disease statistics*, London, 2003, BHF.

British Medical Association Board of Science (BMA): *Alcohol misuse: Tackling the UK epidemic*, 2008, http://www.bma.org.uk/images/Alcoholmisuse_tcm41–147192.pdf accessed 21/8/09.

Cabinet Office Strategy Unit: *Alcohol misuse: how much does it cost?*, London, 2003, COSU.

Cabinet Office Strategy Unit: *Alcohol harm reduction strategy for England*, London, 2004, COSU.

Canadian Cancer Society Manitoba Division: *Effective school-based physical activity interventions*, Winnipeg, 2008, Canadian Cancer Society.

Central Office for Information (COI): *Drugs: protecting families and communities: the 2008 drug strategy*, COI, London, 2008, HM Government.

Chief Medical Officer: *At least five a week. Evidence on the impact of physical activity and its relationship to health*, London, 2004, DH.

Cummins S, Macintyre S: Food environments and obesity: neighbourhood or nation?, *Int J Epidemiol* 35:100–104, 2006.

Davison C, Frankel S, Davey Smith G: The limits to lifestyle: reassessing 'fatalism' in the popular culture of illness prevention, *Soc Sci Med* 34(6):675–685, 1992.

Department of Health (DH): *The health of the nation: a strategy for health in England*, London, 1992, HMSO.

Department of Health (DH) Nutrition Task Force: *Low income, food, nutrition and health: strategies for improvement*, London, 1996, HMSO.

Department of Health (DH): *White paper: smoking kills*, Cm 4177, London, 1998, The Stationery Office.

Department of Health (DH): *Saving lives: our healthier nation*, London, 1999, The Stationery Office.

Department of Health (DH): *National service framework: coronary heart disease*, London, 2000a, The Stationery Office.

Department of Health (DH): *The national strategy for sexual health and HIV – consultation*, London, 2001b, The Stationery Office.

Department of Health (DH) Home Office Department of Education and Department of Culture, Media and Sport: *Safe. Sensible. Social. The next steps in the National alcohol strategy*, London, 2007, The Stationery Office.

Department of Health: *Review of the National Alcohol Harm Reduction Strategy for England Health Impact Assessment*, Leeds, 2007, Ben Cave Associates for the DH.

Doll R, Hill AB: Smoking and carcinoma of the lung: preliminary report, *Br Med J* 143:329–336, 1950.

Doniger AS, Adams E, Riley JS, et al: Impact evaluation of the 'Not Me, Not Now' abstinence-oriented, adolescent pregnancy prevention communications program, Monroe County, New York, *J Health Commun* 6:45–60, 2001.

Doyal L: *What makes women sick?: gender and the political economy of health*, Basingstoke, 1995, Macmillan.

Ezzati M, Lopez AD, Rodgers R, et al: Selected major risk factors and global and regional burden of disease, *Lancet* 360(9343):1347–1362, 2002.

Froggatt P: *4th Report of the Independent Scientific Committee on smoking and health*, London, 1988, HMSO.

Graham H: Disadvantaged lives and women's smoking patterns and policy levers, *MIDIRS Midwifery Digest* 13(2):152–156, 2003, http://hsciweb.york.ac.uk/research/public/Publication.aspx?ID=642

Grandes Gb, Sanchez A, Sanchez-Pinilla RO, et al: Effectiveness of physical activity advice and prescription by physicians in routine primary care, *Arch Intern Med* 169(7):694, 2009.

Health Development Agency (HDA): *Coronary heart disease: guidance for implementing the preventive aspects of the national service framework*, London, 2001, HDA.

HM Government: *Healthy weight, healthy lives: a cross-government strategy for England*, London, 2008, Department of Health and Department for Children, Schools and Families.

HM Government: *The 2008 drug strategy: one year on*, London, 2009, COI.

Home Office: *Updated drug strategy*, Available at http://www.drugs.gov.uk/Reports and Publications/NationalStrategy2002 accessed 30/11/03

King's Fund: *Low-income groups and behaviour change interventions*, London, 2008, King's Fund.

Lang T: Food control or food democracy? Re-engaging nutrition with society and the environment, *Public Health Nutr* 8(1):730–737, 2005.

Lawton BA, Rose SB, Elley CR, et al: Exercise on prescription for women aged 40–74 recruited through primary care: two year randomised controlled trial, *Br Med J* 337:a2509, 2008.

Lupton D: *The imperative of health. Public health and the regulated body*, London, 1995, Sage.

Lupton D: *Risk*, London, 1999, Routledge.

Medical Foundation for AIDS and Sexual Health (MedFASH): Progress and priorities – working together for high-quality sexual health, Review of the National Strategy for Sexual Health and HIV, 2008, www.medfash.org.uk.

Naidoo J, Wills J: *Foundations for health promotion*, edn 3, London, 2009, Baillière Tindall.

NHS Information Centre: *Health survey for England 2007 volume 1: healthy lifestyles, knowledge, attitudes and behaviour*, 2008, http://www.ic.nhs.uk/webfiles/publications/HSE07

NHS Information Centre for Health and Social Care *Statistics on alcohol:* England 2008, London, 2008, NHS.

NICE: *Four commonly used methods to increase physical activity: brief interventions in primary care, exercise referral schemes, pedometers and community-based exercise programmes for walking and cycling*, 2007a, at 2007ahttp://www.nice.org.uk/PH2

NICE: *School-based interventions on alcohol*, 2007b, http://www.nice.org.uk/PH7

NICE: *Smoking cessation services in primary care, pharmacies, local authorities and workplaces, particularly for manual working groups, pregnant women and hard to reach communities*, 2008, at http://www.nice.org.uk/PH10

NICE: *Promoting physical activity, active play and sport for pre-school and school-age children and young people in family, pre-school, school and community settings*, 2009, at http://www.nice.org.uk/PH17

Office for National Statistics: *National food survey 1999*, London, 2000, The Stationery Office.

Press V, Mwatsama M: *Nutrition and food poverty toolkit*, National Heart Forum, 2004.

Riethmuller A, McKeen K, Okely AD, et al: Developing an active play resource for a range of Australian early childhood settings: formative findings and recommendations (Report), *Aust J Early Child* 34(1):43–52, 2009.

Room R, Babor T, Rehm J: Alcohol and public health, *The Lancet* 365(9458):519–530, 2005.

Stead LF, Perera R, Bullen C, et al: *Nicotine replacement therapy for smoking cessation*, Cochrane Database Systematic Review (online), 2008. http://www/ncbi/nlm.nih.gov.pubmed/18253970 Jan 23 (1) CD000146

Swann C, Bowe K, McCormick G, et al: *Teenage pregnancy and parenthood: a review of reviews. Evidence Briefing*, London, 2003, Health Development Agency.

Thomson R, Holland J: Young women and safer sex: context, constraints and strategies. In Kitzinger C, Wilkinson S, editors: *Women and health: feminist perspectives*, London, 1994, Falmer.

UNICEF: *State of the world's children 2008 – child survival*, New York, 2008, UNICEF.

Wang D, Connock M, Barton P, et al: 'Cut down to quit' with nicotine replacement therapies in smoking cessation: a systematic review of effectiveness and economic analysis, *Natl Inst Health Res Health Technol Assess* 12(2):1–156, 2008.

World Health Organization (WHO): *Education and treatment in human sexuality: the training of health professionals*, Technical Report Series 572, Geneva, 1975, WHO.

World Health Organization (WHO): *Framework convention on tobacco control A56/8*, Geneva, 2003, WHO.

Chapter Twelve

Population groups

Key points

- Targeting population groups
- Approaches to targeting:
  - Older people
  - Children
  - Black, Asian and minority ethnic groups
  - Refugees and asylum seekers
- Targeting as a health promotion/public health strategy

OVERVIEW

Targeting interventions towards specific groups such as black, asian and minority ethnic (BAME) groups or young people is often advocated as a means of achieving equity. By directing activities to groups in need, practitioners seek to address health inequalities. This chapter reviews the arguments for targeting particular groups because of their health risks and needs and attempting to create more flexible and responsive services. It discusses different approaches to working with population groups from targeting resources to particular groups to interventions to improve opportunities or strengthen communities. The chapter outlines the health needs of older people, children, BAME groups, refugees and asylum seekers and then discusses some examples of effective interventions or projects that work with these

groups to illustrate a range of health-promoting or health-developing activities.

Introduction

The establishment of the NHS in the United Kingdom as a universal service for everyone, available according to need and free at the point of delivery, has been heralded as one of the great health achievements of the twentieth century. The NHS has enjoyed unparalleled public support, and its achievements in providing high quality care at relatively low cost are undeniable. There have, however, been some criticisms of this universalist model of provision. Whilst it appears equitable, in that the same service is available for all, in reality certain groups fare better than others. This has been evident in the debate around the 'postcode lottery' whereby certain geographical areas provide better services and manage to recruit and retain staff more easily than other more disadvantaged areas. In general, this reflects the socio-economic makeup of the local population, with poorer areas receiving poorer services. Many commentators have argued that the NHS perpetuates sexist, ageist and racist stereotypes and fails to adequately meet the needs of particular population groups (Doyal 1998). In order to meet the needs of specific marginalized, 'harder to reach' groups, targeting has been suggested as an appropriate strategy.

 Box 12.1 **Activity**

What do you understand by targeting? How do you target programmes/services in your practice?

Targeting means identifying particular needs and creating more flexible services in order to meet those needs. Targeting has been proposed as both a more equitable and efficient means of meeting health needs. Opponents argue that targeting involves additional resources being directed at small communities or groups, and that this is inequitable. This fails to take account of the fact that any universal service will appeal more to certain groups than others, and also that certain groups have much greater levels of need than others. Proponents of targeting also argue that linking provision to needs should be done for all groups, and that flexibility is a hallmark of high quality services.

The targeting of population groups has three rationales:

1. an ethical rationale based on equity
2. an economic rationale based on cost-effectiveness
3. a scientific rationale based on the notion of risk.

The ethical rationale argues that on the grounds of equity, targeting is needed to supplement a universal service if the needs of all population groups are to be met equally. For example, homeless people without a fixed address are unable to register with a GP and are therefore denied access to a range of community services. Innovative strategies to meet the needs of homeless people include using public addresses such as park benches in order to register homeless people, and employing staff with a specific remit for this group.

The economic rationale argues that it is more cost-effective to provide resources to meet needs effectively rather than have to spend resources later addressing the multiple social effects (e.g. crime, unemployment, and acute and chronic ill health) resulting from a failure to meet needs. The broad argument that prevention is cheaper than cure has been recognized; it merely needs to be reinforced for specific groups.

The scientific rationale rests on a notion of risk. Epidemiological evidence identifies these groups on the basis of their behavioural risk factors (see Chapter 11) or their health outcomes (ill health or premature death), access to care and services or in relation to particular characteristics such as low income, housing or work (see Chapter 9). For example:

- the prison population suffers high rates of mental illness
- life expectancy among street homeless is mid forties
- infant mortality in social class 5 is double that of social class 1.

Traditionally, analysis of modern society has seen it as divided by class, gender, sexuality and ethnicity and this social stratification as shaping experience and opportunities. Targeted population groups are normally those who share one of these characteristics and are deemed to have special health needs and include men/women, older people/children, homeless, teenage mothers, minority ethnic groups, and lesbian, gay, bisexual, transgender (LGBT) people.

A report by the Health Education Authority on the needs of the homeless provides a common argument for the explicit targeting of a population group: 'due to the wide range of health-related problems that affect homeless people, and their particular living environment and lifestyle, interventions should be targeted to their specific needs, rather than relying only on those aimed at the general population' (HEA 1999, p. 30). Blanket approaches simply cannot cater to everyone.

The term 'vulnerable groups' has been widely adopted to indicate those in need of particular provision. This could be because they have greater health needs; because their health needs are not being adequately addressed; or because they are at risk of social exclusion. Groups such as people with learning disabilities and looked after children might then be seen as vulnerable.

 Box 12.2 **Discussion point**

What are the problems of defining groups in this way?

The use of this term has been criticized for projecting a view of such groups as helpless or dependent. Defining groups as vulnerable ignores the fact that most needs are met privately, and that vulnerable groups in fact possess valuable resources for meeting needs. Recognizing what groups have to offer (assets) rather than seeing them solely as recipients of services, is a more health promoting strategy that builds community self-esteem.

'Social exclusion' is a relatively new term used to describe groups of people who are marginalized and on the outside of society usually because of their lack of access to material and social resources and also because of their isolation from social interactions. The UK government has defined social exclusion as 'what can happen when people or areas suffer from a combination of linked problems such as unemployment, poor skills, low incomes, poor housing, high crime, bad health and family breakdown' (Social Exclusion Unit, www.socialexclusionunit.gov.uk). Refugees and asylum seekers are an example of a group that is seriously threatened with problems of social exclusion. A disproportionate number of refugees become long-term unemployed, no matter what qualifications and experience of work they bring with them and most have problems of housing and community settlement.

 Box 12.3 **Discussion point**

How useful is the term 'social exclusion' in identifying target population groups?

Social exclusion, unlike poverty, includes several dimensions of deprivation and participation and draws attention to the ways in which people's position in society may change over time (Hills et al 2002). It changes the focus of interventions from those to take people out of poverty or ameliorate its effects (see Chapters 5 and 9) to those that focus on involvement and engagement.

Approaches to working with population groups

Targeting risk groups can seem an attractive proposition. Resources may be directed towards groups with the highest level of health needs, which should prove effective and equitable. As discussed in *Foundations for Health Promotion* (Naidoo and Wills 2009), needs assessment is intended to look at unmet needs for services and to provide information that will allow services to be tailored to local populations.

Target groups can be distinguished in two ways:
- geographical groups bound together by locality
- social groups bound together by some other attribute, such as age.

Within any target group such as older people (65 or more years of age) there are some people who have more needs than others, for example:
- those over 80 years of age (mainly women)
- those who live on their own
- those who belong to ethnic minority groups.

Targeting any group is thus problematic. Groups are often assumed to be homogenous for policy interventions when they may share important characteristics such as income or gender. Whilst this is important, behaviour is not simply a matter of following a social script, nor do individuals who share one characteristic such as their age necessarily form one homogenous group. For example, the experience of older women is very different to that of older men (Arber and Ginn 1999).

Understanding health disadvantage is often within a medical model that identifies physical health needs and barriers to accessing primary care services. Homeless people, for example, have marked health needs (see Box 12.4).

Box 12.4 **Example**

Homelessness and health

- People sleeping rough have a rate of physical health problems that is two or three times greater than in the general population.
- The rate of tuberculosis among rough sleepers and hostel residents is 200 times that of the known rate among the general population.
- Rough sleepers aged between 45 and 64 have a death rate 25 times that of the general population.
- Of people sleeping rough, 30–50% suffer from mental health problems.
- About half of the people sleeping rough are heavy drinkers and about 70% use drugs.
- Rough sleepers are 40 times more likely than the general population not to be registered with a GP.

Source: HEA (1999) www.crisis.org.uk ODPM (2002)

Box 12.5 **Discussion point**

What difficulties do marginalized groups face in accessing primary care?

Marginalized groups can have considerable difficulties accessing health services which may be perceived to be:
- intimidating
- stigmatizing
- inaccessible.

Interventions targeted to the needs of marginalised groups thus tend, in acknowledging the wide range of health problems they face, to focus on improving access to primary care services. Many homeless people for example are not registered with a GP and most will go to an A&E department as a consequence. Attempts to improve access to primary care tend to take the following forms:
- outreach workers
- NHS walk-in centres
- Satellite clinics, mobile services, home visits, drop-ins.

This example shows how services can exclude population groups and also the importance, at the practitioner level, of raising the awareness of the nature of that exclusion. A key aspect of work with the homeless is values-training with practitioners – to tackle the attitudes of primary care workers that make access difficult such as views about the deserving and undeserving patient, the perception that homeless patients are violent and the reluctance to treat because of the perception that they are migrants.

Box 12.6 **Activity**

Have you come across views on the 'deserving' and 'undeserving' patient?

Being homeless also encompasses other aspects of health including isolation, insecurity and poverty, and one of the problems of targeting a population group is that these interconnecting needs that are pathways or barriers to health also need to be addressed. This requires partnership working across professional and organizational boundaries, so that social and health needs are met. It also means working *with* (rather than for) people as partners, listening to their views, and acknowledging their areas of expertise. For more discussion of issues relating to partnership working, see Chapter 7.

Carers are an example of a population group (estimated at 5.8 million in the United Kingdom) that has only recently been recognized as having specific health needs in common. The role of caring itself has meant that carers have been invisible in society and the National Carers' Strategy (DH 1998) urges recognition of carers as individuals in their own right separate from those they care for and as a group with distinct needs (see Box 12.7):

Box 12.7 **Example**

Carers and Health

- A large proportion of carers are over 60 and therefore more likely to suffer physical injury such as back injuries.
- 13% had consulted a GP in the past year for anxiety, depression or emotional problems.
- Around a third of carers feel their health is affected by caring.
- Around two-thirds report stress, one-third report depression.
- Around half of carers have periods of depression.

Source: DH 1998; Henwood 1998; Singleton et al 2002

Strengthening the community of carers may mean providing emotional support or help and advice from a support group. Mental and emotional well-being can also result from feeling in control of the situation – which means, for carers, having the information and resources to help them to care. Befrienders projects support isolated carers who have become inactive within the community due to their caring role. The role of the befriender is to provide company either in the carer's home or on social outings and to offer support that is reliable, consistent and dependable. This example shows how a significant mental health issue may remain largely invisible unless a specific population group is targeted. By targeting carers, they are made part of the mainstream health agenda.

Box 12.8 **Discussion point**

What are the advantages and disadvantages of targeting versus a universalist approach?

The example of HIV/AIDS illustrates some of the dilemmas associated with both targeting specific groups for health education and services, and adopting a universal approach. Gay men and intravenous drug users were the initial target of HIV health education messages in the early 1980s. Alongside some success of this approach in reducing the HIV infection rate amongst gay men were the negative effects such as the maintenance of heterosexuals' illusion of invulnerability and a homophobic backlash. Predictions in the late 1980s of a heterosexual epidemic led to a change in emphasis and by 1990 the message was 'it's not who you are but what you do', that is, targeting risk behaviours not risk groups. This was accompanied by a shift in funding from projects for men who have sex with men to professionally led initiatives aimed at the heterosexual population. Whilst this has meant more mainstream funding, the 'de-gaying' of HIV also led to a shift of attention from the group most at risk. The linking of HIV to broader sexual health issues (see Chapters 10 and 11) means that prevention funds are often used to support generic health promotion activities, needle exchange and sexual health promotion aimed at heterosexuals.

National patterns of HIV prevalence, however, and what is known of the existence of priority groups in local communities, would suggest that interventions targeting men who have sex with men, and African communities, should take precedence over interventions targeting groups who are easier to access but at much less risk of HIV such as 'the general public'.

This chapter considers four different population groups – older people, children, Black, Asian and minority ethnic groups (BAMEG), and refugees and asylum seekers – in detail. For each population group, their specific health needs are outlined, followed by examples of different kinds of strategies and interventions targeted at the group to meet their needs.

Older people

The developed world talks of a demographic time bomb in the twenty-first century. The UK census of 2001 revealed that for the first time there are more people aged over 60 than there are under 16. People aged over 60 have risen from 16% of the whole of the population in 1951 to 19% in 2007. There are also 2.7 million people aged over 80. This poses major problems for the care and costs to the state of supporting an ageing population. Reducing mortality and increasing life expectancy is also not seen as an unmitigated public health success. The quality of life is also important. Although chronological age is not synonymous with disease and ill health, nevertheless there is an increase in frailty, chronic illness and greater use of health and social care services with increasing age.

 Box 12.9 **Activity**

How is old age framed in your practice? What language is used?

Any targeting of a population group marks that group as distinctive and 'a problem'. Whilst this can be helpful in drawing attention to marked inequalities, it can also be a source of discrimination. The use of the term 'elderly' has been abandoned in health discourse because it marks out people as being different rather than merely being relatively older than others. Old age is not in itself a problem although in public and professional discourse it is seen as a time of decline, physical and economic dependency, and separation from everyday life.

 Box 12.10 **Discussion point**

Ageism can be defined as legitimising the use of chronological age to mark out classes of people who may receive different care, treatment, services or opportunities. Are there examples of ageism in health and social care?

Organizations such as Age Concern (Age Concern 1999) have consistently highlighted incidences of lower quality care and rationing of services based on age and not individual need. This has been of sufficient concern for the first standard of the National Service Framework for Older People (DH 1999) to be 'Rooting out age discrimination'.

 Box 12.11 **Example**

Inequalities in health: older people

- Older people are more likely to live in poverty, in poorer and older accommodation and as such are at risk of fuel poverty and accidents.
- Access to transport is difficult, which limits access to goods and services and social contacts, which is reflected in a decline in psychosocial health in some older people, especially widows.
- Poverty in older people particularly affects women as there are 3 times as many women as men aged 85 and over and most of these live alone – only 38% of older women live with a partner/husband.

The health of older people does decline with age although there may be little association between chronology and physiological age. Degenerative conditions such as weaker muscles, loss of flexibility in joints, poor vision and hearing and loss of cognitive function may occur in the 'young old' of 60–70 or the 'old old' of 85 plus or not at all. Health problems tend to be related to a number of limited diseases for which the risk factors are well known – coronary heart disease (CHD) and stroke, cancers, respiratory illness and osteoporosis. Dementia affects 1 in 5 people over 85 although its severity varies. Although it is clear that as men and women reach very late life their activities become more circumscribed, in earlier late life their mobility and task capacity are unimpaired and they are well able to be involved beyond their home and household, in work, care giving, sport and recreations. A longer life does not necessarily mean worsening health. As people live longer, most morbidity gets compressed into the later years of life and many people reach 'natural death' without ill health. A review of health status in 1994 found it impossible to conclude whether the health status of the older population had improved, deteriorated or remained the same over the preceding decades of mortality decline (MRC 1994). Although health spending is higher for older age groups (40% of the NHS budget), the economic argument to prioritize older people because of their greater consumption of services and health needs is not the only or most convincing argument. An alternative argument is a rights-based one – to tackle age-based inequalities.

Box 12.12 **Activity**

What does quality of life in older age mean to you?

Standard 8 of the UK National Service Framework for Older People aims to 'extend the healthy life expectancy of older people'. For most older people this means their independence, autonomy and maintaining their functional capacity. Yet disability as measured in relation to activities of daily life tends to rise in those over 70 and is mostly related to locomotor function. Nearly two-thirds of people aged over 65 cannot walk 200 yards without stopping or climb a flight of 12 stairs (DH 2007a). Falls and fractures are associated with high morbidity, mortality and substantial costs. In 1999, there were over 3000 deaths and over 85,000 serious injuries as a result of falls in older people (DH 2001). Hip fracture is the most common serious injury and this can precipitate admission to long-term care. Even those falls that do not result in injury may have psychological consequences of loss of confidence and fear (of a future fall), decreased activity, social isolation and depression.

Encouraging older people to remain physically active is a major priority. This means action in broader areas – ensuring the maintenance of pavements, better lighting in streets and parks, restricting traffic in residential and shopping areas, and improving town centres, as well as developing affordable and accessible public transport through concessionary fares and mobility buses and tackling community safety so that older people feel safe in public areas.

Box 12.13 **Example**

Falls prevention

Many epidemiological studies have explored the causes of falls and over 400 variables have been investigated (National Centre for Reviews and Dissemination 1996). These include nutritional status, environmental hazards such as lighting or loose carpets, and medication and its effect on balance and inactivity. A consistent feature of falls is that the person is likely to be less mobile, in poorer health, and more overweight. A systematic review of interventions for preventing falls in older people (Gillespie et al 2002) and NICE guidance (2004) conclude that interventions likely to be . beneficial are:

- muscle strengthening programmes and balance retraining carried out at home by a trained health professional

- Tai Chi – a programme of at least 15-weeks' duration
- home hazard assessment and modification for people with a history of falling including personal alarms and hip protectors
- gradual withdrawal of psychotropic medication.

The relative importance of different strategies is not known – vision screening and home hazard management, for example, are not markedly effective as single interventions but add value when combined with an exercise programme.

In the acute settings, practice development initiatives have focused on developing best practice guidelines and assessment tools for those at risk of falls and integrated care pathways for fractured neck of femur which is the most common injury.

In this section, we have examined some of the arguments for targeting a population group for specific health promotion interventions. Improving quality of life for an ageing population is important in terms of health improvement and to reduce some of the strain on services.

Children

In 1943, following the publication of Richard Titmuss' *Birth, Poverty and Wealth*, newspapers reported that 'poor folks' babies stand less chance'. More than half a century later, this headline is still true. Evidence shows this is not inevitable, but can be addressed by social and health policies. Parental poverty triggers a chain of social risk which is transmitted to the next generation. Children are therefore identified as a population group having specific health needs that should be targeted. The reasons relate to a commitment to reduce health inequalities whose origins are said to lie in childhood and to provide the basis for health in later years. Intervening in childhood is seen as a key strategy to break the cycle of social disadvantage.

Childhood is a critical stage in health when many diseases such as cardiovascular disease and diabetes have their origin and economic and social circumstances can have lasting effects. Although the infant mortality rate is falling, there has been a dramatic increase in morbidity as measured by self-reported illness. A Health Survey for England that focused on young people found that just over 25% of boys and just under 25% of girls aged 2–15 years reported a long-standing illness, with 10% indicating that it limited their activities in some way (Prescott-Clarke and Primatesta 1998). Psychological disorders in children show similar increases.

There are two arguments that show it is important to focus on children in social policy interventions:

1. the biological rationale
2. the social rationale.

The biological explanation suggests that events such as malnutrition and exposure to smoking, alcohol or infections in utero may 'programme' an individual's risk before encountering other risk factors. For example, infants whose mothers are obese are at greater risk of developing CHD. Those small at birth have a greater risk of developing non-insulin dependent diabetes.

The social explanation is that low birth weight and delayed growth are merely markers for social disadvantages. Socio-economic differences in adult life can be explained by these earlier life processes. Wadsworth and Butterworth (2006) have analysed birth cohorts and shown that family circumstances influence later health status. The cycle of deprivation includes poor physical development and low educational attainment, and leads to a raised risk of unemployment or low status/low control jobs and perceived social marginality. Roberts (1997) argues that family structure, whether lone, reconstituted or intact, has less influence on health status than family centredness (time spent in family activities). Conflict between young people and their parents is related to poor health and social outcomes such as smoking and alcohol consumption, delinquency and contact with the police.

 Box 12.14 **Discussion point**

What types of policy intervention may follow from this analysis?

One element of policy interventions may focus on the protective factors for childhood – optimizing growth before birth and early education interventions. Policy interventions also need to be safety nets to prevent the accumulation of further disadvantage, be springboards to help young families onto a more advantageous trajectory, and need to occur at critical social transition points such as the early years and starting of secondary school.

Tackling childhood disadvantage has tended to be through early intervention programmes offering social and emotional support and interventions to improve health status. Roberts (2000) looks at evidence of effective interventions providing social and emotional support; early detection of

Box 12.15 **Example**

Food supplementation

Addressing the nutritional health of pregnant women is a priority in tackling health inequalities. In many countries this is tackled through food supplementation programmes. In the United States, for example, the Special Supplementation Programme for Women, Infants and Children (WIC) is a huge federally funded nutrition programme targeted at low income women who are pregnant or who have just had a baby and children up to 5 years. A cheque or food token is issued which allows the purchase of foods (e.g. cereals, milk, cheese, eggs, peanut butter, fruit or vegetable juice, carrots, tuna and pulses). The WIC programme has shown increases in birth weight and fewer pre-term deliveries but what is not clear from the evidence is whether it is the addition of the food supplements, nutrition education or contact with health and social care professionals that makes a difference.

Box 12.16 **Example**

Inequalities in health: children

- A child from social class 5 (8.1 per 1000 births) is twice as likely to die before 15 as a child in social class 1. Infant mortality among babies of mothers born in Pakistan is 12.2 per 1000 live births.
- Babies with fathers in social classes 4 and 5 have a birth weight that is on average 130 grams lower than babies with fathers in social classes 1 and 2.
- Children in poorer families are more likely to experience illness, especially respiratory infections, gastroenteritis, *Helicobacter pylori* and TB.
- A child from social class 5 is five times as likely to die from injury or poisoning as a child from social class 1.
- 3.5 million were living in poverty in 2004, mostly in urban areas.
- 33% children from lower socio-economic groups gained higher grades at GCSE compared to 76% children from higher socio-economic groups.

Source: Roberts (2000), Northern and Yorkshire Public Health Observatory (2001), DH (2007b), DWP (2006)

postnatal depression; policies to increase the initiation and maintenance of breastfeeding; policies which improve the health and nutrition of women of childbearing age and their children; and preschool education.

In the United Kingdom, a welfare food scheme has been in place since 1940, originally providing cod liver oil and orange juice. 'Healthy Start' (DH 2002), the current scheme, has widened its nutritional base to include fruit, vegetables and cereal-based foods as well as liquid milk or formula. It reaches around half a million pregnant women and children under four in low income and disadvantaged families. Initiatives such as this bring families into contact with the NHS in the early years of life and can link them with other schemes such as food co-ops and community kitchens aimed at improving food access.

Sure Start is a programme that was targeted at preschool children and their families initially in disadvantaged areas of England, and Children's Centres are

Box 12.17 **Example**

Young people and social disadvantage

- One in five children in the United Kingdom grows up in a workless household.
- One in 16 young people leaves school with no qualifications each year and the numbers of excluded pupils is rising (2000 in London in 1996–1997), disproportionately affecting Black children.
- One in six 16–24-year-olds is the victim of a violent offence each year. Five in 100 teenagers in London have been accused of a crime (theft 37%, drugs 11%, criminal damage 11%).
- 10% of children under 18 lived at a different address 1 year before the 1991 census.

Source: Acheson (1998)

being rolled out to every community. The objectives are to:

- improve social and emotional development
- improve health
- improve the ability to learn
- strengthen families and communities (DfEE 1999).

Sure Start was developed following evidence from the United States High Scope programme, a pre-school intervention based on child-initiated learning. It started 30 years ago in Michigan and has been comprehensively evaluated. By the age of 19, those who took part in the programme were more likely to have completed their schooling, be in paid employment, and girls were less likely to have become pregnant. At 27 years, participants had higher monthly earnings, were more likely to own their own home, and were less likely to have been arrested for crimes including drug taking or dealing.

 Box 12.18 Discussion point

Do early intervention programmes improve health?

Initial targets were set (e.g. 5% reduction in low birth-weight babies) which have been difficult to achieve but there is evidence from evaluations of Sure Start that it has resulted in:

- a reduction in emergency hospitalizations for severe injury or respiratory infection
- increases in access to routine health care
- increase in smoking cessation among pregnant women.

Sure Start began as an area-based initiative. Whilst this is a means of targeting disadvantage and social exclusion, it can mean less impact on neighbouring areas. Area-based initiatives can also result in a proliferation of projects, many on short-term funding with consequent problems of sustainability.

In this section, we have seen a different response to the targeting of a population group that includes a rounded approach to child health which

 Box 12.19 **Discussion point**

'Joined up thinking' is a familiar phrase in UK government policy but to what extent is it evident in tackling childhood poverty? What needs to be addressed?

encompasses anti-poverty and social exclusion strategies. Early intervention programmes provide education, care and improved nutrition. Supporting education and tackling 'the poverty of expectation' is a major plank of UK policy. As Wilkinson (1998) has pointed out, 'The problems being experienced by families today are rooted in economic stress and in family disintegration. Any progressive family policy must address both these issues'.

Black, Asian and minority ethnic groups

Ethnic minority disadvantage cuts across all aspects of deprivation. Taken as a whole, ethnic minority groups are more likely than the rest of the population to live in poor areas, be unemployed, have low incomes, live in poor housing, have poor health, and be the victims of crime.

Social Exclusion Unit (1998, 1.26)

BAME groups are an attempt to move away from the medicalized concept of 'race' referring to biological and physical differences between human groups, such as skin colour. This concept of 'race' has now become discredited, due to the lack of significant separation of biological characteristics between different 'racial' groups, and its association with racism, or discrimination based on 'racial' attributes. The concept of BAME groups prioritizes notions of culture rather than race, and highlights the importance of social rather than biological characteristics. Ethnicity refers to a shared cultural heritage including language, religion, history and customs, and as such can be applied to the majority White population in Britain as well as minority groups.

Ethnicity was first measured in the 1991 census. In the 2001 census in England and Wales, people assigned themselves to one of 16 ethnic categories. The term BAME group is used in the United Kingdom and refers to those in Mixed, Asian or Asian British, Black or Black British, Chinese or Other ethnic groups. It therefore includes a number of very different ethnic groups with different experiences of health, education, employment and income. However, there is a unity due to a common experience of being discriminated against and overall there is evidence of higher than average health and social care needs (Gill et al 2003; Nazroo 1997).

Box 12.20 **Activity**

Do you use the term 'Black and ethnic minority groups' in your practice Why do you think this term has been adopted? The term 'Black, Asian and minoity ethnic groups (BAME) is now used in the UK. Why do you think this term is used?

There is a substantial body of evidence demonstrating differences in health status between ethnic groups and a complex picture of high or low rates of specific conditions among ethnic groups. South Asians have high mortality rates from diabetes and CHD. Caribbean people have low death rates from CHD but a relatively high mortality from stroke, linked to high prevalence of diabetes and hypertension. There is a higher than average infant mortality rate for most BAME groups, and a particularly high rate among babies of Pakistan-born mothers. People from Pakistani, Bangladeshi and Caribbean communities perceive their health to be significantly poorer than does the average population. On the plus side, there is generally lower than average mortality due to breast and lung cancer amongst people from BAME groups, although there is some evidence that these patterns may be changing (Bhopal 2007).

The diversity of health experience between different BAME groups may be caused by several different factors, or a combination of these factors:

- Different causes of poor health, especially social and environmental factors and also cultural and genetic factors, for example low income, sickle cell disease.
- Different susceptibility to poor health caused by social factors, for example social isolation, stress due to migration, and experiences of racism.
- Reduced access to health and social services due to institutional and/or individual racism.

Box 12.21 **Discussion point**

What is the main focus of health promotion interventions targeted at Black, Asian and minority ethnic groups?

Whilst many health promotion programmes targeting ethnic minority groups have focused on cultural differences, often using stereotyping rather than concrete evidence, it seems likely that, just as with social class inequalities, it is material factors that are most significant in causing excess ill health and mortality.

Box 12.22 **Discussion point**

Is it appropriate to focus on culture as the key to tackling BAME group health inequalities?

Cultural essentialism, or a focus on cultural norms as the key to health inequalities, has been a feature of much of the activity directed towards improving the health of people from BAME group. Culture is assumed to affect health through health-related behaviours (such as smoking, exercise, diet, sexual behaviour) and the organization of families affecting child rearing and gender roles. Cultural practices in ethnic minority groups are compared to the ethnic majority. Frequently these are seen as accounting for health inequalities and thus viewed as 'problematic'. Cultural essentialism is a form of victim blaming at the community level, and has strong parallels with victim blaming at the individual level. In both cases, universalist and structural strategies which would affect health, such as higher incomes through employment or benefits, are overlooked in favour of targeted campaigns advocating lifestyle changes such as not eating betel nut which has been linked with mouth cancer.

Positive features of the lifestyles of people from BAME groups, such as the low rates of women smoking amongst Asian women, and the generally low levels of alcohol consumption for men and women from BAME groups, tend to be ignored. A salutogenic approach focusing on what enables people from disadvantaged communities to cope without recourse to recreational drugs might enhance our understanding of health. The focus on health care for a diverse society has tended to concentrate on improving access, removing language barriers and providing culturally sensitive information.

Box 12.23 Discussion point

What are the main barriers for BAME groups in accessing and using primary care?

A range of factors may influence access:
- Culture and gender.
- Differential presentation due to somatization of symptoms leading to incorrect referrals.
- Linguistic competence and literacy level.
- 'Newness' to the country or user ignorance.

Box 12.24 Practitioner talking

Equal opportunities is not an issue here. There are very few people from BMEGs living locally. We provide a 'colour-blind' service that is the same for everyone irrespective of their colour or culture.

Commentary

This is a common response from service providers, even in areas with large communities of people from BAME groups. Whilst on one level it encapsulates an ideal, in reality holding this view is likely to be associated with providing a relatively poorer service for people from BAME groups. This is because factors that are taken for granted within the majority White population, such as easy communication and a broad consensus on cultural norms, may be problematic for people from BAME groups.

Box 12.25 Example

Young Asian women and suicide

Making assumptions and stereotyping ethnic minorities is common. A study in Newham, an area of London with a large Asian population, found that service providers believed that the main reason for self-harm was culture conflict (balancing family traditions against influences of Western culture). Young Asian women, however, identified lack of information about mental health services and not being understood by primary care professionals. A focus on culture conflict meant that health services did not examine the scope for other interventions or service improvements.

Source: Arora et al (2000)

Other factors relate to the service itself:
- Lack of provision where there may be isolated minorities.
- Staff lacking cultural competence.

The desire to reflect a multicultural society in service provision has led to an emphasis on practitioners being more 'culturally aware', understanding the customs, traditions and religious beliefs of different ethnic communities. Increasingly, the term 'cultural competence'

Box 12.26 Discussion point

In 2005, Ann Cryer, MP for Keighley in West Yorkshire, called for an end to first cousin marriages and was widely criticised (see Dyer 2005). She said 'As we address problems of smoking, drinking, obesity we say it's a public health issue, and therefore we all have to get involved with it in persuading people to adopt a different lifestyle. I think the same should be applied to this problem in the Asian community'.

Is it appropriate to respect other cultures if there is a risk to public health?

is used to describe an organization that has a clear understanding of how it addresses issues of diversity.

Box 12.27 **Activity**

Have you attended any cultural competence or diversity training? What is your reaction to such training?

The targeting of any population group assumes a homogeneity of the group. The beliefs associated with any ethnic group will be adhered to with varying degrees and 'they are constantly refashioned within a culture, especially after migration when people have access to the resources of two different cultures' (Davey Smith et al 2000, p. 400).

Box 12.28 **Example**

Indigenous peoples

Indigenous peoples are those whom 'on account of their descent from the populations which inhabited the country, or a geographic region to which the country belongs, at the time of conquest or colonization or the establishment of present state boundaries and who, irrespective of their legal status, retain some or all of their own social, economic, cultural and political institutions'.

ILO (1989)

In Australia, promoting health in indigenous communities starts from a concept of health which is 'a matter of determining all aspects of their life, including control over their physical environment, of dignity, of community self esteem, and of justice. It is not merely a matter of the provision of doctors, hospitals, medicines or the absence of disease or incapacity'.

NAHS (1989, p. ix)

Separate interventions targeting BAME groups inevitably risks marginalizing minority ethnic issues. It also implies that the health problems in minority ethnic groups are different from those in the ethnic majority, with different causes and different solutions, whereas in fact the similarities are greater than the differences. However, unless specific consideration is given to minority ethnic issues, interventions may unintentionally favour the ethnic majority. Thus policies to consider inequalities in health should include consideration of the application of these policies to minority ethnic groups as a matter of course, including ways of ensuring that racial prejudice and harassment are overcome. This requires that the structures and processes of policy making are sensitive to the position and needs of people from minority ethnic groups. One way of ensuring that the needs of BAME groups are integral to programme planning and policy making is to ensure that minority ethnic groups are represented, consulted and involved in planning and delivery. As with all excluded groups, their visibility can help to reduce the sense of exclusion.

Refugees and asylum seekers

Refugees and asylum seekers are an example of a population group that may be targeted for interventions because they have specific health needs and can be amongst the most vulnerable and excluded groups in society, facing poverty and lack of cohesive social support.

Box 12.29 **Discussion point**

What is the difference between a refugee and an asylum seeker?

The UN convention of 1951 defines a 'refugee' as someone who 'owing to a well founded fear of being persecuted for reasons of race, religion, nationality, membership of a social group, or political opinion is outside the country of his nationality and is unable, or owing to such fear, is unwilling to avail himself of the protection of that country; or who, not having a nationality and being outside the country of his former habitual residence, as a result of such events is unable to or owing to such fear, is unwilling to return to it'. Asylum seekers are those who have applied for refugee status. In order to be admitted to countries such as the United Kingdom it is necessary to have first applied for asylum.

There are 21 million refugees worldwide with a further 25 million people displaced within their own countries. The vast majority of refugees remain in countries close to their own. The number of asylum seekers in Europe is falling and although the United Kingdom ranks third in number of applications, compared to its total population it is only about mid table (www.unhcr.org).

As we have seen in this chapter, targeting any population group means assuming a degree of homogeneity. Refugees and asylum seekers like older people or people from BMEG are not a homogenous group and may come from a wide range of countries, ethnic groups, social backgrounds and have different histories. War, conflict and economic poverty have resulted in rising numbers of refugees across Europe, often leading to negative media reports and racist attacks. Of the 21 million refugees worldwide, 86% originate from developing countries and 72% remain in a developing country.

Box 12.30 **Discussion point**

What are the likely health problems of refugees on arrival?

For most refugees immediate concerns are safety, food and shelter. Some may have experienced war, rape, torture and other traumatic events as well as displacement and a difficult journey to a new country resulting in complex mental health needs (trauma, stress and depression). Most will have experienced anxiety or depression but do not have a mental illness. Those fleeing for safety may arrive with physical disabilities such as amputations or may have come from refugee camps where nutrition and sanitation have been poor (HEA 1998). Most refugees arriving in the United Kingdom are young and physically fit and the health problems experienced are similar to those of deprived groups and excluded groups who are isolated and unable to feel part of a community.

Box 12.31 **Discussion point**

Health problems may even worsen after arrival. Why might this be?

The practice of dispersal, accommodation in poor housing and public hostility in some areas exacerbate isolation. Current regulations in the United Kingdom mean asylum seekers cannot be employed and are eligible only for 70% rate of income support benefits. Asylum seekers therefore have reduced access to many of the basic determinants of health such as good housing or an adequate income.

The health needs of refugees, in common with homeless people, have been seen within a medical model that prioritizes physical health. Burnett and Peel (2001, p. 544) suggest that 'refugee health in many areas of Britain has become the responsibility of communicable disease departments, giving the impression that refugees are vectors of infection, but refugees with infectious diseases needing care and treatment are the minority'. On arrival many refugees may have untreated conditions but screening on arrival seems more to protect the host population than benefiting the health of the refugee. HIV prevalence mirrors the country of origin and TB, although rising in areas with high numbers of refugees such as some London boroughs, is not common in new arrivals. A Home Office pilot scheme in Kent screened 5000 refugees for TB but all tested negative according to a report in the *Guardian* newspaper on 7 February 2003. Because refugees live in poor, overcrowded conditions the possibility of infection developing and then spreading is likely.

Whilst the health needs of refugees and asylum seekers are similar to those of the host population, many experience difficulties accessing health care. Many refugees have problems registering with a GP either because the patient list is closed, or sometimes because of a lack of awareness by primary care staff about the rights and entitlements of refugees. According to a High Court ruling in 2008, asylum seekers whose claims had failed can be classed as 'ordinarily resident' and therefore entitled to NHS treatment. Language difficulties, in both personal contact with practitioners and in filling out forms, is another barrier for many refugees and asylum seekers. The onus is nevertheless on the refugee to use services but for many, health problems are not a priority and remain untreated until they become chronic or an emergency.

 Box 12.32 **Example**

Interventions to meet refugee health needs have focused on:

- developing networks of support
- using link workers to provide better integration with mainstream services
- providing interpreters and advocates to ensure available services are accessed
- providing better information on arrival
- offering specialist locality-based services on mental health, women's services, genitourinary medicine and TB screening
- 'one stop shops' for recent arrivals at initial accommodation centres
- Training and resources to support healthcare workers, for example Health for Asylum Seekers and Refugees Portal at http://www.harpweb.org.uk/index.php.

Many health professionals have difficulty working with marginalized groups, seeing them as an excessive burden on the NHS or adopting stereotyped attitudes. Many areas have produced information packs for practitioners working with refugees that provide basic information on:

- understanding refugee support needs
- exile and identity
- cultural differences
- communication in health care
- issues of women (sexual health, possible survivors of rape and as main healthcare provider in families)
- working with survivors of torture and rape.

Communication is essential to the delivery of services. There are three broad categories of interventions used to improve communication (Sanders 2000):

1. A linguistic model that assumes the barrier to communication is language and uses interpreters or telephone language link.

2. A professional-centred model that attempts to build service teams with knowledge and understanding of target communities. They may use link workers or bilingual workers as 'intercultural mediators' and focus on developing culturally appropriate materials.

3. A client-centred or advocacy model that focuses on the client, communicates their wishes, and acts as an advocate to ensure that their needs are met in an appropriate and accessible manner.

In this section, we have seen how health promotion may target a population group on the basis of specific health needs but this can be problematic. The laudable attempts to meet those needs can appear stigmatizing with the singling out of particular conditions whilst the health needs that are shared with the rest of the population may be ignored.

Conclusion

Targeting health promotion at specific population groups is based on several different rationales, including a scientific notion of risk, an ethical notion of equity, and an economic notion of cost-effectiveness. The scientific notion of risk is problematic in practice, focusing on biological, genetic or lifestyle factors that have less impact on health status than basic structural factors such as education and income. In addition, this notion of risk can very easily become victim blaming, assuming that the responsibility for poor health lies with the individual or group and their chosen lifestyles. For BAME groups in particular, this ignores the importance for overall health of following cultural and religious norms, and also the reality of a mixed cultural heritage for second generation migrants. Using a notion of risk also focuses on what are perceived to be problematic behaviours and neglects the health-promoting aspects of the lifestyles of people from BAME groups.

Targeting is more strongly based on ethical notions of equity. Certain marginalized groups in society have both high levels of health needs and low access to services. In order to provide an equal service for all, such groups need specific targeted services to enable them to have the same access as the general population. Examples of such groups are homeless people and people from BAME groups. Other groups, such as mothers and children, are targeted because they are pivotal in breaking the cycle of disadvantage that perpetuates inequalities from one generation to the next. Groups such as older people and people with learning disabilities are targeted because society in general, including health and social care provision, is often guilty of discrimination due to reduced expectations of the health potential of people in these groups. Without specific targeting these groups are likely to have problems accessing relevant services and reaching their full health potential.

There is also an economic rationale for targeting. Providing additional resources to proactively meet the health needs of marginalized groups is likely to be far more cost-effective than waiting to meet the costs of a range of health and social needs resulting from increased marginalization and corresponding ill health and social exclusion.

There are therefore sound reasons for targeting specific groups as a public health and health promotion strategy. However, there are also problems and challenges attached to using targeting as a strategy. Targeting may reinforce, instead of challenging, stereotypes by labelling specific groups as dependent and problematic. Targeting is often used as a substitute for universalism and may become a means of avoiding, instead of supplementing, mainstream provision. People with learning disabilities, for example, may have particular health needs (higher incidence of sensory impairment and epilepsy), but in many other ways their needs are the same; yet they experience poor access to services and limited social and economic opportunities.

Identifying groups with unmet health needs is a key aspect of reducing health inequalities but is not always the most effective way to achieve equity. Targeting groups may be linked to short-term funding and limited resourcing, leading to uncertainty and an inability to plan ahead.

Further discussion

- How might health promotion interventions be targeted at specific population groups to avoid falling into the traps of cultural essentialism and stereotyping?

- Is targeting population groups an effective way to achieve equity?

- Who stands to gain most from targeting specific population groups – organizations, clients or practitioners?

Recommended reading

- Department of Health (DH): *Addressing inequalities – reaching the hard to reach groups. National Service Frameworks: a practical aid to implementation in primary care*, London, 2002, DH.

    A resource pack providing guidance for reaching 'hard to reach' groups together with case studies of good practice.

- Kai J: *Ethnicity, health and primary care*, Oxford, 2003, Oxford University Press.

    A practical guide to some of the challenges of providing health care in the diverse ethnic communities in the United Kingdom.

References

Acheson D: *Independent inquiry into inequalities in health*, London, 1998, The Stationery Office.

Age Concern: *Turning your back on us: older people and the NHS*, London, 1999, Age Concern.

Arber S, Ginn J: Gender differences in health in later life: the new paradox?, *Soc Sci Med* 48(1):61–76, 1999.

Arora S, Coker N, Gillam S, et al: *Improving the health of black and minority ethnic groups: a guide for PCGs*, London, 2000, King's Fund.

Bhopal RS: *Ethnicity, race, and health in multicultural societies*, Oxford, 2007, Oxford University Press.

Burnett A, Peel M: Health needs of refugees and asylum seekers, *Br Med J* 322:544–547, 2001.

Davey Smith G, Chaturvedi N, Harding S, et al: Ethnic inequalities in health: a review of UK epidemiological evidence, *Crit Public Health* 10(4):375–408, 2000.

Department for Education and Employment: *Sure Start: making a difference for children and families*, London, 1999, DfEE.

Department for Work and Pensions: *Making a difference; tackling poverty – a progress report*, London, 2006, DWP.

Department of Health (DH): *National carers' strategy*, London, 1998, DH.

Department of Health (DH): *Saving lives: our healthier nation*, London, 1999, The Stationery Office.

Department of Health (DH): *Accidental injury task force working group: priorities for prevention*, London, 2001, DH.

Department of Health: *Healthy start: proposals for reform of the welfare foods scheme*, London, 2002, DH. www.dh.gov.uk/healthystart.htm.

Department of Health (DH): *Health survey for England: 2005: health of older people*, London, 2007a, DH.

Department of Health (DH): *Review of the health inequalities: infant mortality PSA target*, London, 2007b, DH.

Doyal L: *Women and health services: an agenda for change*, Maidenhead, 1998, Open University Press.

Dyer O: MP is criticised for saying that marriage of first cousins is a health problem, *BMJ* 331:1292, 2005.

Gill PS, Kai J, Bhopal RS, et al: *Health care needs assessment of black and minority ethnic groups in NHS health needs assessment, the fourth series of epidemiologically based reviews*, Oxford, 2003, Radcliffe. www.hcna.radcliffe-oxford.com/bmegframe.htm.

Gillespie LD, Gillespie WJ, Robertson MC, et al: *Interventions for preventing falls in elderly people*, Cochrane Review, Issue 3, Oxford, 2002.

Health Education Authority (HEA): *Promoting the health of refugees*, London, 1998, HEA.

Henwood M: *Ignored and invisible? Carers' experience of the NHS*, London, 1998, Carers' National Association.

Hills J, Le Grand J, Piachaud D: *Understanding social exclusion*, Oxford, 2002, Oxford University Press.

International Labour Organisation: *Convention concerning indigenous and tribal peoples in independent countries*, 1989 Convention 169.

Medical Research Council (MRC): *The health of the UK's elderly people*, London, 1994, MRC.

Naidoo J, Wills J: *Foundations for health promotion*, edn 3, London, 2009, Baillière Tindall.

National Aboriginal Health Strategy Walking Party: *National strategy*, Canberra, 1989, Department of Aboriginal Affairs.

National Centre for Reviews and Dissemination: *Effective health care: preventing falls and subsequent injury in older people*, York, 1996, NCRD.

Nazroo J: *The health of Britain's ethnic minorities: findings from a national survey*, London, 1997, Policy Studies Institute.

NICE: *Falls: the assessment and prevention of falls in older people*, London, 2004, NICE. Available at www.nice.org.uk/nicemedia/pdf/CG02NICEguideline.pdf.

Northern and Yorkshire Public Health Observatory: *Inequalities in the health of children and young people*, 2001. Occasional Paper No. 3 at www.nypho.org.uk.

ODPM: *Addressing the health needs of rough sleepers*, London, 2002, ODPM.

Prescott-Clarke P, Primatesta P: *Health survey for England: the health of young people 1995–97*, London, 1998, Dept Epidemiology and Public Health, University College London, The Stationery Office.

Roberts H: Socio-economic determinants of health: children, inequalities and health, *Br Med J* 314: 1122–1129, 1997.

Roberts H: *What works in reducing inequalities in child health*, London, 2000, Barnardo's.

Sanders M: *As good as your word: a guide to interpreting and translation services*, London, 2000, Maternity Alliance.

Singleton N, Maung NA, Cowie J, et al: *Mental health of carers*, London, 2002, London Office of National Statistics.

Social Exclusion Unit: *Rough sleeping*, London, 1998, Cabinet Office.

Wadsworth M, Butterworth S: Early life. In Marmot M, Wilkinson RG, editors: *Social determinants of health*, edn 3, Oxford, 2006, Oxford University Press.

Wilkinson H: The family way: navigating a third way in family policy. In Hargreaves I, Christie I, editors: *Tomorrow's politics: the third way and beyond*, London, 1998, Demos.

Note : Page numbers followed by *f* indicates figures, *b* indicate boxes and *t* indicates tables.

retrospective (case-control) studies, 26
risk of disease and illness, 159f
  estimating, for an individual, 26
  HIV/AIDS
    risk behaviour, 202
    risk groups, 202
  mental health problems in older people, tackling risk
    factors, 200
  perception, 208, 209
  social factors affecting, 158–159
  see also behaviour; lifestyle
road traffic accidents, 176, 177–178, 195
role culture (in organisations), 128
role models, risk perception influenced by, 209
Romp and Chomp initiative, 215
Round Table on Sustainable Development, UK, 174

S

safety, vaccine, 54, 189–190
safety measures
  community, 169
  road safety cameras, 177
  see also Health and Safety at Work Act
salutogenic approach, 154, 184
  ethnic minority groups, 240
Saving Lives: Our Healthier Nation, 110, 184
schistosomiasis, China, 143
schools
  food in, 155–156
    breakfast clubs, 43
    fruit and vegetable scheme, 214
  Healthy Schools Partnership, 133
  walk to, 218
scientific rationale of population group targeting, 230
Scotland, suicide prevention, 198
screening, 186–189
  cancer see cancer
  types, 186
searching for evidence, 47–48
self-efficacy, enhancing, 141–142
self-employment, start-up loans, 167
self-management plans for patients, 110
Sentinel Site for Obesity Prevention, 215
services
  centralized vs devolved, 74
  extent of their meeting needs, assessing, 26
  operation, assessing, 26
  partnerships improving delivery of, 125

services (Continued)
  rationing of, vs needs, 73–74
  tackling health inequalities and, 94
    helpful vs unhelpful services, 94t
  users see users
sex see gender
sexual health, 223–224
  Chlamydia screening, 188–189
  definitions, 223
  HIV and see HIV disease
sexually-transmitted infections (STIs), 188–189,
    223, 224
shared goal, finding a, 127–132
sin, risk replacing notion of, 208
single assessment process for older people,
    implementation, 63
Single Equality Scheme 2009–2012, 89
skills
  client, to make changes in life, developing, 142–143
  professional, 8–10
    evidence-based practice (EBP), 44
skin cancer, 193–194
sleeping positions of babies and sudden death, 54
small business start-up loans, 167
smoking (and tobacco), 86b, 91–92, 210–213,
    222–223
  cessation, 45b
    cost-effectiveness, 53
    evidence of effective methods, 212
    in pregnancy, 51–52
  epidemiology, 210b
    reducing death rates, 91–92
  mixed methods research, 34b
  peoples' views about, 86b
  South Asian men, 192
social class
  and child health inequality, 237
  and male life expectancy, 85f
  and smoking, 211
Social construction of risky behaviours and
    risk perception, 208
social determinants of health, 157–181
  epidemiological studies, 26
  social inequalities linked to health inequalities, 81, 82,
    160–161
  WHO recommendations on tackling, 160
social exclusion (marginalization) and health inequality
    (social production of health model), 86, 231, 232
social justice and community development, 116